A.C.E.S for P.A.C.E.S.

Advanced Clinical Evaluation System for
Practical Assessment of Clinical
Examination Skills

DR. AJITH JAYASEKERA

M.B., B.S. (Colombo, Sri Lanka) M.R.C.P. (U.K.)

The London Press

© Dr. B.A.S. Jayasekera 2005

Published in the United Kingdom by The London Press Ltd.

Cover Design: The Digital Canvas Company, Scotland (www.digican.co.uk)

Typeset: Decent Typesetting (www.decenttypesetting.co.uk)

A CIP catalogue record of this book is available from the

British Library

ISBN: 1-905006-04-7

While every attempt has been made to ensure that the information provided in this book is correct, the author and publishers make no representation, express or otherwise, with regard to the accuracy of the information contained herein and cannot accept any legal responsibility or liability for any errors or omissions that have been made or for any loss or damage resulting from the use of the information.

Contents

Preface

From the dawn of history, mankind has used stories to enable people to understand and remember concepts. The major world religions have used this method with admirable effect. Following in this tradition, this book begins with a story.

The Royal Tusker

In South Asia over 500 years B. C. a king wished to have an elephant to use as a royal mount. He wanted a large tusker as he felt that this would enhance his status both within and without his kingdom. He enlisted the services of an experienced and wise tracker to track down a suitable elephant in the jungle and arrange its capture.

The tracker began his search and soon came upon a large elephant's footprint. Now the tracker could have said to himself, "Here is a large footprint and this would indicate that it has been made by a large bull elephant. If these tracks are followed they should lead to the large bull elephant." However, the experienced and wise tracker realised that a large female elephant too could have made these footprints and he continued to follow the tracks.

He then came across a tree that had branches broken high up on the tree. Noting the height at which the branches were broken he thought that it was probably a large bull-elephant that was responsible for this damage. But being experienced and wise, the tracker realised that a large she-elephant too may have broken these branches high up on the tree.

He continued to follow the tracks of the elephant until he came upon a tree that had scratchings on its bark. He thought that the teeth of a large bull-elephant could have caused these scratchings but being experienced and wise he realised that a large female too could have caused these scratchings.

He continued to follow the tracks of the elephant until he came to a tree where the trunk had been damaged by the tusks of an elephant. He knew that this definitely indicated that it was indeed a large bull-elephant that had made these marks. However, since he was experienced and wise he realised that the tusks of this elephant may be crooked or damaged and that this elephant may not be suitable for a royal mount.

He continued to follow the tracks of the elephant until he finally came across a large tusker foraging in the jungle. The elephant was a large, magnificent specimen with fine tusks and was most suitable for a royal mount.

Being experienced and wise, the tracker realised that arrangements for capturing the elephant depended upon the environment in which the elephant resided, the temperament of the animal and whether it was a lone bull or part of a herd. He made a note of all these features and went back to his village and made arrangements to capture this elephant.

To capture an elephant the *kraal* or pen into which the animal would be herded should be constructed of suitable, high-quality materials. The people involved must be knowledgeable in the art of elephant capture and they should be experienced. Hence, he recruited suitable individuals for the task and made arrangements for the supply of suitable materials to build the *kraal* and for experienced personnel to construct the *kraal*.

Following capture the elephant should be cared for. It should be fed, watered, bathed and housed in a suitable environment. The mahouts responsible should be knowledgeable, experienced and caring individuals who have a sense of duty. Hence, the tracker made arrangements for suitable individuals to be recruited to care for the elephant and the necessary facilities to be made available to house the elephant.

Finally, the elephant must be trained to carry out its duties as a royal mount. A knowledgeable, experienced, dutiful mahout should carry out this training. The tracker made arrangements for such a mahout to train the elephant.

After all the arrangements had been made, the elephant was captured and trained and the king was provided with a magnificent royal mount.

One may ask what relevance this story has to the practice of medicine.

In the management of patients the first thing one should do is make a diagnosis. The way (method) of making a diagnosis is similar to the method used by the tracker to find the elephant. One begins by speaking to the patient and after asking a few questions a preliminary idea comes to mind. One then follows this train of thought, always bearing in mind the alternatives, and after acquiring more information from history taking, physical examination and investigation one narrows down the possibilities till one finally finds enough evidence to conclusively prove a diagnosis.

After making a diagnosis one plans management bearing in mind the particular requirements of the patient in question. One always bears in mind that throughout this process the patient should be cared for and that the patient should be educated about his or her illness in particular and health in general. Patients should be trained to care for themselves if possible.

This is similar to the way in which the elephant was cared for and trained.

Thus, one will realise that the parable of the royal tusker and the knowledge passed down for generations is still relevant to us physicians of today.

Finally, if one thinks that the functions of a king are not relevant to doctors of today please bear in mind an ancient Singhala saying, "*Rajakama Nethnam Vedakama,*" which means, "If one cannot be a king, then be a doctor instead."

How to use this book

This is a book on clinical skills. It aims to help the reader develop a system that will improve his or her day-to-day practice and enable the reader to succeed in professional examinations. To do so one should be proficient in:

♣ Diagnosis

♦ Skills to make a diagnosis

♥ Knowledge to make a diagnosis

♠ Retrieval of the knowledge required in making a diagnosis

♣ Communication

Diagnosis

The major part of this book deals with diagnosis. There are many ways in which a physician may reach a diagnosis. They are pattern recognition, the use of algorithms, the exhaustive method (going through every aspect of history, examination and investigation) and the hypothetico-deductive method. The method that most use is the hypothetico-deductive method where an initial idea comes to mind and this idea is followed seeking more information either for or against until one finally acquires enough information to reach a conclusive diagnosis. In other words one follows the elephant's footprint.

Skills

To use the above method one requires the skills to acquire this information and secondly one requires knowledge of the likely symptoms and signs and the causes of these symptoms and signs.

To acquire the clinical skills follow the methods given in this book and practice endlessly. Read the methods, practice and then read again to make sure that the methods are being applied correctly. Enlist the help of a senior colleague to observe one's technique and make the necessary constructive criticism. This will be immensely helpful.

If one is teaching remember, to teach clinical skills the teacher should use the DISC method; Demonstration, Instruction, Supervision, Constructive Criticism (correction)

DISC

♣ Demonstrate the method

♦ Instruct the learner on how to perform the method

♥ Supervise as the learner performs the method

♠ Criticise in a constructive manner (Correct)

Knowledge

To acquire knowledge of the symptoms and signs that occur in disease and their causes, again, seeing more and more patients is the best method. This book has given many examples of the clinical features that occur in diseases affecting the various systems and they have been placed in the order in which history taking and physical examination are usually carried out. Read this and attempt to visualise the clinical scenario taking place. Again repetition is of utmost importance.

vii

Retrieval of Knowledge

In performing any task it is essential that all the instruments or implements that are used in the task are readily available. Ideally, all these instruments or implements should be labelled and stored in an orderly fashion so that retrieval is easy when required. Similarly, knowledge should be stored in an orderly fashion so that retrieval is facilitated. In each chapter a section on lesions of the relevant system has been included. This has been designed to collate information regarding lesions of each system so that retrieval of knowledge would be facilitated.

Communication

The section on communication skill has been designed to help the reader develop a system of communication. Read it and practice the methods. Again enlist the help of a colleague to observe and feed back with constructive criticism, as this would be immensely helpful.

In writing this book I have drawn from the extensive literature available, the experience of the various excellent clinicians I have had the opportunity to learn from and from my own experience as a clinician. I hope that I have come close to fulfilling my aim of preparing a concise textbook that gives a pragmatic approach to clinical method that is suitable for both professional examinations and day-to-day practice.

Finally, I would be grateful for feedback in particular with regard to any errors or omissions for which I apologise.

AJITH JAYASEKERA

www.acesforpaces.com

www.ydr.org.uk

Chapter 1

The P.A.C.E.S. Examination

Examinations are, and in all probability will always be, an integral part of a career in the medical profession. From schooldays, examinations are used in the process of selecting those deemed suitable to progress to the more intellectually demanding fields of study.

The question will arise whether this is necessary and whether there are less demanding and less stressful methods by which this selection process may be carried out. If one were to look at nature one would see that evolution is based on the process of natural selection. It is the stress of adverse conditions that acts as the selection pressure required for the eradication of the less suitable and the survival of those more suitable. Without these adverse conditions and their resultant selection pressures, evolution would cease.

Examinations are one of the aspects of this process of natural selection and maintain an important part in the evolution of the medical profession. Seen in this context one would appreciate the fundamental role played by the adverse conditions and stress associated with examinations. This function is in addition to the primary objective of examinations being the assessment of knowledge and skills.

What is examined?

To answer this one must first define the attributes of a good physician. Most would agree they are:

- ♥ Knowledge Base
- ♠ Clinical Skill
- ♦ The Art of Medicine

Knowledge Base

A sound knowledge base is essential if one aspires to be a physician. Anatomy, Physiology and Biochemistry are the foundations of this knowledge. To this foundation, which should be solid, one should add the study of Pathology and Microbiology (the term microbiology is used in an inclusive sense, encompassing all organisms that cause disease in mankind). On the basis of these sciences one would gain an understanding of the pathogenesis of disease and the resultant structural changes that occur in cells, tissues, organs and organ systems. In addition, these basic sciences would help one understand pathophysiology and the resultant disturbances in function of organs and organ systems. Thus, knowing the normal structure and function of the human body and combining this knowledge with an understanding of the evolution of the underlying structural and functional changes in disease, one would be able to understand and work out for oneself how clinical features develop and what they would be. In the same way, this would enable one to understand and work out for oneself the natural history of disease. When studied in this way a dynamic, mental image of how disease affects the human body is built up in one's mind.

This all important knowledge base may be represented diagrammatically in the form of a pyramid. (Fig 1.1) Like a pyramid, knowledge built up in this manner would be robust and long lasting. However, like the building of a pyramid acquiring this knowledge would entail a lot of hard work and time.

In clinical practice the process occurs in reverse. After eliciting clinical features, one works backwards to understand what the underlying changes in structure and function are. This understanding and the mental picture that one builds up of the underlying structural and functional changes that occur in the patient, allows logical planning of relevant investigations and subsequent management.

Once this basic knowledge is acquired one should also study the various methods of investigation that one may apply in further evaluation and documentation of disease.

Finally, the methods of treating illness should be studied. That is, pharmacology and the principles of surgery and radiotherapy should be studied. Methods of supporting the various systems when they malfunction due to disease should be learned. Lifestyle changes that have an impact on disease should be studied.

Studying medicine in this way, learning the basics and then using these basics to develop one's understanding of the principles of pathogenesis, pathophysiology, diagnosis and treatment, will give one a well grounded, rational approach that will stand the test of time.

Wisdom

Wisdom is the realisation of knowledge. Realisation comes from experience. For example one knows that toothache is painful but if one experiences a toothache then one would realise how painful it could be.

Figure 1.1

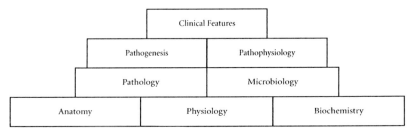

Similarly knowledge of a disease becomes realisation when one sees patients who suffer from it. The same applies to treatment, knowing about a form of treatment is knowledge but after actually using it on patients one realises its effects.

In studying any subject one goes through a learning curve. From this one may derive an acronym to help one remember the stages one would go through in acquiring wisdom. The acronym is **KERW**, *which stands for* **K***nowledge,* **E***xperience,* **R***ealisation,* **W***isdom.*

Clinical Skill

There are two aspects of clinical skill. They are:

♣ Diagnostic Skill

♥ Therapeutic Skill

The major part of this book is devoted to discussing diagnostic skill. Therapeutic skill is a very important part of being a good physician but only one aspect of therapeutic skill is discussed in later chapters.

The Art of Medicine

One would define the Art of Medicine as the use of knowledge, skill, imagination and creativity to ensure that the interaction between the doctor and the patient inspires confidence, is pleasant, rewarding and an aesthetic experience.

Like any art this is difficult to teach. A large part of it depends on the personality of the practitioner and his or her attitude to medicine. That is, whether one regards the practice

of medicine as employment or vocation.

The basis of developing the art of medicine is to acquire a sound knowledge base, develop one's clinical skills and develop one's personality through mental, physical and social discipline.

In short, by:

Being a physician rather than doing medicine.

The attributes of a good physician may be summarised in the acronym **MASKK** *where* **M** *stands for* **M***edicine,* **A** *for the* **A***rt of medicine,* **S** *for clinical* **S***kills,* **K** *for* **K***nowledge and the second* **K** *for Kaizen. The meaning of the Japanese word* **K***aizen will be explained in the chapter on clinical skills.*

The Art of Medicine

As an aide memoire one could use:

The sick pray that they are treated by a doctor who is well versed in the art of medicine.

Here **SICK** stands for **S**kill, **I**magination, **C**reativity, **K**nowledge

PRAI stands for **P**leasant, **R**ewarding, **A**esthetic experience, **I**nspires confidence

Medical Examinations

Various types of examinations are used to test the knowledge and skill of medical practitioners. Basically they are tests of the individual's knowledge base and tests of clinical diagnostic skills. At present no satisfactory examinations are available to test an individual's therapeutic skill.

Tests of Knowledge Base

The types of test vary. Long, essay type answers have largely been replaced by multiple-choice formats, structured essays, image recognition, data interpretation and case history based questions. Viva voce examination is not as commonly used as before.

Tests of Clinical Skills

This type of examination has sought to test the skills required by a physician in day-to-day practice. These skills are:

♠ Long Case Skills

♦ Short Case Skills

Long Case

An important aspect of day-to-day practice is the ability to see a patient for the first time, take a history, examine the patient, make an adequate assessment, reach a diagnosis and formulate a management plan. These skills are tested using a Long Case where a candidate has a specified time to see a patient, take a history, examine the patient and make a diagnosis and management plan.

Short Case

Another important aspect of day-to-day practice is the ability to make a quick assessment of a relevant system such as the assessment that one may make when a patient is reviewed following initial diagnosis, either in the outpatient or inpatient setting. These skills were tested using Short Cases where the candidate examined several patients, with conditions affecting the various organ systems, and the examiners assessed the candidate whilst he or she performed the examination. This was the only direct assessment of a candidate's clinical examination skills.

One of the drawbacks of this type of examination (long case and short case) was that the candidate's history taking skills were not assessed directly. The indirect assessment made by the examiners listening to the candidate describing the patient's history was a poor reflection of the candidate's history taking skill, the most important skill a physician should acquire.

In addition, although the viva voce assessed communication skill, the art of communicating with the laity was not examined in either the long or short cases.

The P.A.C.E.S examination may overcome these deficiencies.

The P.A.C.E.S. Examination

The examination takes the form of a carousel divided into five main stations, three of them being further subdivided.

The stations are:

♠ **Station 1**

Respiratory System

Abdominal Examination

♥ **Station 2**

History Taking Skills

♠ **Station 3**

Cardiovascular System

Central Nervous System

♦ **Station 4**

Communication Skills and Ethics

♣ **Station 5**

Endocrine, Eyes, Locomotor, Skin

Timing

Each station will be for a precise period of twenty (20) minutes. This is controlled by a timekeeper and will be signalled by the sounding of a bell.

At stations 1 and 3 ten minutes will be allocated for each system. At station 5 approximately five minutes will be allowed for each system. Station 2 and 4 will allow fourteen minutes for interaction with the patient, one minute for reflection and five minutes for discussion with the examiners.

A period of five minutes will be given between stations for changing over. During this period the examiners will independently complete the mark-sheets. The candidates will prepare for the next station by going through the instruction sheets at that station.

At each station two examiners will be present throughout the duration of the cycle.

Station 1

Respiratory System and Abdominal Examination

At this station an assessment will be made of the candidate's ability to examine the respiratory system and the abdomen and interpret the findings.

Ten minutes will be allowed for each system. During this period the candidate will be expected to make a systematic and thorough examination of the relevant system and discuss the findings with the examiners.

A notice will be displayed by the side of the patient. This will give a short history and the instructions to the candidate regarding the system to be examined.

The examiners will be looking for a demonstration of a systematic and thorough examination. Correct method should be used. Skill should be evident. The ability to correctly elicit physical signs will be assessed. Following this, the discussion will focus on the accurate interpretation of the findings on examination. If time permits a sensible management plan may be discussed. The plan should demonstrate clear, appropriate and professional clinical thinking.

Station 2

History Taking Skills

At this station an assessment will be made of the candidate's ability to take a good clinical history and interpret the information obtained.

5

Before entering the station the candidate will be given information regarding the situation. The information will be as follows:

♥ The first part of the information will be regarding the role played by the candidate. It will detail level of seniority and environment in which the scenario takes place. For example it could be as a Senior House Officer in a clinic or on an admissions unit.

♠ The second part of the information will be a short introduction to the patient and the problem. This will usually be in the form of a referral letter.

Five minutes will be available to study this information and then the bell will signal the candidate to enter the room and begin the consultation.

The consultation will take fourteen minutes and this will be followed by one minute where the candidate may pause for reflection and after this there will be five minutes of discussion with the examiners. At the end of twelve minutes the candidate will be reminded that only two minutes remain. The examiners will be present throughout the period of history taking.

At this station the examiners will be looking for the candidate to demonstrate a structured but flexible manner. Language should be intelligible and avoid jargon. The candidate should be confident, establish rapport with the patient and demonstrate empathy. When discussing clinical issues the candidate should be sensible. Where the patient demonstrates areas of doubt or ignorance the candidate should demonstrate the ability to acknowledge this and explain. The candidate should demonstrate an awareness of patient concerns and should demonstrate the ability to negotiate.

Station 3

Cardiovascular and Central Nervous Systems

This station involves an assessment of the candidate's ability to examine the cardiovascular system and the central nervous system.

This is similar to Station 1 except that it is two different systems that are being assessed. The same format will be followed.

Station 4

Communication Skills and Ethics

This station involves an assessment of the candidate's ability to communicate and his or her knowledge of medical ethics.

Before entering the station information regarding the situation will be available to the candidate. This information will define:

♦ **Role**

The role played by the candidate will be defined. For example this could be as the Senior House Officer on a Care of the Elderly Ward.

♣ **Subject Definition**

Information regarding the person with whom the candidate will discuss the issue. This could be either the patient or a relative.

♥ **Problem**

The candidate will be given a short outline of the problem that will be encountered and should be dealt with.

♠ **Scenario**

The scenario will be defined. This will include information regarding the patient's diagnosis, personal, family and social details and the issues to be discussed.

Five minutes will be available to study this information and then the candidate will enter the station and begin discussion with the subject.

Fourteen minutes will be available for discussion with the subject and this will be followed by a one-minute period of reflection by the candidate and then five minutes of further discussion with the two examiners who will be present throughout the period allocated to the station. At the end of twelve minutes the candidate will be informed that only two minutes remain.

The examiners will be looking for the candidate to demonstrate the same qualities as in the history taking station.

They are:

♦ Confidence

♣ Structured but flexible manner

♥ Language intelligible and avoidance of jargon

♠ Establishment of rapport

♦ Demonstration of empathy

♣ The ability to discuss issues in a sensible manner

♥ Ability to recognise areas of doubt or ignorance on the part of the subject

♠ Ability to recognise areas of concern for the subject

♦ Ability to explain

♣ Ability to negotiate

Ethics

Medical ethics is a difficult area as all issues that may be raised are not clearly defined. The law does not clearly define what can or cannot be done in several instances. However, this does not matter, as the candidate's knowledge of law and legal process is not being examined.

As morals, philosophy and religion play a part in these issues, they are fraught with controversy and should be approached in a delicate manner.

A few basic principles should be followed. They are:

♥ Duty

♠ Respect

♦ Law

Duty

The candidate should demonstrate an awareness of a sense of duty as a physician.

Respect

The candidate should demonstrate respect for the patient as an individual and respect for the patient's or relative's concerns.

Law

The candidate should follow the law where applicable.

Station 5

Endocrine, Eyes, Locomotor, Skin

This station involves an assessment of the ability of the candidate to examine the endocrine system, the eyes, the locomotor system and the skin.

This is very similar to Stations 1 and 3. The difference is that only five minutes will be allowed for each system. Four patients will be examined, each patient having a problem related to the relevant system. A printed card by the patient will give a short introduction to the patient and instructions for the candidate to follow. Two examiners will watch the candidate perform the relevant examination and then engage in a short discussion.

The examiners will be looking for the abilities outlined in Station 1.

Figure 1.2

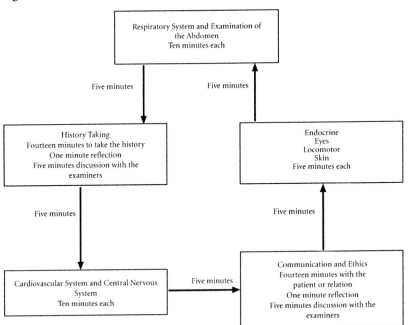

Chapter 2

Clinical Skills

In the strictest sense clinical skills means bedside skills as the word clinical is derived from the Greek word *kline*, which means bed or couch. That is, the skills that are necessary for a successful doctor-patient interaction. The laity describe these skills as bedside manner and they have always been appreciative of, and admired, good bedside manner.

Clinical Skills

Clinical skills may be broadly divided into two categories:

- ♥ Diagnostic Skills
- ♠ Therapeutic Skills

Diagnostic Skills

The major part of this book is devoted to this aspect of clinical skill. These skills are the ability to take a good history or **History Taking Skills** and the ability to perform a thorough physical examination or **Physical Examination Skills**. The ability to arrange and interpret **Relevant Investigation** is not a clinical skill in the strictest sense. It will be dealt with, very briefly, in a later chapter.

Therapeutic Skills

These are wide ranging skills. The art of communication is the most basic of these skills and without this all else is irrelevant. If one were unable to communicate effectively and explain the nature of their illness to patients in terms that they will understand easily then, it is unlikely that compliance with management strategy would be achieved. This aspect of therapeutic skill will be dealt with in this book.

Other therapeutic skills vary from the ability to venesect and introduce an intravenous cannula to the ability to perform complex surgery. The development of these skills is outside the scope of this book.

The Importance of Clinical Skills

Many people question the importance of clinical skills arguing that with advancing technology the need for clinical skills diminishes. The equivalent would be that with the development of the wheel walking would have become obsolete! On the contrary one may put forward the argument that with advancing technology even better clinical skills are required. In other fields, where technology has advanced greatly, this is indeed the case. One may cite examples such as piloting aircraft and motor sport where advanced technology has required more skilled pilots and drivers to safely handle these machines. It would be easy to realise that better clinicians are needed today to select the relevant investigations from the batteries of advanced tests available, thus reducing both the costs and risks associated with a blanket or shotgun approach. In addition, good clinical skills and the rational approach that follows is exceedingly important in formulating an effective management plan for the patient. This reduces the time taken for the patient to benefit from interventions, it reduces morbidity and mortality and it is the only way to reduce healthcare costs that are at present rising in an uncontrollable fashion.

An analogy will help to clarify the concept. If one were to arrange investigations and reach a diagnosis without taking a good history and performing a thorough physical examination, it would be like reading only the last page of a book or watching only the end of a movie or play. One would know the answer to the question, who was the culprit or who won the heroine's heart, but one would not appreciate or understand the atmosphere, the background, the characters and the scenario nor would one have an understanding of the plot. In other words this is a sure way to lose the plot!

Benefits of Clinical Skills

The benefits of clinical skills could be categorised as:

♦ Benefits to the Practitioner

♣ Benefits to the Patient

♥ Benefits to the Doctor-Patient Relationship

♠ Benefits to the Service

Benefits to the Practitioner

The benefits to the practitioner are:

♦ Personal Development

♣ Pleasure

♥ Pride

♠ Profit

Personal Development

Development of clinical skill by continuous clinical practice is one of the finest forms of mental development. Clinical practice stresses and thereby develops retentive memory, analytical skill and imagination. In addition continuous clinical practice enhances one's sensory and motor capabilities. Interaction with patients and exposure to people's problems helps one to develop character. Ultimately, clinical practice will lead one to have better understanding and insight and this will culminate in realisation of knowledge and wisdom.

Pleasure

The practice of clinical medicine does give rise to pleasure. The reasons for this are manifold. One may derive pleasure from the challenge of elucidating a diagnosis or from recreating the story of a patient's illness. Or, it may simply be the altruistic joy of being able to deal with a patient's problems. Whatever the reason, if one does not derive pleasure from the practice of clinical medicine then, some other avenue of specialisation should be sought.

Pride

One should derive pride from the fact that this skill is unique to the profession and the ability to perform well is greatly appreciated; at least by the patients.

Profit

Dare one mention the fact that everyone gains a financial benefit from the practice of medicine? In days gone by in South Asia, the rich practised medicine free of charge. But, this was so they could acquire merit for their next life. Today everyone practices medicine for a living, either fee for service or for a salary. The best way to develop a practice is to be a skilled clinician as good clinical skill provides immense benefit to patients and this encourages repeat visits and referrals.

It will be seen that all the reasons given above begin with the letter P. Denying these reasons could be viewed as taking the Pees out of medicine!

Benefits to the Patient

The benefits the patient will derive from good clinical skill are first and foremost, quicker and more accurate diagnosis. This will lead to less exposure to costly and sometimes risky investigations. Secondly, good clinical skill results in better management with more focused treatment strategies and this will result in quicker benefit and lower morbidity and mortality.

Benefits to the Doctor-Patient Relationship

Good clinical skill is the only way to establish rapport with the patient. It lays the foundation for a good doctor-patient relationship, which is essential for a successful outcome for both the patient and the doctor.

Benefits to the Service

Whatever the type of health service that is provided, be it state controlled, insurance funded or self-funded by the patient, cost is an important consideration. Good clinical skill is the only way of reducing cost. It reduces the burden of costly and sometimes risky investigation. In addition, the better, more focused management that results from good clinical skill speeds up the achievement of benefit thus reducing cost. It also reduces complications that result in an increase in morbidity, mortality and financial cost.

Development of Clinical Skills

Development of clinical skills will require instruction in correct method followed by endless practice.

In the following chapters an endeavour has been made to provide instruction in correct method. Endless practice is up to the reader.

In developing clinical skills attention should be paid to three aspects. They are:

♥ Development of form

♠ Development of clinical sense

♦ Repetition

Form

Form is a word more commonly associated with sportsmen than with medical practitioners. One may wonder what form has to do with the practice of medicine.

To clarify this an analogy will be made with the practice of the martial arts. Martial arts have been chosen as they have played an integral role in the evolution of mankind and human civilisation.

In the study of the martial arts, practitioners develop a form. The form is a predetermined sequence of attacking and defensive movements and they encompass all the requirements for attack and defence. Practitioners undertake endless practice until the form becomes reflex or second nature to them. When this state is reached these practitioners can easily respond to any attack with the appropriate defensive or attacking move.

In addition to practice, continuous assessment and refinement of technique is also a feature of the martial arts. This process of continuous assessment and improvement is known, in Japan, as *Kaizen.*

Kaizen

This Japanese term is derived from **KAI**, *which means change or modify, and* **ZEN**, *which means to improve. Thus, Kaizen means gradual, orderly, never-ending, continuous improvement.*

In clinical medicine it is essential to develop such a form, a sequence of history taking and examination techniques that will encompass all situations. When one has learned such a form and practised it to the extent that it has become reflex or second nature to oneself, then one would be considered to be an advanced clinical examiner or ACE.

Cultivate form and one will harvest success.

Clinical Sense

Hopefully, one would have had the opportunity to work with or study under practitioners who were gifted with clinical sense. Then, one would have observed their, almost magical, ability to ask the correct question and demonstrate the appropriate physical sign to clinch a diagnosis. One would have noted their ability to appreciate the most subtle clues in the history or examination and their ability to put everything together to make a coherent whole. In addition, the unerring accuracy with which these individuals target the appropriate investigations and treatment would have been noticed.

Is it possible to develop clinical sense? This has not been studied in medicine but in the field of sports science this has been studied extensively. Successful sportsmen in all fields from motor-racing drivers to cricketers and rugby players demonstrate similar skills. That is the ability, with unerring accuracy and speed, to play the correct stroke or make the appropriate move in response to a particular situation.

This "sense" of the game or sport is thought to arise from the ability of these individuals to detect very subtle clues, in the environment or in the actions of opposing players, that guide their decisions. In addition, these individuals have the ability to attain a state of heightened awareness or mindfulness, the so-called "zone". This enables these sportsmen to sense these clues, come to a split second decision and implement an action without interference from intruding and distracting thought processes. One should realise that development of this sense of a game or sport is not an ability that arises spontaneously. These sportsmen have certain characteristics in common namely, they are highly disciplined and they engage in hours of dedicated practice.

Thus, one may deduce that clinical sense is the ability to detect the most subtle clues in the history and examination and put them together to arrive at a coherent diagnosis and combine this with a logical approach to investigation and management. Reaching a heightened state of awareness or mindfulness is essential for this process to occur.

All practitioners may develop clinical sense provided they pay attention to the development of form and practice endlessly.

Like becoming skilled in the art of medicine, the development of clinical sense is achieved by *being a clinician rather than doing clinical medicine.*

Repetition

One would acknowledge that the key to the development of clinical skill is practice; in other words repetition. If one were to consider a situation where a route is travelled on constantly, one would note that with time a well-defined path would appear. This would make travel along this route easy and one would be unlikely to lose one's way. On the other hand if one were to stop travelling along this path and if it were to be left in disuse, grass and weeds would grow and obliterate the path thus hindering travel and increasing the chance of losing one's way. The same applies to the development of any skill, clinical skill being no exception. Repetition would develop and sharpen one's skill whereas lack of use will allow the skill to degenerate and disappear.

Arguments may be made that repetition ad infinitum is boring. This may be so but please remember that the word **BORE** *is an acronym for* **B**rilliance is **O**btained by **R**epetition *and* **E**ndurance.

Chapter 3

Diagnosis

The process of ascertaining a diagnosis or identifying the disease process affecting the patient is fundamental to the management of the patient.

This was considered so important that medical students were expected to say it thrice when asked what three important inferences should be reached before a patient could be managed effectively. The first question on a clinical teaching round would be, "When considering a patient, what three important inferences (deductions) should one reach (be made) before one may manage a patient effectively?"

The answer was:

- ♥ Diagnosis
- ♠ Diagnosis
- ♦ Diagnosis

To this one should add a fourth point. That point being **Diagnosis**!

The reason for repeating the word diagnosis four times is not only to stress the importance of the diagnosis but, to establish that a diagnosis has four components.

The Four Components of a Diagnosis

The four components of a diagnosis are as follows:

- ♣ Anatomical Diagnosis
- ♥ Pathological Diagnosis
- ♠ Physiological Diagnosis
- ♦ Aetiological Diagnosis

Anatomical Diagnosis

Anatomical diagnosis refers to identification of the anatomical site, organ or organ system affected by the disease process.

Pathological Diagnosis

Pathological diagnosis refers to identification of the main pathological process underlying the disease.

Physiological Diagnosis

Physiological diagnosis refers to identification of any functional abnormality caused by the disease process.

Aetiological Diagnosis

Aetiological diagnosis refers to identification of the aetiological agent or agents responsible for the disease process.

A few examples will help to clarify the concept.

If one were to say that a patient has pneumonia a limited amount of information is given but this is insufficient to manage the patient. If however, one were to say that the patient has a right, lower lobe pneumonia caused by *Streptococcus pneumoniae* and there is evidence of respiratory failure then adequate information is available to effectively manage the patient as all the components of the diagnosis have been identified.

Quite often a name is given to identify a disease. This is often simpler than giving all the details but the information supplied by this method is usually inadequate. For example saying that a patient has Crohn's disease is easier than saying that the patient has a chronic inflammatory disorder of unknown aetiology, affecting both the small and large bowel and causing nutritional failure and partial small intestinal obstruction. But, the information supplied by the latter method is much more useful in planning further management.

Aide Memoire

*The acronyms **APPA** or **PAPA** may be used as an aide memoire for **A**natomy, **P**athology, **P**hysiology and **A**etiology. Interestingly both words, in different languages, mean father. It makes this method different in that it is not the mother of all diagnoses but the father of all diagnoses!*

Diagnostic Techniques

There are three techniques that are used to make a diagnosis. In diminishing order of importance they are:

♣ **History Taking**

A Good History

♥ **Physical Examination**

A Thorough Physical Examination

♠ **Investigation**

Relevant Investigations

History Taking

History taking is the most crucial of the techniques. A good history will result in a diagnosis in the majority of patients and indeed some so-called functional disorders are diagnosed on the basis of history alone. It is also on the basis of the history that one directs subsequent physical examination and investigation. However, it is not an easy technique to master and most flounder at this the most basic of diagnostic skills. In the next chapter an attempt will be made to provide an understanding of the technique and on the basis of this understanding, develop a structure or form that may be used in any situation.

Physical Examination

Physical examination is next in importance. One should understand the basic concepts, develop good methods and be thorough. This will be studied in depth in the following chapters.

Investigation

Investigation would seem to be the easiest technique. One could be facetious and say it is only the ability to fill in a form! The skill here is to use common sense and arrange relevant investigations, the results of which will guide further action. This aspect will be dealt with when discussing the communication and ethics station.

In conclusion to summarise technique:

A diagnosis is made on a good history, it is confirmed by a thorough physical examination and documented by relevant investigations.

Checklists

The use of checklists (sieves) is a method that helps enormously in difficult situations; both clinical situations and professional examinations. As knowledge and experience increase reliance on checklists decreases but it is useful to have them as a safety net.

The following checklists are given to aid diagnosis.

* Anatomy Checklist
* Pathology Checklist
* Aetiology Checklist
* Physiology Checklist

Anatomy Checklist

The best checklist is a good knowledge of anatomy but for finer definition the following checklist would be useful.

All organs are or have been derived from hollow structures. Therefore the structure has a lumen, a wall and exterior relationships. Hence, when defining the anatomical site of a lesion, one could consider lesions within the lumen, lesions within the wall and lesions exterior to the structure.

To this one should add systemic lesions and thus consider manifestations of systemic disease. To consider systemic lesions one should refer to a list of systems; cardiovascular (CVS), respiratory (RS), gastrointestinal (GIT), kidneys and urinary (KUS), reproductive and genitals (RAG), locomotor (LMS), nervous (CNS), endocrine and metabolic (E&M), haematological (HS), integumental (IS)

The checklist would thus be:

* Luminal or Internal
* Mural
* External
* Systemic

Aide Memoire

As an aide memoire one may use the acronym **PIPES**. *This would stand for* **P**onder *the* **I**nternal, *the* **P**eripheral, *the* **E**xternal *and* **S**ystemic *where internal would mean luminal, peripheral would mean mural, external would be local external factors and systemic would refer to the various systems of the body.*

Pathology Checklist

It is useful to have a checklist of pathological conditions when tackling a difficult diagnostic problem. It is useful in practice and in professional examinations when one's mind may suddenly go blank.

This checklist is a modification of the sieve that was taught by surgeons many years ago.

Pathology Checklist

The pathology checklist would be as follows:

- ◆ Developmental
- ♣ Traumatic
- ♥ Inflammation (Acute or Chronic)
- ♠ Neoplasia (Benign and Malignant)
- ◆ Dysplasia
- ♣ Vascular (Thrombosis, Embolism, Haemorrhage)
- ♥ Necrosis
- ♠ Degeneration
- ◆ Interstitial Infiltration
- ♣ Hypertrophy
- ♥ Metabolic
- ♠ Functional

One must realise the fact that it is the most dominant pathological feature that is taken into account, as it is common for different pathological entities to co-exist; for example necrosis and inflammation.

Aetiology Checklist

Similarly an aetiological checklist may be developed for use in difficult situations in practice and in professional examinations.

The checklist is as follows:

- ◆ Biological Agents
- ♣ Physical Agents
- ♥ Chemical Agents

Biological Agents

Biological agents may be:

- ♠ External Agents
- ◆ Internal Agents

External Agents

External agents could be:

- ♣ Bacteria
- ♥ Fungi
- ♠ Viruses
- ◆ Prions
- ♣ Parasites

Internal Agents

Internal agents could be:

- ♥ Immune reactions (cell mediated and humoral)
- ♠ Genetic mechanisms

Physical Agents

Physical agents could be agents such as:

- ◆ Mechanical force or trauma
- ♣ Heat
- ♥ Light
- ♠ Radiation

Chemical Agents

Chemical agents may cause problems by:

- ◆ Toxicity
- ♣ Deficiency

Toxicity

Toxicity may be caused by substances that are inherently noxious or by excessive amounts of substances normally present in the body.

Deficiency

Deficiency of essential nutrients such as vitamins or elements like iron may cause disease.

Types of Chemical Agents

Chemical agents may be:

♥ Elements such as lead, iron

♠ Compounds, which may be organic or inorganic

Physiology Checklist

Disease may cause increased function, decreased function or aberrant function of the affected organ or organ system. Hence one should consider:

◆ Hyperfunction

♣ Hypofunction

♥ Dysfunction

Chapter 4

History Taking

The history is the story of the patient's illness or condition. All good stories have a detailed and vivid description of the setting in which the story occurs. The characters are well described and colourful. An appropriate atmosphere is conveyed. The story line is coherent.

In a similar fashion, the clinical history should describe the patient and the environment in which he or she lives. The symptoms should be described in detail and placed in a coherent structure, which is usually in chronological order. Additional information including relevant negative findings should be given to make the story complete. Information regarding the patient's beliefs, expectations and anxieties or concerns regarding the illness or condition should be provided to convey the appropriate atmosphere.

The above refers to the manner in which a patient's case history should be presented but before presentation one must first undertake the process of history taking. It is an area of confusion as many different styles of history taking are described. One method commonly described is to ask the patient to relate his or her story and listen whilst extracting the relevant features. This would be fine in an ideal world. Unfortunately, practically, in a clinical situation or in professional examinations, time is a constraint. Thus, this Utopian method is not suitable for everyday use. Instead, one should carefully direct the interview so that the necessary information is obtained from the patient whilst he or she is not stifled but is yet, gently, prevented from rambling. Remember that the technique is known as history taking **not** history listening!

Whilst taking the history one should bear in mind that the objective is to make a diagnosis. That is the four components of a diagnosis should always be borne in mind. Remember, one is using the history to try and answer a number of questions.

Questions to be answered by taking a history

When taking a history one should endeavour to find the answer to the following questions:

- ♥ What anatomical site, organ or organ system is involved?
- ♠ What type of pathology is involved?
- ♦ Is there a functional abnormality and if so how severe is it?
- ♣ What is the underlying aetiology?

21

The path to finding the answers to these questions is to initially describe and analyse what the patient feels. In other words, analyse the symptoms. This should give clues that will help in answering the questions posed above. From the analysis of symptoms one should be able to identify the anatomical site, organ or organ system involved. Then, one would move on to analyse that system for further clues to try and answer the questions posed above. Following this a review of the other systems will give further information in relation to the disease process and, or, the presence of any other disease or condition. After this one should proceed to obtain details regarding past illnesses, drugs used and allergies. Personal and family details should be obtained and the relevant social circumstances should be defined. In addition one should enquire about the patient's beliefs and expectations regarding the illness or condition. One should also ask about any anxieties (concerns) the patient may have regarding the causes and effects of the disease and any anxieties (concerns) the patient may have regarding survival. Throughout the process one should bear in mind that taking the history must be done with a sense of purpose, that purpose being, finding the answers to the questions posed above.

Identification (Introduction)

Probably the most important aspect of clinical medicine is the development of the bond between the doctor and the patient. Without this it is difficult to achieve a successful outcome. In the development of this bond the first step is identification of each other. In most settings the patient would have been identified prior to first contact by the availability of notes. If not one should introduce oneself and then ask the patient the relevant information, which would be the patient's name, address, date of birth and any relevant identification number or code. Remember, even if the patient's details are available one must always introduce oneself and it is wise to confirm the patient's identity.

Aide Memoire

To summarise history taking; **I**dentification *then* **P**urposefully **A**nalyse **S**ymptoms *and* **S**ystems, **E**licit **D**etails *and ask about* **B**eliefs, **E**xpectations *and* **A**nxieties (concerns) *regarding* **C**auses, **E**ffects *and* **S**urvival.

This gives the acronym **I PASSED B**y **E**mploying **ACES**. *Hopefully this system should help one to achieve success at professional examinations.*

Analysis of Symptoms

When analysing symptoms one could consider each symptom as a separate entity and attempt to remember the details that should be obtained regarding every one of them. On the other hand, it would be easier and more logical to develop a structure that would enable one to obtain details regarding any symptom and analyse any symptom.

Take the symptom pain. This is a symptom that is commonly encountered and tends to make patients seek treatment early. The details obtained are set out below:

Symptom: Pain

When analysing the symptom, pain, one would enquire about the following:

- ♥ **Site:** Anatomical site where the pain is felt.

- ♠ **Radiation:** Area to which the pain spreads.

- ♦ **Character or Nature (Quality):** The patient's description of what the pain feels like.

- ♣ **Severity (Quantity):** An estimate of how severe the pain is

- ♥ **Associated Features:** A description of any associated features such as sweating, nausea and vomiting

- ♠ **Precipitating Factors:** A description of anything that brings on the pain

- ♦ **Aggravating Factors:** A description of what makes the pain more severe

- ♣ **Relieving Factors:** A description of what reduces the intensity of the pain

- ♥ **Onset:** How quickly the pain develops

- ♠ **Progress:** The pattern of further development of the pain

- ♦ **Duration:** How long the pain lasts

- ♣ **Cessation:** If the pain subsides the mode or rate of cessation

- ♥ **Periodicity:** In the case of pain that recurs the pattern of recurrence

These features may be grouped together as in the format for examination of function that will be discussed later. Thus the grouping will be:

- ♠ **Position:** Site and Radiation

- ♦ **Character:** Nature

- ♣ **Quantity:** Severity

- ♥ **Transmission:** Associated features (associated features may be seen as symptoms that are transmitted to a remote region from the area affected by the index symptom)

- ♠ **Modifying Factors:** Precipitating, Aggravating and Relieving Factors

- ♦ **Rate:** Onset, Progress, Duration, Cessation (these are grouped under rate as they deal with timing)

- ♣ **Rhythm:** Periodicity

This structure or form is ideal for describing and analysing the symptom pain. The question is whether the same structure or form may be used to analyse other symptoms.

One may take the example of diarrhoea to test whether this structure or form may be used to obtain details about and analyse this totally different symptom.

Symptom: Diarrhoea

One would ask about the following:

- ♥ **Site:** Not applicable. The exception would be a patient with a stoma.

- ♠ **Radiation:** Not applicable.

- ♦ **Character or Nature (Quality):** Watery, semi-formed, mucoid, bloody, steatorrhoea.

- ♣ **Quantity (Severity):** Number of motions per day.

- ♥ **Associated Features:** Tenesmus, pain, incomplete evacuation
- ♠ **Precipitating Factors:** Such as a meal
- ♦ **Aggravating Factors:** Meals or particular constituents of a meal
- ♣ **Relieving Factors:** Usually drugs
- ♥ **Onset:** Rate of onset.
- ♠ **Progress:** Nature of and rate of progression
- ♦ **Duration:** Period of time the patient has diarrhoea
- ♣ **Cessation:** Rate of and mode of cessation
- ♥ **Periodicity:** If recurrent, frequency and pattern

From the above one may infer that this structure or form would be suitable for analysis of the symptom of diarrhoea.

Similarly, this structure or form may be used to obtain details about and analyse any symptom. It would be too time and space consuming to detail its use in every symptom that may occur. However, the reader may use it as an exercise to go through other symptoms using this structure or form to describe and analyse them. It will help greatly in understanding the principle and in development of form.

Aide Memoire

- ♥ **P**osition *(Site and Radiation)*
- ♠ **C**haracter or Nature *(Quality)*
- ♦ **Q**uantity *(Severity)*
- ♣ **T**ransmission *(Associated Features)*

- ♥ **M**odifying **F**actors *(Precipitating Factors, Aggravating Factors, Relieving Factors)*
- ♠ **R**ate *(Onset, Progress, Duration, Cessation)*
- ♦ **R**hythm *(Periodicity)*

A mnemonic will help one remember.

Please **C**arefully **Q**uestion **T**hese **M**ethods **F**or **R**eliability **a**nd **R**esilience

Analysis of Systems

Unfortunately no single structure has been developed to suit every system. But, knowledge of basic anatomy and physiology will allow one to analyse any system and determine sites of involvement, pathology and functional deficit.

As an example one may use the digestive system excluding the hepato-biliary component. This is the easiest to analyse as it has clearcut beginning and end points. One may commence at the mouth and proceed caudally.

Analysis of the Digestive System

One would ask about the following:

- ♥ Appetite
- ♠ Mastication
- ♦ Pain or soreness of the mouth
- ♣ Swallowing:

  Enquire about difficulty in swallowing or pain.
- ♥ Heartburn
- ♠ Reflux
- ♦ Belching

♣ Abdominal Pain

♥ Early Satiety

♠ Bloating or Distension

♦ Swelling

♣ Bowel Movements:

Number of motions

Consistency

Blood

Mucous

♥ Evacuation of Faeces:

Enquire about rectal sensation, continence and adequacy of evacuation (complete or incomplete evacuation). Ask about ease of commencement of evacuation and whether there is a need to strain.

♠ Prolapse of rectum

♦ Perianal Problems:

Discharge, pain, lump

Similarly, using knowledge of anatomy and physiology, one may develop methods to analyse the other organ systems of the body. This will be done at the beginning of each relevant chapter.

Elicit Details

This is the easiest part of history taking but still remains important. The details to be obtained are those regarding the following:

♥ Past Illnesses

♠ Drug History

♦ Drug Intolerance

♣ Allergies

♥ Personal History

♠ Family History

♦ Social History

♣ Beliefs

♥ Expectations

♠ Anxieties (Concerns)

Past Illnesses

Define any significant illnesses that have been experienced by the patient and place them in chronological order.

Drug History

Obtain details of drugs in use by the patient and those that have been used by the patient. Both prescription and non-prescription drugs should be included.

Drug Intolerance

Obtain details of any drugs that the patient is intolerant of and the reason for this intolerance.

Allergies

Obtain details of allergies to drugs and other substances.

Personal History

Obtain details regarding the patient's:

♦ Diet

♣ Exercise

♥ Alcohol intake

♠ Smoking history

Family History

Obtain details of any relevant illness in the family.

25

Social History

Obtain details regarding the patient's:

- ◆ Family
- ♣ Work
- ♥ Housing
- ♠ Activities of Daily Living (Washing, Dressing, Eating, Going to the Toilet, Shopping, Preparation of Food)
- ◆ Support (Patients may receive support from family, friends, neighbours, Religious Organisations, Non-Governmental Organisations, Social Services)
- ♣ Leisure Activities
- ♥ Sexual History (where appropriate). This may be included here or in the review of the reproductive and genital system

Beliefs

Make enquiries about the patient's beliefs regarding the illness or condition. Ask about:

- ♠ **Thoughts**

  What they think is wrong with them
- ◆ **Knowledge**

  What they know about the illness

Expectations

Make enquiries about the patient's expectations regarding the disease or condition and his or her expectations regarding investigations and treatment.

Anxieties (Concerns)

Find out if the patient has any anxieties or concerns regarding the disease or condition. These anxieties may be regarding the following:

- ♣ **Causes**

  What caused the disease or condition.
- ♥ **Effects**

  The effects the disease or condition may have on the patient, his or her lifestyle and on the patient's relatives, friends and colleagues. The patient may also have concerns regarding the effects of any tests that may be performed and regarding the effects of treatment.
- ♠ **Survival**

  The patient may have concerns regarding the chances of survival from the disease or condition and the expected duration of survival.

At the conclusion of the clinical encounter one should be able to generate a problem list. A problem list should be more extensive than a list of diagnoses. The problem list should include the patient's beliefs and expectations and any anxieties (concerns) the patient may have regarding causes, effects and survival.

Listening

The skill of listening is a very important skill to acquire. The secret of becoming a good listener is to keep one's mind in a state of awareness and not allow it to wander.

This is easier said than done but may be achieved by constant practice.

Chapter 5

Physical Examination

This refers to examination of the patient in order to obtain clues that will lead one to determine the underlying diagnosis. One uses the sensory modalities of the body with enhancement by instruments such as stethoscopes and ophthalmoscopes.

The senses used are the visual, tactile and auditory senses and from these one derives the techniques of inspection, palpation, percussion and auscultation. The olfactory sense is used more rarely, an example being the detection of foetor hepaticus. Taste is not used now but in the past, before the development of chemical reagents, this was the only method of detecting sugar in the urine.

In the east a less unpleasant technique was used. Patients were asked to void urine in the yard and the practitioner would then observe whether ants were attracted to the site by the presence of sugar in the patient's urine.

Concept of Examination

Knowledge of anatomy and physiology enables one to recognise the normal structure and function of the body. When one examines a patient, one observes whether normal structure and function are preserved and, if not, one takes note of the degree of deviation from normal. In addition, one takes note of any features of underlying pathology such as the cardinal signs of inflammation; rubor, tumor, calor, dolor, functiolaesa (for the less pompous; redness, swelling, heat, pain, loss of function). Clues to aetiology may sometimes be found on examination.

In short, physical examination is examination of **Structure** and examination of **Function** using the four basic techniques of **Inspection, Palpation, Percussion** and **Auscultation.** However, bear in mind the rare use of the olfactory sense. Deviations from normal structure and function enable one to locate the anatomical site of the disease, clarify the functional abnormality and obtain clues to the underlying pathology and sometimes the aetiology.

In each region of the body it would be best to examine structure first and then move on to examine function although this may be reversed in certain instances.

One should always bear in mind that in addition to the primary function of examining the patient for the purpose of finding clues to the diagnosis, this physical contact between the doctor and the patient helps to establish the bond that is such an essential part of a good doctor-patient relationship.

System of Examination

As in every aspect of clinical medicine, when performing physical examination of a patient it is best to utilise a system that is thorough, robust and versatile.

In developing such a method or form two important points must be made. First, the method should be thorough so that every part of the body is examined and secondly, when examining each part of the body every feature should be noted and any deviation from the normal characterised. That said, the method cannot be too time consuming, as in professional examinations and in clinical practice time is limited.

In summary the method should enable the practitioner to:

♥ Examine every part of the body

♠ Examine every feature of the part examined

Examining Every Part

If one were to examine a map, a picture or a photograph, the way to make sure that every detail is examined would be to start off with a general or global look at the whole. One would then divide the whole using a grid and then examine every individual square on the grid. The more detailed one would like to make the examination the smaller the grid would be. If particular parts were of greater interest than the others then those areas would have more grid lines thus allowing examination in finer detail.

Examination of the patient is performed in a similar fashion. After an initial look in general or taking a global look, one would divide the body into regions or systems and then examine these regions or systems thus allowing a more detailed examination to be performed. Depending on the area concerned, greater division will allow examination in greater detail. However, one must balance repeated division and the examination of finer details against the constraints of the time available.

Some parts of the body are best examined by dividing into sub-regions whereas other parts are best examined by dividing into systems. As examples one may use the examination of two regions; the head and the hands.

When examining the head one would take a general or global look and one would then divide the head into regions, which are the nose, eyes, face, mouth and ears. The eyes may be further divided into the orbits, the globe in general, the eyelids, the conjunctiva, the sclera, the cornea, the anterior chamber, the iris, the lens, the vitreous and the fundus. The same could be done for the mouth. Thus, it would become obvious that examination in greater detail may be achieved by further division of each area. Time would be the only constraint.

In the case of the hands after taking a general look at the hands division may be performed. However, when considering the hands, instead of dividing them into sub-regions it would be more practical to divide them into systems as this lends itself to a more logical method of examination. Thus, the hands would be better divided into the integument that is the nails and skin, the locomotor system that is the bones, joints, tendons and muscles and the cardiovascular system that is the peripheral circulation and the radial pulse. Next, one would look for involuntary movements and examine the nervous system and examine function of the locomotor system if required.

Examination of Features

Next, one should develop a method of ensuring that every feature of the part in consideration will be examined. This would enable one to determine whether these features are normal and if not characterise the deviation from normal.

One would examine features of:

♦ Structure

♣ Function

Structure

As a starting point in developing a method or form for examination of structure one may take the examination of a lump or swelling.

Examination of a Lump

Using   inspection,   palpation,

percussion and auscultation, the features that are defined in the examination of a lump are the following:

♥ Site

♠ Size

♦ Shape

♣ Edge or margins

♥ Colour

♠ Surface

♦ Crepitus or Rub

♣ Consistency

♥ Temperature

♠ Tenderness

♦ Mobility

♣ Attachments

♥ Percussion note

♠ Blood vessel pattern

♦ Pulsations

♣ Bruit

♥ Hum

The above is a comprehensive list but it is a lot and cumbersome to use. It could be classified further into:

♥ **Dimensions**

   Site

   Size

   Shape

   Margins or Edge

♠ **Cover**

   Colour

   Surface

   Crepitus or Rub

♦ **Contents**

   Consistency

Temperature

Tenderness

Percussion note

♣ **Connections (Contacts)**

Mobility

Attachment

Percussion note (helps to determine overlying structures)

♥ **Circulation**

Blood vessels

Pulsations

Bruit

Hum

This further classification makes it easier as instead of the sixteen subdivisions presented earlier it is reduced to just five. That is **Dimensions, Cover, Contents, Connections and Circulation.**

Aide Memoire

As an aide memoire it could be simplified to DC₄ or Diagnostic Clues x 4

Although the system may appear time consuming at first, if one practices regularly, using the short form DC₄ to screen and moving on to the longer form, the multiple subdivisions, only when required, the technique will soon become second nature to one and become established as part of one's form.

Examination (or Assessment) of Function

As in examination of structure, in examination of function it would be beneficial to develop a system that could be applied to any situation. To do this advantage may be taken of the fact that bodily functions have several features in common. These features are the following:

♠ **Position**

A starting position may usually be defined.

♦ **Quantity**

Bodily functions perform defined quantities of work and these quantities fall within a certain range.

♣ **Characteristics or Patterns**

Bodily functions usually follow well-defined patterns or display well-defined characteristics.

♥ **Transmission**

Movement is a characteristic of most bodily functions. Thus movement of substrates or energy can be recognised.

♠ **Modifying Factors**

Bodily functions may be modified by voluntary or involuntary actions

♦ **Repetition**

Bodily functions are usually cyclical events that are repeated endlessly. The rate of repetition usually falls within a defined range.

♣ **Rhythm**

Bodily functions follow fairly well-defined biorhythms.

From the above a system may be developed. Take the examination of the arterial pulse.

Examination of the Arterial Pulse (Radial)

When examining the radial arterial pulse one examines the following:

♥ Rate

♠ Rhythm

♦ Volume (Quantity)

♣ Character (Quality)

♥ Condition of the vessel wall

♠ Radio-Femoral delay

This system may be modified to examine function in multiple situations. Condition of the vessel wall may be deleted, as strictly speaking this is examination of the structure of the arterial wall. Instead of radio-femoral delay one may substitute the word transmission to define this characteristic of bodily function. Add in starting position or position at rest, as this will be important in several situations. In addition one should also consider factors that modify bodily functions. Hence the new format will be as follows:

Examination of Function

♦ Position

♣ Character

♥ Quantity

♠ Transmission

♦ Modifying Factors

♣ Rate

♥ Rhythm

Aide Memoire

*A mnemonic will help one to remember this. It is: **P**lease **C**arefully **Q**uestion **T**hese **M**ethods **F**or **R**eliability and **R**esilience. This stands for Position, Character, Quantity, Transmission, Modifying Factors, Rate, and Rhythm.*

One must bear in mind that these divisions, into examination of structure and examination of function, are not absolute. For example in acromegaly, large hands, a structural change, reflect a change in function of the pituitary gland. Radio-femoral delay may reflect coarctation of the aorta, a structural change.

Summary of Examination

In summary begin by applying the system generally and then re-apply the system locally. It will be too time consuming to go through each and every area and sub-division of the areas and each and every item on the list of features, especially as quite a few of them are not applicable in every instance. A balance must be reached between slavishly sticking to the system thus spending too much time and being careless by skipping over items too quickly. It is however important to keep to an order.

Aide Memoire

*All this can be remembered using the acronym **GLOBE** i.e. from **G**eneral to **L**ocal **O**rderly **B**alanced **E**xamination*

Examination of Systems and Examination of Regions

Physical examination may be carried out by specifically examining an organ system or by examining an anatomical region. When teaching clinical method and in professional examinations, it is the method of examining systems that is used. In practice, however, physical examination is performed by examining anatomical regions. It would be obvious that examining a patient by examining each system in turn would be quite tedious and would subject the patient to great inconvenience as it would entail multiple changes in position as each region is examined on repeated occasions in relation to different systems.

In the chapters that follow an attempt will be made to provide a method that will allow one to get the best of both techniques.

Chapter 6
Regional Examination

In clinical teaching the standard method employed is to teach examination of the systems. Each system is considered as a separate entity and a method of examination is taught for every one of them. This is a good method and allows a thorough examination of each system. However, in most clinical situations more than one system has to be examined and then this method is found to be lacking in versatility. It is easy to see that slavishly following this method will waste time and be tiring for the patient as the same region is examined on multiple occasions in different systems.

In practice one tends to examine the patient by region rather than by system. This method is better for the patient but it is more difficult for the clinician. Most clinicians would compromise by performing a regional examination but leaving out examination of the central nervous system and the locomotor system and performing these as separate systems at the end.

In this chapter a system of regional examination will be presented. This will attempt to provide a method that is comprehensive enough to cover every situation although this makes it time consuming. In practice one would leave out sections deemed to be of lesser importance clinically.

A brief outline of the method will be given in this chapter with a few examples for clarity. A more detailed explanation of method, possible findings and their causes will be given in the chapters on the various systems.

Each region or sub-region should be examined in two stages. The stages are examination of structure and examination of function. In the first stage, which is examination of structure, one should examine the features of relevance to that area. That is whatever is relevant from Dimensions, Cover, Contents, Connections and Circulation.

Next, one should examine the relevant aspects of function. That is, whatever is relevant for that particular function from the list of Position, Character, Quantity, Transmission, Modifying Factors, Rate and Rhythm.

At first this type of examination, by division into regions and examination of each region in detail before moving on to the next , may seem time-consuming and laborious. But, it is only by examining each area thoroughly that one will avoid missing important clinical findings and initially one will need to sacrifice speed for the sake of completeness. However, with continued practice this method will become second nature to one and the speed of examination should increase.

Clothing

It would be ideal to examine the patient stripped down to the minimum clothing required to maintain modesty. However, this is not always practical and one usually resorts to asking the patient to remove clothing as and when required during the course of the examination.

♥ **Clothing and Grooming**

Before commencing examination of the patient one should make an assessment of the patient's clothing and grooming, as this would give important information regarding the patient. One should then move on to examine the patient. (The word grooming has been used in an all-inclusive sense to encompass cleanliness and neatness)

General Examination

One should commence examination by taking an overall impression of the patient. This is done by inspection from a distance usually the foot end of the bed. From this one would derive a lot of information but it is important not to try and do too much at this point. Instead, pay attention to a few particular areas of interest. This will mainly concern the endocrine and metabolic system and the

integument. Hence, the main emphasis would be on the dimensions of the patient, the colour and surface of the skin, the distribution of hair, any major change in the cutaneous circulation and the body temperature. Thus, what will be covered are the state of growth and development, the state of metabolism and any gross changes in the integument.

The method of examination would be as follows:

Dimensions

Pay particular attention to the following:

♠ Position

♦ Height and Proportions

♣ Weight and Shape

Position

First, one should look at the site or position of the patient. This would give a lot of information regarding the patient's general state of health. A patient who walks into a consultation room or who is seated comfortably in bed is much less likely to be seriously ill than a patient who is unable to do so because of breathlessness or pain or who is bed bound.

Height and Proportions, Weight and Shape

Next, pay attention to the height and weight of the patient. This will assess growth and development of the patient and the state of metabolism. Height and weight should be ascertained and anthropometric measurements made where indicated. A note should be made of the patient's linear proportions and shape.

Integument (Skin)

Note the following:

- ♣ Cover
- ♥ Circulation

Cover

Changes in the colour of the skin and the surface of the skin may be obvious at this point or would be noted during the course of the regional examination. The same applies to the distribution of body hair.

Circulation

Any dramatic changes in the state of the patient's cutaneous circulation should be noted. These are features such as flushing, cyanosis or pallor.

Body Temperature

The body temperature should be ascertained as this will give important information regarding the metabolic state of the patient.

This would conclude general examination, as most other observations would be made during the course of the regional examination.

Regional Examination

After performing general examination one should proceed with regional examination. Clinicians differ in the sequence used to perform regional examination. Some prefer to start by examining

the hands others prefer to start by examining the head. In this text regional examination commences with examination of the head. The examination would proceed as follows:

- ♥ Head
- ♠ Upper limbs
- ♦ Neck
- ♣ Chest
- ♥ Back
- ♠ Abdomen
- ♦ Inguinal region
- ♣ Genitals
- ♥ Lower limbs
- ♠ Perianal region
- ♦ Per rectal examination
- ♣ Spine
- ♥ Gait
- ♠ Romberg's sign
- ♦ Standing from a seated or squatting position

Examination of the Head

This is probably the most difficult part of the regional examination. It would be impossible to attempt this as a single entity and it would be advisable to divide the head into regions and examine these regions individually.

Mental State (Cerebral Cortex)

As both structure and function are being evaluated it would be advisable, at this stage of the examination, to pause and consider examination of the cerebral hemispheres. Most of the examination of the mental state should have been performed whilst taking the history but if any part of it has not been done then this would be a suitable juncture at which to complete this examination. Detailed examination of the cerebral hemispheres will be dealt with in the chapter on the central nervous system.

Head

Next, move on to take a general or global view of the head. Pay attention to the dimensions; the size and shape of the head. Note any gross changes in the integument. Note any abnormal movements of the head as a whole. In summary:

♥ Dimensions

♠ Integument

♦ Movement

Following this move on to examine the regions of the head. It would be best to consider the following regions:

♠ Nose

♦ Eyes

♣ Face

♥ Mouth

♠ Ears

The reason for the order of examination of the regions of the head being as outlined above is so that one may efficiently combine examination of structure and function. More detail will follow and make this clearer.

Nose

Examine the structure of the nose and then test function. The functions of the nose are twofold. They are the sense of smell and the function of breathing. If indicated test the sense of smell. Note any abnormal smell in the breath of the patient such as foetor hepaticus or the smell of ketones. Look for any evidence of respiratory distress.

Eyes

The eyes give a great deal of clinical information and should be examined carefully and in depth.

Commence examination by testing visual acuity and then assess the visual fields and look for sensory inattention. Test for visual agnosia if required.

Follow this by examining the structure of the eyes. Examine the orbits and then the eyes. Note the position of the orbits in relation to one another.

Take a global view of the eyes paying particular attention to site and size. Site would be the position of the eyes in relation to the orbit. An apparent change in the size of the eyes may occur depending on the position of the globe in relation to the orbit and on the position of the eyelids. A real change in the size of the eyeball, is rare.

Next, move on to examine the eyelids, the conjunctiva, the sclera, the cornea, the anterior chamber, the iris, the lens, the vitreous, and the fundus.

Conclude examination of the eyes by testing eye movements and the pupils.

Face

The face could be further divided into the scalp, the forehead, the eyebrows, the cheeks or the malar region and the chin.

◆ **Scalp**

On examination of the scalp one would be mainly concerned with the quantity, distribution and characteristics of the hair on the scalp. These features will be affected by both local and systemic disease.

♣ **Forehead**

The forehead does not give a great deal of clinical information but nevertheless it should not be neglected.

♥ **Eyebrows**

The eyebrows give limited clinical information but still should not be neglected.

♠ **Malar Region** (the cheeks)

Examine the structure of the cheeks. Pay particular attention to the integument.

◆ **Chin**

Note the structure of the chin paying particular attention to the integument.

Function

In relation to function of the face one would examine functions of the facial and trigeminal nerves. When examining function of the face pay attention to the site of the naso-labial fold and the angle of the mouth. Look for wasting and involuntary movements. Then test facial movement that is, test the function of the facial nerve. Test the corneal reflex. Elicit Chvostek's sign if required. If required test sensation in relation to the trigeminal nerve. Usually this would be left to be performed at the end of the examination of the lower limbs so that sensory examination of the entire body may be carried out in a sequence.

Mouth

When examining the mouth one should consider the following:

♣ Jaw

♥ Lips

♠ Teeth

◆ Gums

♣ Buccal mucosa

♥ Tongue

♠ Palate

◆ Fauces

♣ Salivary glands

Structure and function may be examined together. Examine the structure of the jaw. Look for wasting and involuntary movements. Ask the patient to clench the teeth together and feel for contraction of the masseter and the temporalis muscles. Ask the patient to open the mouth whilst offering resistance. This will test the pterygoids. Test the movements of the temperomandibular joint and feel for any clicks and note any pain on movement.

Test the jaw jerk if required. Examine the lips, evaluating structure in detail. Ask the patient to open the mouth.

Now examine the open mouth. Examine the structure of the teeth, the gums, the buccal mucosa, the tongue, the hard and soft palates and the fauces.

Look for wasting and involuntary movements and then test movements of the soft palate and the tongue. Test the gag reflex. The sensation of taste may be tested if required.

Evaluate the functions of the mouth. Remember that the mouth has many functions; as part of the digestive tract, as part of the respiratory tract and it is used in speech.

Look at the use of the lips in breathing. The abnormalities in relation to digestion and speech would have been elicited in the course of history taking. Examine the structure of the salivary glands.

Ears

Examine the structure of the ears and test hearing.

This will conclude examination of the head. It would be best to move on now and examine the upper limbs rather than the neck, as this would allow the examination to flow better.

Upper Limbs

Start off by taking a general or global view of the upper limbs. Note the dimensions and any changes in the integument. Then proceed to evaluate the regions. Start with the hands.

Hands

The hands are also a complex region but definitely easier to examine than the head. For convenience it is best to divide the hands into systems as this makes examination more methodical, easier to perform and reduces the likelihood of missing important clinical signs.

The systems into which one should divide the hands are the integument that is the nails and the skin, the locomotor system, the vascular system and the nervous system.

♥ **Dorsum of the Hand**

Begin examination by taking a general or global view of the dorsum of the hands paying particular attention to the size and shape of the hands. Then move on to examine the nails and the skin. After this examine the bones, the joints, the tendons and the musculature.

♠ **Palmar Aspect of the Hands**

Ask the patient to turn the hands over and repeat the above process for the palmar aspect. Examine the skin, the bones, the joints, the tendons and the muscles. Evaluate the peripheral circulation by palpating the hands. Test capillary refill. Next, examine the radial pulse. Following this, ask the patient to stretch his or her arms out in front of him or her and analyse any involuntary movements that may be evident. Ask the patient to extend the wrists, spread the fingers apart and look for a flapping tremor. Then test active and passive movements of the hands and evaluate muscle strength, reflexes, coordination and sensations.

Depending on the situation one may defer examination of movements, power, reflexes, coordination and sensations until the end of the examination of the upper limbs thus allowing one to examine all limb functions together.

Forearms

Examine the structure of this region. Defer testing of function to the end of the examination of the upper limb.

Elbows

Examine structure; defer examination of function till the end of the examination of the upper limb.

Upper Arm

Perform examination of the upper arm in detail. Examine the brachial artery. Remember to measure the blood pressure.

Shoulders

Examine the structure of the shoulders

Axillae

Examine the axillae paying particular attention to the skin and examination of the lymph nodes.

Functions of the Upper Limbs

Now analyse any involuntary movements that may be present. Test the tone of the muscles in the upper

limb and then examine movements of the upper limb both active and passive. Test muscle strength. Examine the tendon reflexes and examine coordination.

Examination of the sensory system may be performed now or deferred until the end of the examination of the lower limb so that the entire body may be tested in sequence.

This concludes examination of the upper limbs.

Now move on to examine the neck.

Neck

Take a general view of the neck. Note the size and shape of the neck. Note any changes in the integument. Look for enlargement of the thyroid gland. Note any abnormality of the sternocleidomastoid muscle. After this examine the jugular venous pressure, the carotids and the trachea. The thyroid gland and the lymph nodes should be palpated when the patient changes position to examine the back.

Examine the structure of the neck musculature. Move on to analyse any involuntary movements that may be present and then examine active and passive movements of the neck. Test muscle strength.

In the appropriate situation look for neck stiffness.

Now move on to examine the chest.

Chest

Begin by examining the structure of the chest wall. Then analyse respiration. After this examine the contents of the chest that is the lungs and the heart. Detailed description of these aspects of examination will be given in the relevant chapters.

Now ask the patient to sit up and lean forward and examine the patient from the back.

Back

Take a general or global view of the back with special emphasis on the structure of the spine. Then examine the neck in detail. The thyroid gland and the lymph nodes should be palpated at this stage.

Examine the back of the chest. Note any abnormality of the scapula. Examine the chest wall. Examine the lungs.

Now examine the lower back.

When this is complete ask the patient to lie down and examine the abdomen.

Abdomen

Examine the abdominal wall. Analyse the movements of the abdominal wall with respiration and look for visible peristalsis. Perform neurological examination of the abdominal musculature if required and test the superficial reflexes.

Examine the contents of the abdominal cavity, the liver and spleen, the kidneys and bladder, the uterus and the ovaries, the aorta, the para-aortic lymph nodes, the intestines and any intra-abdominal masses.

Examine for any free intra-abdominal fluid. Listen for a succussion splash. Auscultate the bowel sounds, listen for bruits and a venous hum.

Inguinal Region and Genitals

Now examine the inguinal region and the genitals. Remember that the male genitalia are best examined with the patient standing. Examination of the female genitalia is not performed routinely. If required one should perform this with the patient correctly positioned and with the necessary equipment.

Test the cremasteric reflex if required.

The next step would be examination of the lower limbs.

Lower Limbs

Begin with a general or global view of the lower limbs. Note the dimensions and the state of the integument. Then move on to examine the regions. Start with the hips.

Hips

Examine the structure of the hips. Movements would be best examined at the end when all movements may be examined in sequence

Thighs

Next examine the structure of the thighs.

Knees

Examine structure in detail. Do not forget to examine the popliteal fossa and the popliteal pulses.

Lower Leg

Examine the structure of the lower leg.

Feet

The same method that was that used for the hands may be used. Start with the dorsum of the feet. Note the dimensions. Examine the nails and the skin, the bones, the joints, the tendons and the musculature. Next, examine the plantar aspect in the same way. Note the dimensions; examine the skin, the joints, the tendons and the muscles. Feel the skin and note the state of the peripheral circulation. Test capillary refill. Feel the dorsalis pedis and posterior tibial pulses.

Functions of the Lower Limbs

Look for any involuntary movements of the lower limbs, test the tone of the muscles and then examine both active and passive movements of the lower limb. This will include compression and distraction of the sacro-iliac joints, movements at the hips, knees, ankles and feet. Test muscle strength. Test the reflexes both the deep tendon reflexes and superficial reflexes. Test coordination.

Sensory System

This would be the best time to perform examination of the sensory system in full. Start at the head and move down examining all the senses over the entire body.

Peri Anal Region and Per Rectal Examination

Now ask the patient to turn onto the left lateral position and examine the buttocks, the perianal region, test the anal reflex and perform rectal examination if required.

Spine

The spine is examined in several stages. Some aspects of examination of the spine have already been carried out when examining the back, others are carried out with the patient in the supine position, some with the patient in the prone position, a small part with the patient seated and most of the examination is performed with the patient standing.

Spine in the Supine Position

Do the straight leg-raising test and look for Kerning's sign if required.

Spine in the Prone Position

Ask the patient to roll over onto the prone position and examine structure from the back. Examine movements of the erector spinae if required.

Perform the femoral stretch test.

Popliteal Fossa

Take this opportunity to examine the popliteal fossa in detail.

Spine in the Seated Position

Ask the patient to sit on the edge of the bed or couch and look for truncal ataxia

Spine with the Patient Standing

Now ask the patient to stand. Examine the structure of the spine in detail and test movements of the spine.

Gait

Now asses gait. Assess tandem walking.

Romberg's Sign

Look for Romberg's sign if required.

Trendelenburg's Test

Perform Trendelenburg's test if required.

Standing from a Seated or Squatting Position

If required, assess the patient's ability to stand from a seated or squatting position.

This concludes a comprehensive examination of the patient. It would not be practical to perform such a detailed examination every time and depending on the situation parts of the examination may be omitted. Remember that not examining structure or function of any region or sub-division of a region should be an active decision that one can rationalise and defend. Forgetting to do so would not be acceptable.

The method described, commences with examination of the head, as this is most conducive to a thorough physical examination of both structure and function. Some clinicians prefer to begin by examining the hands and this is up to individual choice.

Chapter 7

Examination of Systems

Traditionally one evaluates the different systems of the body. This enables one to evaluate disease processes that predominantly affect a particular system. However, systems do not exist in isolation either structurally or functionally. In addition causes and effects of disease processes that predominantly affect a particular system are often reflected in other systems. Thus, in the strictest sense, it is a fallacy to discuss evaluation of systems.

In history taking, when one analyses the systems the process cannot be strictly limited to a particular system as this will leave out very important information. For example in analysis of the gastrointestinal tract, if one were to leave out evaluation of weight, temperature control and energy, evaluation would be incomplete. But, in the strictest sense the latter are part of the evaluation of metabolism.

Similarly, in physical examination the procedure is not limited to a system in the strictest sense. For example in examination of the cardiovascular system, the nails and skin are inspected for important signs such as clubbing.

In summary when evaluating systems one takes a history and examines the patient for:

♥ Abnormalities in structure and function in relation to the system under consideration

♠ Abnormalities in structure and function in other systems that reflect the causes and effects of the disease process that predomi-nantly affects the primary system under consideration.

In the chapters that follow a method of evaluation of each system will be described in detail. This will be followed by a discussion of the lesions that are likely to occur in that system. Finally, the abnormalities that may be detected and their causes will be discussed.

The reader is advised to use these chapters as follows:

♦ Use the first part of the chapter to develop one's clinical skills. Read the section, practice when seeing patients, read again and correct technique. Repeat *ad infinitum.*

♣ Use the second section to go through the pathology that is likely to be seen in practice and in professional examinations.

♥ Use the third section to famil-iarise oneself with the findings that one may encounter. When reading please try and visualise the scenario in one's mind. This is a very good method of learning and practising for examinations.

Please remember that in each chapter a description has been given of a thorough examination of the relevant system. In professional examinations such as PACES time would be a constraint and only the relevant sections of the examination should be carried out. A summary of the techniques required for professional examinations has been given in the appendix.

Chapter 8

The Endocrine and Metabolic System

Endocrinology and metabolism are considered together as they are inextricably linked. In analysis of this system, the balance of anabolism and catabolism should be considered together with their effects on growth, development and body composition. Energy production with its resultant release of heat and control of body temperature should be studied. The balance of other constituents of the body such as salt and water and mineral metabolism should also be considered. Nutrition has a pivotal place in metabolism and this will be reflected in the study of metabolism and endocrinology.

The causes and effects of conditions that affect this system may be reflected in other systems. Hence, they should be analysed as well.

Thus, one would infer that evaluation of this system is performed in two parts. That is evaluation of the endocrine and metabolic system and secondly evaluation of other systems looking for evidence of the causes and effects of conditions that affect the primary system. However, this poses the question of what makes up the endocrine and metabolic system? This would be difficult to define. It would be logical to use the overall appearance of the patient or general examination, that is the state of growth and development of the patient, the metabolic state, the integument and temperature control, as the basic assessment of the metabolic and endocrine system and add on evaluation of the endocrine glands that may be performed clinically. This second stage, that is evaluation of the glands, would be performed in the course of the regional examination.

History Taking

Analysis of the Endocrine and Metabolic System

In analysis of the endocrine and metabolic system one should enquire about:

- ♥ Size of the Body
- ♠ Energy Production

Size of the Body

With regard to the size of the body one should enquire about:

- ♦ Height
- ♣ Size of Extremities
- ♥ Weight

Height

Enquire about the patient's height. Rate of change in height would be important in patients who have not completed growth. Where extremes of height are concerned comparison to the height of the parents and siblings would be important.

Extremities

Enquire about any change in the size of the extremities. This may be reflected by a change in shoe, glove or hat size.

Body Weight

Enquire about any change in body weight. If a change has occurred the rate of change is important.

Energy Production

With regard to energy production one should enquire about:

- ♠ Body Temperature
- ♦ Sweating
- ♣ Energy

Body Temperature

Enquire about fever.

Enquire about heat or cold intolerance

Sweating

Enquire about excessive sweating, reduced sweating or night sweats.

Energy

Ask whether the patient feels energetic or lethargic

In the strictest sense these are the only true features of metabolic and endocrine function. The other features are a reflection of the causes and or effects on other organ systems of disease that primarily affects the endocrine and metabolic system. These features will be evaluated by performing a review of systems.

It will be seen that analysis of related systems or review of systems becomes as important as analysis of the metabolic and endocrine system. This is so in all systems and that is the reason why it is recommended that analysis of other systems or review of systems should be performed at this point and should not be left to the end of the history. If the review were to be left to the end it would probably mean retaking the entire history.

Examination

Examination of the endocrine and metabolic system follows the same pattern as the examination outlined in the chapter on regional examination. However, as that was a comprehensive examination and time consuming, emphasis will be placed on the aspects of examination most likely to yield a result and thus the extent of examination will be greatly reduced.

The aspects on which most emphasis will be placed are the general examination, the anatomical regions where there is an increased likelihood of detecting evidence of a structural change in an endocrine gland and the systems that are most likely to be affected by the causes and effects of pathology in the endocrine and metabolic system.

General Examination

The major functions of the endocrine and metabolic systems are growth and development and production of energy. These aspects are reflected in the general examination.

Method of General Examination

As in any aspect of examination structure and function should be evaluated.

Structure

Commence examination of structure by noting:

♥ Dimensions

♠ Integument

Dimensions

When evaluating the dimensions of the patient consider:

♦ Position

♣ Growth, Development and Metabolic State

Position

Consider the position adopted by the patient. This will give an early indication of how unwell the patient is.

Growth, Development and Metabolic State

An important objective of examination is to determine the state of growth and development of the patient and to assess the metabolic state of the patient. This will be reflected by the relative quantities and distribution of bone, lean tissue, fat and fluid in the body. Hence, one should determine the state of growth and development and assess the metabolic state of the patient by noting the height and linear proportions of the patient and the weight and shape of the patient. One should assess:

♥ Height and Proportions

♠ Weight and Shape

Height and Proportions

Determine the patient's height. Ideally this should be measured in metres. Determine the linear proportions of the patient. That is, the length of the limbs in relation to the trunk. This is assessed by measuring the upper and lower segments of the body and the arm span.

Upper and Lower Segments

The lower segment is the distance from the upper border of the symphysis pubis to the floor. The upper segment is the height minus the lower segment. Normally the upper segment is equal to the lower segment.

Arm Span

The arm span is the distance from the tip of the middle finger of one hand to the tip of the middle finger of the other hand with the arms held wide apart. The arm span is greater than the height in patients who have eunuchoid proportions. The arm span should be more than 5 cms greater than the height of the patient to be significant.

An eunuch is a castrated male

Weight and Shape

Note the weight and shape of the patient.

Weight

Determine the patient's weight (ideally in kilograms) and relate this to the height as the body mass index. Other anthropometric measurements may be required in the evaluation of nutritional status.

Shape

Observe the shape of the patient. This will give very important clues to the metabolic state of the patient as the relative proportions and distribution of bone, lean tissue, fat and fluid determine the shape of the patient.

Integument

The cover of the patient, the integument, may show changes. These changes would be best observed in the course of the regional examination but some may be strikingly obvious such as changes in the colour of the skin or changes in the surface characteristics of the skin.

In addition one may assess the state of the cutaneous circulation and note any gross changes such as generalised flushing or severe vasoconstriction. In summary assess:

♦ Colour

♣ Surface

♥ Circulation

Examination of Function

Body Temperature

The function that will be evaluated during the general examination is control of body temperature. Body temperature is a very important measurement. For fever, routine thermometry is adequate but in the assessment of hypothermia special, low reading instruments are required to assess core temperature (the rectal temperature).

Regional Examination

Commence regional examination by starting with the head. Some may prefer to begin regional examination by examining the hands.

Head

Assessment of function of the cerebral cortex should have been performed already during history taking. If not assess the mental state now. This would not be required in a professional examination. Note the dimensions of the head. Examine the nose, eyes, face (scalp, forehead, eyebrows, malar region, chin) mouth (jaw, lips, teeth, gums, buccal mucosa, tongue, palate, fauces, salivary glands) and ears. When examining the face look for Chvostek's sign if required.

Upper Limbs

Perform a quick general examination of the upper limbs noting the dimensions and the state of the integument.

Hands

Note the dimensions. Then examine the dorsum of the hands; the nails and skin, the bones, joints, tendons and muscles. Ask the patient to turn the hands over and examine the palms; the skin, the bones, joints, tendons and muscles. Palpate the hands and note the state of the peripheral circulation and then examine the radial pulse. Ask the patient to stretch the arms out and look for a tremor. If the tremor is minimal, place a sheet of paper on the patient's outstretched hands. This will help, as the oscillations of the paper will accentuate the tremor. Next, ask the patient to extend the wrists with fingers spread wide apart. Look for a flapping tremor. Examine the nervous system and function of the locomotor system of the hands if required.

Forearms, Upper Arms, Shoulders and Axillae

Examine the rest of the upper limbs, the forearms, the upper arms, the shoulders and the axillae. A detailed examination is not usually required. It is important to measure the blood pressure. Look for Trousseau's sign if necessary. Active and passive movements of the upper limb and neurological examination should be performed only if required.

Neck

Note the dimensions of the neck and the state of the integument. Then examine the thyroid gland, the sternocleidomastoid muscles, the jugular venous pressure, the carotids, the trachea and the lymph nodes.

Thyroid Gland

Examination of the Thyroid Gland

Technique

Begin examination by inspecting the neck. This should be performed whilst standing in front of the patient. Look for enlargement of the gland. Ask the patient to swallow and see whether the gland moves upwards. A glass of water should be provided for this purpose. To perform palpation, stand behind the patient who should be seated comfortably in an upright chair. One should gently flex the patient's neck so that the sternocleidomastoid muscle is relaxed. One's thumbs should be behind the patient's neck and palpation should be performed with the pulp of the fingers, movement being mainly at the metacarpophalangeal joints. Perform a thorough palpation of the gland noting the dimensions, the cover (surface), the contents and the connections. The patient should be asked to swallow in order to define the lower margins of the gland. Palpate the carotids and the cervical lymph nodes. After completing palpation of the thyroid, go to the front of the patient and palpate the trachea. Percussion over the manubrium sterni may be used to define any retrosternal extension of the thyroid gland but this is an unreliable sign. Auscultate for bruits over each lobe and listen for stridor.

Complete examination of the thyroid gland by looking for Pemberton's sign. Ask the patient to raise both arms over the head as high as they can. In the presence of thoracic inlet obstruction due to retrosternal extension of the thyroid gland this manoeuvre would result in venous congestion and cause congestion of the patient's face, cyanosis and sometimes signs of respiratory distress and stridor.

Chest

Examine the chest wall and the contents of the chest; the lungs and the heart.

Ask the patient to sit up and lean forward.

Back

Examine the posterior aspect of the chest and the lower back.

Abdomen

Ask the patient to lie supine and examine the abdomen.

Lower Limbs

Examine the lower limbs in general then examine the hips, thighs, knees, lower legs and the feet. Active and passive movements and examination of the nervous system should be performed if required.

Buttocks, Perianal Region and Per Rectal Examination

Examine the buttocks and peri anal region and perform per rectal examination if required.

Spine

Examine the spine if required.

Gait, Romberg's Sign, Standing from a Seated or Squatting Position

Examine gait and look for Romberg's sign if required. Perform the Trendelenburg test and assess the patient's ability to rise from a seated or squatting position if indicated.

A method of performing a complete examination of the endocrine and metabolic system has been described. In a professional examination one should restrict examination to the areas of concern.

Lesions of the Endocrine System

Lesions of the endocrine glands should be analysed on the basis of their hierarchy as shown in figure 2.1.

Fig 2.1

One should consider lesions of the following endocrine glands:

- ♥ Pituitary
- ♠ Thyroid
- ♦ Parathyroid
- ♣ Adrenal
- ♥ Pancreas
- ♠ Testes
- ♦ Ovaries

In addition one should consider:

- ♣ Multiple Endocrine Neoplasia
- ♥ Polyglandular Failure

Pituitary Gland

One should consider lesions of the:

- ♣ Anterior Pituitary
- ♥ Posterior Pituitary

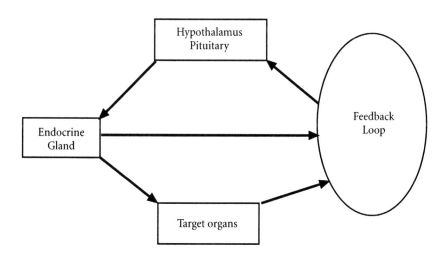

Anterior Pituitary

Lesions of the anterior pituitary may cause:

- ♠ Hypopituitarism
- ♦ Hyperpituitarism

Hypopituitarism

Decreased pituitary function may affect:

- ♣ All the hormones released by the pituitary gland (panhypopituitarism)
- ♥ Affect individual hormones causing isolated deficiencies

Panhypopituitarism

The causes of panhypopituitarism may be classified according to the pathology affecting the gland:

- ♠ **Developmental**

  Hypopituitarism may be caused by developmental abnormalities:

  Craniopharyngioma.

- ♦ **Trauma**

  The pituitary gland may be affected by trauma in:

  Skull trauma, hypophysectomy, radiation injury

- ♣ **Inflammation**

  The pituitary gland may be affected by inflammation in:

  Lymphocytic hypophysitis, tuberculosis, sarcoidosis, syphilis

- ♥ **Tumours**

  Tumours that may occur in the pituitary gland are:

Chromophobe adenoma, ectopic pinealoma, secondary deposits, meningioma, glioma

- ♠ **Vascular Lesions**

  Vascular lesions that may affect the gland are:

  Sheehan's syndrome (post-partum pituitary infarction) and pituitary apoplexy (haemorrhage into or infarction of the pituitary gland)

Isolated Deficiencies

Isolated deficiencies of the pituitary hormones are the following:

- ♦ Isolated gonadotrophin deficiency may occur. Kallman's syndrome refers to hypogonadotrophic hypogonadism associated with anosmia and sometimes with bony, renal, cerebral abnormalities, cleft palate, colour blindness
- ♣ Isolated ACTH deficiency is very rare
- ♥ Isolated TSH deficiency almost never occurs
- ♠ Isolated growth hormone deficiency may rarely occur in association with pituitary adenoma or following irradiation.

Receptor Abnormalities

Abnormalities of the receptors to the anterior pituitary hormones are uncommon.

Growth Hormone Receptor

Laron's syndrome refers to a condition in which the growth hormone receptor is abnormal. It is characterised by failure of growth and a distinct phenotype (hypoplasia of the base of the skull with a small face and mandible, delayed closure of the fontanelles, saddle nose, hypotrichosis, delayed dentition, tooth discolouration, crowding of defective teeth, high pitched voice, acromicria, infantile genitalia, thin and underdeveloped muscle, osteoporosis). In this condition growth hormone levels are high but insulin like growth factor I levels are low. Inheritance is autosomal recessive.

Hyperpituitarism

Hyperpituitarism usually causes an increase of a particular hormone resulting in a clearly defined syndrome. The syndromes that result are the following:

- ◆ Acromegaly
- ♣ Hyperprolactinaemia
- ♥ Cushing's Disease
- ♠ Nelson's Syndrome
- ◆ Thyrotroph Adenoma
- ♣ Gonadotroph Adenoma

Acromegaly

Acromegaly could be due to:

♥ **Pituitary Lesions**

Pituitary adenoma

♠ **Hypothalamic Lesions**

Rarely acromegaly may be due to increased growth hormone releasing factor, which may be of hypothalamic or ectopic origin.

Hyperprolactinaemia

Hyperprolactinaemia may be due to:

◆ **Pituitary Lesions**

The most likely cause is a prolactinoma.

Pituitary disease other than prolactinoma may cause hyperprolactinaemia. These are conditions such as acromegaly, Cushing's disease, other tumours such as metastases, non-secreting tumours, gonadotroph adenoma, meningioma and inflammatory disease. This is due to pituitary stalk compression resulting in a lack of inhibition of prolactin secretion. (Pseudoprolcactinoma)

♣ **Hypothalamic Lesions**

Hypothalamic lesions that result in hyperprolactinaemia are:

Chronic inflammatory disease, tumours, benign intracranial hypertension, radiation injury

♥ **Systemic Lesions**

Systemic diseases that result in hyperprolactinaemia are conditions affecting the:

E&M hypothyroidism

KUS chronic renal failure

GIT cirrhosis of the liver

RS chest wall lesions

CNS spinal cord lesions

Drugs mainly dopamine receptor antagonists, antihypertensives, oestrogens and opiates

Cushing's Disease

Cushing's disease is caused by increased production of ACTH from a pituitary adenoma

Nelson's Syndrome

Nelson's syndrome is caused by autonomous production of ACTH following bilateral adrenalectomy.

Thyrotroph Adenoma

Thyrotroph adenoma results in thyrotoxicosis

Gonadotroph Adenoma

Gonadotroph adenoma usually results in overproduction of FSH. The common presentation is with hypogonadism.

Posterior Pituitary

Lesions of the posterior pituitary may result in either:

♠ Hyperfunction

♦ Hypofunction

Hyperfunction of the Posterior Pituitary

Hyperfunction of the posterior pituitary results in SIADH

SIADH (Syndrome of Inappropriate Anti Diuretic Hormone Secretion)

The syndrome of inappropriate antidiuretic hormone secretion may occur due to:

♣ Cranial Lesions

♥ Systemic Lesions

Cranial Lesions

Cranial lesions that cause SIADH are the following:

♠ **Trauma**: head injury

♦ **Inflammation**: meningitis, encephalitis, Guillain-Barre syndrome, cerebral abscess

♣ **Tumours**: brain tumours either primary or secondary

♥ **Vascular lesions**: cerebrovascular events, subarachnoid haemorrhage

♠ **Functional lesions**: acute psychosis

Systemic Lesions

Systemic lesions that result in SIADH are conditions affecting the:

♦ **RS** pneumothorax, pneumonia, tuberculosis, empyema, asthma, positive-pressure ventilation

♣ **HS** lymphoma, leukaemia, thymoma

♥ **E&M** ACTH deficiency, porphyria

♠ **Drugs** arginine vasopressin, chlorpropamide, chlorpromazine, cytotoxics

Hypofunction of the Posterior Pituitary

Hypofunction of the posterior pituitary results in diabetes insipidus.

Diabetes Insipidus

Diabetes insipidus may be:

♣ Cranial

♥ Nephrogenic

Cranial Diabetes Insipidus

The causes of cranial diabetes insipidus are:

♠ **Inherited Disorders**

Inherited disorders are usually autosomal dominant, recessive disorders are rare.

DIDMOAD syndrome refers to diabetes insipidus, diabetes mellitus, optic atrophy, deafness

♦ **Trauma**: head injury, surgery

♣ **Inflammation**: meningitis, encephalitis, granulomas, cerebral abscess

♥ **Tumours**: pituitary tumours, hypothalamic tumours, secondary deposits, lymphoma

♠ **Vascular**: cerebral infarction

♦ **Idiopathic**

Nephrogenic Diabetes Insipidus

Nephrogenic diabetes insipidus may be caused by conditions affecting the:

♣ **E&M** hypercalcaemia, hypokalaemia

♥ **KUS** renal failure, renal tubular acidosis, idiopathic

♠ **Drugs** demeclocycline, gliben-clamide

Thyroid

Disorders of the thyroid gland may present as:

♦ Hypofunction

♣ Hyperfunction

♥ Goitre

Hypothyroidism

Hypofunction of the thyroid hormones may be due to:

♣ Primary hypothyroidism

♦ Secondary hypothyroidism

♣ Peripheral resistance (tissue resistance)

Primary Hypothyroidism

Primary hypothyroidism is due to problems within the thyroid gland and may be caused by conditions that are:

♥ **Congenital**: thyroid agenesis, thyroid maldescent, dyshormonogenesis

♠ **Traumatic**: post-thyroidectomy hypothyroidism

♦ **Inflammatory:** Hashimoto's thyroiditis, lymphocytic thyroiditis, Riedl's fibrosing thyroiditis

♣ **Metabolic:** iodine deficiency or excess

♥ **Drugs**: anti-thyroid drugs, lithium, amiodarone, radioiodine therapy

Secondary Hypothyroidism

Secondary hypothyroidism is caused by pituitary disease:

♠ Panhypopituitarism

♦ Isolated TSH deficiency almost never occurs

Tissue Resistance to Thyroid Hormone

Tissue resistance to the action of thyroid hormone is rare and is usually inherited in an autosomal dominant pattern.

Hyperthyroidism

Hyperfunction of the thyroid hormones may be due to:

♥ Primary thyroid disease

Or it may be:

♠ Secondary to extra-thyroid disease

Primary Thyroid Disease

Primary thyroid diseases that result in hyperthyroidism are the following:

♦ Grave's disease

♣ Toxic multinodular goitre

♥ Toxic solitary adenoma

♠ Thyroiditis may result in thyrotoxicosis.

 The types of thyroiditis are:

 Sub-acute, viral, de Quervain's

 Silent, painless

 Post partum

Extra-Thyroid Disease

Extra-thyroid diseases that result in thyrotoxicosis are:

♦ **E&M** TSH secreting pituitary adenoma, metastatic thyroid carcinoma (follicular)

♠ **RAG** hydatidiform mole, choriocarcinoma, struma ovarii (teratoma that contains thyroid tissue)

Goitre

The causes of goitre are discussed in the section on examination findings.

Parathyroid

Diseases of the parathyroid gland may result in:

♣ Hyperparathyroidism

♥ Hypoparathyroidism

Hyperparathyroidism

The causes of hyperparathyroidism may be classified as:

♥ Primary hyperparathyroidism

♠ Secondary hyperparathyroidism

♦ Tertiary hyperparathyroidism

♣ Pseudohyperparathyroidism

Primary Hyperparathyroidism

Primary hyperparathyroidism may be due to:

♥ Adenoma (single or multiple)

♠ Carcinoma

♦ Hyperplasia of the parathyroid gland

Secondary Hyperparathyroidism

Secondary hyperparathyroidism occurs as a result of:

♣ Hypocalcaemia

Tertiary Hyperparathyroidism

Tertiary hyperparathyroidism refers to:

♥ Autonomous functioning of parathyroid tissue following secondary hyperparathyroidism

Pseudohyperparathyroidism

Pseudohyperparathyroidism refers to the production of:

- ♠ PTH like substances from malignant tissue especially lung

Hypoparathyroidism

The causes of hypoparathyroidism are:

- ◆ Primary Hypoparathyroidism
- ♣ Pseudohypoparathyroidism

Primary Hypoparathyroidism

Primary hypoparathyroidism is caused by disease of the parathyroid gland. It may be due to conditions that are:

- ♥ **Congenital**: Di George's syndrome refers to the absence of parathyroid tissue and the thymus. These children usually die in childhood.
- ♠ **Trauma**: following thyroid or parathyroid surgery
- ◆ **Inflammatory**: autoimmune hypoparathyroidism
- ♣ **Metabolic**: Wilson's disease, haemochromatosis

Pseudohypoparathyroidism

Pseudohypoparathyroidism refers to resistance to the peripheral action of parathyroid hormone (PTH). It is associated with distinctive somatic features, which are short stature, a round face, short neck, short metacarpals and metatarsals.

Pseudpseudohypoparathyroidism

In pseudpseudohypoparathyroidism the somatic features of pseudohypoparathyroidism occur without the biochemical features. PTH and calcium levels are normal.

Adrenal

Diseases of the adrenal may result in:

- ♠ Hypoadrenalism
- ◆ Hyperfunction of individual hormones

Hypoadrenalism

Hypoadrenalism may be:

- ♣ Primary Hypoadrenalism
- ♥ Secondary Hypoadrenalism

Primary Hypoadrenalism

Primary hypoadrenalism is the result of conditions affecting the adrenal gland. They may be:

- ♠ Congenital Lesions
- ◆ Addison's Disease

Congenital Lesions

Congenital lesions that result in hypoadrenalism are:

- ♣ Congenital adrenal hyperplasia. This may be due to multiple enzyme defects resulting in a variety of syndromes
- ♥ Hereditary adrenocortical unresponsiveness to ACTH

Addison's Disease

Addison's disease may be due to conditions caused by:

♠ **Inflammation**

The cause of inflammation of the adrenal gland may be:

Autoimmune disease, which could be:

♦ Sporadic

♦ Polyglandular deficiency type 1 (Addison's disease, chronic mucocutaneous candidiasis, dental enamel hypoplasia, alopecia, primary gonadal failure)

♦ Polyglandular deficiency type 2 (Addison's disease, primary hypothyroidism, primary hypogonadism, insulin-dependent diabetes mellitus, pernicious anaemia, vitiligo)

Inflammation of the adrenal gland may also occur in tuberculosis, sarcoidosis, fungal infections, cytomegalovirus infection, AIDS

♦ **Trauma**: bilateral adrenalectomy

♣ **Neoplasia**: secondary deposits, lymphoma

♥ **Vascular Lesions**: meningococcal septicaemia, adrenal haemorrhage, adrenal vein thrombosis

♠ **Degenerative**: adrenoleucodystrophy, adrenomyeloneuropathy

♦ **Metabolic**: haemochromatosis

♣ **Interstitial Infiltration**: amyloidosis

Secondary Hypoadrenalism

The causes of secondary hypoadrenalism are:

♥ Hypothalamic Lesions

♠ Pituitary disease

♦ Systemic factors

Hypothalamic Lesions

Hypothalamic lesions that result in secondary hypoadrenalism are those due to:

♣ **Trauma**: surgery, head injury, irradiation

♥ **Developmental**: craniopharyngioma

♠ **Inflammation**: granulomatous disease

♦ **Tumours**: third ventricle tumour, secondary deposits

Pituitary Disease

Pituitary diseases that result in secondary hypoadrenalism are conditions such as:

♦ **Trauma**: surgery, irradiation

♠ **Vascular lesions**: pituitary apoplexy (hemorrhage into or infarction of the pituitary), Sheehan's syndrome (postpartum pituitary necrosis)

♥ **Neoplasms**: large adenoma

♠ **Isolated ACTH deficiency** which is very rare

Systemic Factors

Systemic factors that result in hypoadrenalism are:

♥ **Drugs**: treatment with steroids

Hyperfunction of Individual Hormones of the Adrenal Gland

Hyperfunction of individual hormones may affect the hormones of the:

♥ Adrenal cortex

♠ Adrenal medulla

Adrenal Cortex

Disorders of the adrenal cortex are the following:

♠ Cushing's Syndrome

♦ Primary hyperaldosteronism

Cushing's Syndrome

Cushing's syndrome could be due to lesions in the following:

♣ **Adrenal**

Adenoma, which may be part of MEN type 1, adrenocortical carcinoma

♥ **Pituitary or Hypothalamus**

Cushing's disease

♠ **Systemic Lesions**

Systemic lesions that result in Cushing's syndrome are conditions affecting the:

RS ectopic ACTH secretion from oat cell carcinoma, bronchial adenoma, carcinoid

Drugs: treatment with steroids

Pseudocushings Syndrome

Pseudocushings syndrome occurs in:

♦ Alcoholism

♣ Depression.

Primary Hyperaldosteronism

Primary hyperaldosteronism could be due to:

♥ Adrenal adenoma (Conn's syndrome)

♠ Adrenal carcinoma (rare)

♦ Bilateral adrenal hyperplasia

♣ Glucocorticoid remediable aldosteronism GRA (dexamethasone suppressible hyperaldosteronism)

Adrenal Medulla

Lesions that occur in the adrenal medulla are:

Phaeochromocytoma

Phaeochromocytoma could be due to an:

♦ Adenoma, which may be adrenal or extra-adrenal

♣ Rarely it may be due to a carcinoma.

Pancreas

The conditions that occur as a consequence of disorders of the pancreas are the following:

Hypofunction:

♥ Diabetes mellitus

Hyperfunction:

♠ Insulinoma

♦ Glucagonoma

♣ Gastrinoma

♥ Vipoma

♠ Somatostatinoma

Diabetes mellitus

Diabetes mellitus refers to an absolute or relative decrease in insulin and its consequences.

Insulinoma

Insulinoma causes excessive production of insulin resulting in hypoglycaemia

Glucagonoma

Glucagon producing tumours are rare. They cause diabetes mellitus and a migratory necrolytic erythematous rash.

Gastrinoma

Gastrinoma produces gastrin resulting in peptic ulceration and diarrhoea.

Vipoma

Vipoma causes diarrhoea and dehydration

Somatostatinoma

Somatostatinoma causes diabetes mellitus, steatorrhoea and cholelithiasis

Testes

Hypofunction of the Testes

Hypofunction of the testes results in hypogonadism. The causes are:

♦ **Pituitary/Hypothalamic Lesions (Hypogonadotrophic hypogonadism)**

Panhypopituitarism, hyperprolactinaemia, Idiopathic hypogonadotrophic hypogonadism, Kallman's syndrome, Prader-Willi syndrome, Laurence-Moon-Biedl syndrome

♣ **Testicular Lesions**

Testicular lesions may be:

Congenital anorchia, Klinefelter's syndrome

Trauma torsion, orchidectomy, direct trauma

Neoplasm testicular tumours

♥ **Target Organ Lesions**

Testicular feminisation syndrome

♠ **Systemic Disease**

Hypogonadism may occur in conditions affecting the:

GIT cirrhosis of the liver

KUS chronic renal failure

E&M thyrotoxicosis, uncontrolled diabetes mellitus,

CVS chronic heart failure

Disseminated neoplasia

Ovaries

Hypofunction of the Ovaries

Hypofunction of the ovaries may be due to lesions in the:

♦ **Hypothalamus and Pituitary**

Panhypopituitarism, Idiopathic hypogonadotrophic hypogonadism, Kallman's syndrome, Hyperprolactinaemia

Functional hypogonadotrophic hypogonadism

Functional hypogonadotrophic hypogonadism occurs in the following situations:

Weight related (emaciation) due to decreased body fat content

Exercise related (in females who engage in strenuous exercise), again related to decreased body fat content

Starvation, voluntary or involuntary

♣ **Ovarian Lesions**

Turner's syndrome, primary ovarian failure (which has multiple causes including autoimmune disease, surgery, chemotherapy, and radiotherapy), polycystic ovarian syndrome

Hyperandrogenisation

Hyperandrogenisation refers to increased production of androgens in a female. The manifestations are seborrhoea, acne, male pattern of body hair distribution, clitoromegaly and increased muscle bulk.

The causes of hyperandrogenisation are:

♥ **Ovarian Lesions**

Polycystic ovarian syndrome, tumours such as hilar cell, lipoid cell, Sertoli-Leydig cell, adrenal rest lesions

♣ **Adrenal Lesions**

Cushing's syndrome, congenital or late onset adrenal hyperplasia

Multiple Endocrine Neoplasia (MEN)

Multiple endocrine neoplasia refers to familial conditions with autosomal dominant inheritance.

There are two types MEN1 and MEN 2

♦ **MEN 1** causes lesions in the pituitary, parathyroid and pancreas (less commonly thyroid, adrenal)

♣ **MEN 2** causes lesions in the thyroid (medullary carcinoma) and phaeochromocytoma

MEN 2 A

Parathyroid hyperplasia in addition to the above

MEN 2 B

MEN 2B refers to MEN 2A with additional somatic features such as Marfanoid habitus, mucosal neuromas. Rarely peripheral nerve involvement and involvement of autonomic nerves may occur.

Aide Memoire

*Type **one** has lesions in three glands that all begin with **one** letter the letter P. Type **two** involves **two** glands*

Polyglandular Failure (Autoimmune)

Two types of autoimmune polyglandular failure occur. They are:

♥ Polyglandular deficiency type 1 (Addison's disease, chronic mucocutaneous candidiasis, dental enamel hypoplasia, alopecia, primary gonadal failure, hypoparathyroidism, other endocrine and non-endocrine disorders). This usually presents in childhood.

61

♠ Polyglandular deficiency type 2 (Addison's disease, primary hypothyroidism, primary hypogonadism, insulin-dependent diabetes mellitus, pernicious anaemia, vitiligo). This occurs primarily in adults.

Findings On History

The findings that one may obtain on taking a history are as follows:

Height

It is essential to relate the patient's height to the height of his or her parents and siblings and other members of the same race. This is important, as genetics and nutrition are important determinants of a patient's height. The causes of variations in height will be dealt with in detail under examination.

Body Weight

The weight of the patient will depend to a large extent on the state of nutrition. Hence, assessment of body weight should always be performed in the light of the state of the patient's appetite and intake of food. Normally appetite and weight are closely related. An inverse relationship occurs in thyrotoxicosis where an increase in appetite is associated with loss of weight. The causes of changes in weight will be dealt with under examination.

Body Temperature

Fever will be dealt with in the section on examination.

♦ Cold intolerance is a feature of hypothyroidism

♣ Heat intolerance is a feature of hyperthyroidism

Sweating

Variations in the production of sweat are the following:

♥ Reduced sweating is a feature of hypothyroidism.

♠ Increased sweating is a feature of conditions affecting the:

E&M acromegaly, thyrotoxicosis, phaeochromocytoma, diabetes mellitus, hypoglycaemia

CNS autonomic dysfunction (gustatory sweating)

♦ Increased sweating may be a normal variant in which case the onset is usually in childhood or adolescence and there may be a family history.

♣ Sweating is a feature of fevers especially tropical fevers.

♥ Night sweats occur in chronic inflammatory disease such as tuberculosis and in lymphomas.

Energy

The production of energy may be altered in dysfunction of any organ system. In relation to the endocrine and metabolic system the main determinants of production of energy are the thyroid gland, the adrenal glands, the pancreas and potassium and calcium metabolism.

Lack of Energy

A feeling of lack of energy may be a feature of conditions affecting the:

- ♥ **Thyroid**: hypothyroidism, rarely hyperthyroidism (apathetic thyrotoxicosis)
- ♠ **Adrenal**: hypoadrenalism, Cushing's syndrome
- ♦ **Pancreatic disease**: diabetes mellitus
- ♣ **Electrolyte imbalance**: lack of energy may occur in hypokalaemia, hypercalcaemia

Over Energetic

The patient may be over energetic in:

- ♥ Thyrotoxicosis

Findings on Examination

The abnormalities that one may detect on physical examination of patients are as follows:

General Examination

On general examination of the patient one may note abnormalities in relation to the following:

- ♦ Dimensions
- ♣ Integument
- ♥ Body temperature

Dimensions

On assessing the dimensions of the patient one would note:

- ♠ Position
- ♦ Height and proportions
- ♣ Weight and shape

Position

On examination of the position of the patient one may note:

- ♦ In thyrotoxicosis the patient may be hyperkinetic and fidgety.

Height and Proportions

The height of an individual is determined by many factors. They are genetic, nutritional and endocrine. In addition chronic childhood disease too plays an important part in determining the height of an individual. The abnormalities that one may detect are:

- ♣ Short stature
- ♥ Loss of height
- ♠ Tall stature

Short Stature

Assessment of short stature may be divided into the assessment of:

- ♦ Short stature with normal proportions
- ♣ Short stature with abnormal proportions

Short Stature with Normal Proportions (Proportionate Dwarfism)

Proportionate dwarfism may occur in a number of conditions. They may be divided into:

- ♥ Familial conditions
- ♠ Acquired conditions

Familial Conditions

The familial conditions that result in proportionate dwarfism are:

- Genetic abnormalities
- ♣ Chromosomal abnormalities

Genetic Abnormalities

The genetic abnormalities that result in short stature with normal proportions are:

- ♥ Prader-Willi syndrome, the mucopolysaccharidoses, Laurence-Moon-Biedl syndrome, Noonan's syndrome

Chromosomal Abnormalities

The chromosomal abnormalities that result in proportionate dwarfism are:

- ♠ Down's syndrome, Turner's syndrome

Acquired Conditions

The acquired conditions that result in proportionate dwarfism are:

- Endocrine abnormalities
- ♣ Chronic disease affecting any system

Endocrine Abnormalities

Endocrine abnormalities that result in proportionate dwarfism are conditions involving the following:

- ♥ **Pituitary**: hypopituitarism, diabetes insipidus
- ♠ **Thyroid**: hypothyroidism.
- ♦ **Parathyroid**: pseudohypoparathyroidism
- ♣ **Calcium Metabolism**: disorders of vitamin D metabolism
- ♥ **Pancreas**: diabetes mellitus

- ♠ **Adrenal**: Cushing's syndrome, congenital adrenal hyperplasia
- ♦ **Gonads**: precocious puberty may cause dwarfism due to premature fusion of epihyses.

Disorders of Vitamin D Metabolism

Disorders of vitamin D metabolism may be due to:

- ♣ **Luminal Factors** (this refers to the lumen of the gut)

Low dietary intake

High phytate intake

High phosphate intake

- ♥ **Mural Factors** (reference to the gut)

Malabsorption

- ♠ **External Factors** (reference to the gut)

Vitamin D dependent rickets (pseudo vitamin D deficiency) Type I, which is due to a defect in hydroxylation of 25 hydroxy cholecalciferol

Vitamin D dependent rickets type II. Several forms that are caused by absent or defective receptors for 1,25 dihydroxy cholecalciferol

- ♦ **Systemic Factors**

Conditions involving the:

GIT advanced parenchymal liver disease, cholestasis

Drugs prolonged use of anticonvulsants

KUS chronic renal failure, familial hypophosphataemic (vitamin D resistant) rickets which is due to a renal tubular defect in phosphate transport, Fanconi's syndrome, renal tubular acidosis

Chronic Disease

Chronic disease is also a cause of proportionate dwarfism. It may be disease affecting the:

- ♣ **KUS** renal tubular acidosis, chronic renal failure.

- ♥ **CVS** cyanotic congenital heart disease, congestive cardiac failure

- ♠ **RS** cystic fibrosis, asthma

- ♦ **GIT** nutritional failure

- ♣ **LMS** rheumatoid arthritis

- ♥ **HS** sickle cell disease, thalassaemia

External Features

Short stature with normal proportions may be due to conditions in which the external features are:

- ♠ Dysmorphic

- ♦ Normal

Dysmorphic features result from recognisable clinical syndromes that are inherited.

Short stature with normal features is due to chronic disease affecting the various systems.

Short Stature with Abnormal Proportions

Short stature with abnormal proportions may be divided into:

- ♣ Short stature with short limbs

- ♥ Short stature with short trunk

Short Stature with Short Limbs

The common causes of short stature with short limbs are:

- ♠ Achondroplasia

- ♦ Hypophosphatasia

- ♣ Osteogenesis imperfecta

There are many more rare syndromes that are encountered in paediatric practice but they will not be dealt with here.

Short Stature with Short Trunk

These are very rare. Several syndromes have been described. They will not dealt with here.

Loss of Height

The patient may lose height and become shorter as a result of bone loss in:

- ♠ Severe osteoporosis

- ♦ Hyperparathyroidism

- ♣ Paget's disease of bone

Tall Stature

In a similar fashion to the classification of short stature one may divide those with tall stature into:

- ♣ Tall stature with normal proportions

- ♥ Tall stature with abnormal proportions

Tall Stature with Normal Proportions

Tall stature with normal proportions may be:

- ♠ Normal variant

- ♦ Gigantism due to excessive production of growth hormone

65

Tall Stature with Abnormal Proportions

Eunuchoid proportions are those in which the limbs are disproportionately long in comparison to the torso. Arm span is more than 5 cms greater than the patient's height; the lower segment is longer than the upper segment. Eunuchoid proportions may occur in:

♣ **Inherited Disorders**

Marfan's syndrome, Homocystinuria, Marfanoid habitus in MEN type 2 B

♥ **Hypogonadism**

Hypogonadism may be due to:

Primary Gonadal Failure: Klinefelter's syndrome, 47 XYY syndrome, Soto's syndrome

Secondary Gonadal Failure: isolated gonadotrophin deficiency, Kallman's syndrome

Weight and Shape

Body weight should not be considered in isolation. It should be related to the patient's height as in the body mass index or serial weights should be considered.

Body Mass Index = Weight in kilograms / Height in metres^2

The changes that may be observed are:

♠ Decreased weight

♦ Increased weight

Decreased Weight

A pathological decrease in body weight occurs when catabolism becomes greater than anabolism.

This may be due conditions affecting the:

♠ **GIT** nutritional failure

♦ **E&M** endocrine disease may result in decreased weight and this may be a feature of:

Thyroid disease: thyrotoxicosis

Pancreatic disease: diabetes mellitus

Adrenal disease: Addison's disease

♣ Chronic disease and malignancy result in a decrease in weight. It is caused by the release of cytokines (cachexins)

♥ Surgery and trauma may result in decreased weight

Shape

In nutritional failure and cachexia, a skeletal shape would result. With decompensation and decrease in plasma albumin, oedema and ascites occur. This would result in a skeletal appearance of the upper body with a potbelly and swollen legs.

Increased Weight

A pathological increase in weight may be due to:

♠ An increase in adipose tissue (obesity)

♦ Salt and water retention

Obesity

Obesity may be due to:

♣ **Simple obesity**, which is caused by an increased intake of food and lack of exercise

♥ **Genetic disorders**: Prader-Willi syndrome, Laurence-Moon-Biedl syndrome

♠ **Hypothalamic damage**

♦ **Endocrine disorders** that result in obesity are:

Thyroid disorders: hypothyroidism

Adrenal disorders: Cushing's syndrome

Ovarian disorders: polycystic ovarian syndrome

Shape

Obesity causes characteristic changes in shape depending on the distribution of fat deposition. This may be:

♣ Female Type Distribution

♥ Male Type Distribution

Female Type Distribution

In the female type of fat distribution, the fat has a peripheral distribution resulting in a pear shape. Here the bi-trochanteric diameter is greater than the bi-humeral diameter. This shape is seen in patients with:

♠ **Simple obesity**

♦ **Genetic disorders:** Prader-Willi syndrome, Laurence-Moon-Biedl syndrome

♣ **Hypothalamic lesions**

Male Type Distribution

In the male type of fat distribution, the fat has a central distribution resulting in an apple shape. Here the bi-humeral diameter is greater than the bi-trochanteric diameter. This has a greater association with

diabetes mellitus and atherosclerotic vascular disease. It occurs in:

♥ **Simple obesity** (metabolic syndrome)

♠ **Adrenal disorders**: Cushing's syndrome

♦ **Ovarian disorders**: polycystic ovarian syndrome

Salt and Water Retention

An increase in weight may also be due to salt and water retention. This occurs in failure of organ systems:

♣ Heart failure

♥ Liver failure

♠ Renal failure

♦ Intestinal failure

Shape

Changes in the content of salt and water within the body may also result in characteristic changes in shape. They are:

♣ Dependent oedema characteristically increasing towards evening. This is the common pattern of oedema due to organ failure.

♥ In renal disease, oedema may affect the   face preferentially

♠ End stage organ failure of any type results in a state of cachexia where dependent oedema and ascites is seen in association with gaunt facies, thin neck and thin upper limbs.

Integument

After assessing the dimensions of the patient, one should consider the cover or the integument. This will be assessed further in the course of the regional examination but some features may become obvious at this stage. Abnormalities may be detected in:

- ♦ Colour
- ♣ Surface
- ♥ Consistency
- ♠ Circulation

Colour of the Integument

Changes in the colour of the skin occur in disease states. This may become more obvious when performing regional examination although marked changes may be seen when performing general examination Pigmentation of the skin is dependent on the hormonal environment and metabolism. Hyper or hypopigmentation may result. Pathological conditions related to the underlying disease process may also alter pigmentation. The abnormalities that may be detected are:

- ♦ Increased pigmentation
- ♣ Decreased pigmentation

Increased Pigmentation

Pigmentation is increased by melanocyte stimulating hormone, which is produced by the anterior pituitary. Adrenocorticotrophic hormone, ACTH, is similar in structure to MSH and therefore conditions in which ACTH levels are high result in increased pigmentation. Iron overload too causes increased pigmentation.

- ♦ **Diffuse Pigmentation**

  Diffuse pigmentation is seen in adrenal insufficiency (Addison's disease), Cushing's disease, ectopic ACTH production, Nelson's syndrome, haemochromatosis

- ♣ **Pigmented Macules**

  Pigmented macules are seen in neurofibromatosis, which is associated with phaeochromocytoma.

Decreased Pigmentation

Decreased pigmentation may be:

- ♥ **Diffuse Hypopigmentation**

  Diffuse hypopigmentation occurs in hypopituitarism

- ♠ **Hypopigmented Macules** (Vitiligo)

  Vitiligo may be associated with autoimmune endocrine disease

Surface of the Skin

Here one may detect abnormalities in regard to the following:

- ♦ Quantity and quality of body hair
- ♣ Quantity of sebum
- ♥ Presence of and quantity of sweat

Hair

When analysing the quantity and distribution of hair one should consider:

- ♥ Hirsutism
- ♠ Lanugo Hair
- ♦ Decreased Body Hair

Hirsutism

Hirsutism refers to an increase in growth of hair in the beard, moustache, chest, axillary, abdominal, pubic and thigh areas where growth of hair is sex hormone dependent. It occurs in:

- ◆ **Ovarian disorders**: polycystic ovarian syndrome
- ♣ **Adrenal disorders**: Cushing's syndrome, congenital and late onset adrenal hyperplasia, adrenal androgen secreting tumours.

Lanugo Hair

Lanugo hair is the soft, fine hair on newborn babies. In adults, it occurs in:

- ♥ Anorexia nervosa where it is seen over the back, the arms, the sides of the face

Decreased Body Hair

Decreased body hair occurs in the following conditions:

- ♠ **Pituitary disorders**: panhypopituitarism
- ◆ **Adrenal disorders**: adrenal failure in females
- ♣ **Gonadal disorders**: testicular failure

Sebum

The production of sebum may be:

- ♥ Increased
- ♠ Decreased

Increased Sebum

Increased production of sebum causing an oily skin and acne occurs in:

- ◆ **Adrenal disorders**: glucocorticoid excess
- ♣ **Pituitary disorders**: acromegaly

Decreased Sebum

Decreased production of sebum occurs in:

- ♥ Hypothyroidism

Sweat

The production of sweat may be:

- ♠ Increased
- ◆ Decreased

Increased Sweat

Increased sweating occurs in:

- ♣ Thyrotoxicosis
- ♥ Fevers

Decreased Sweat

Decreased sweating resulting in a dry skin occurs in:

- ♠ Hypothyroidism
- ◆ Heat stroke

Consistency of the Skin

Variations in the consistency of the skin are:

- ♣ The skin would be soft and wrinkled in hypopituitarism.
- ♥ In total lipoatrophy there is complete loss of subcutaneous fat. It is associated with diabetes mellitus.

Circulation of the Skin

Changes in the blood vessels would be best seen during the regional examination. However, gross changes may be obvious during the general examination. One may note:

- ♥ Flushing
- ♠ Telangiectasia

♦ Pallor

Flushing

Dilatation of blood vessels giving a flushed appearance is a feature of:

♠ Fevers

♦ Carcinoid syndrome

Telangiectasia

Telangiectasia occurs in:

♣ Cushing's syndrome

Pallor

Pallor may be due to:

♥ Constriction of blood vessels

♠ Anaemia

This concludes the structural component of general examination. Next, one should consider function. The function that should be considered at this point is control of body temperature.

Body Temperature

In evaluation of body temperature one should make note of the following:

♥ Position

♠ Quantity

♦ Rate

♣ Rhythm

♥ Associated features

Position

The position at which the body temperature is recorded should be mentioned. Temperature may be measured as oral temperature, rectal temperature or temperature may be recorded in the ear.

Quantity

The normal body temperature varies between 36.6 to 37.2 degrees centigrade (Celsius). Variations that may occur are:

♥ Fever

♠ Hypothermia

Fever

The common causes of fever are:

♦ **Infections** fever usually occurs due to infections, which may be acute or chronic.

The other causes of fever are conditions affecting the:

♣ **HS** lymphoma, leukaemia, haemoglobinopathies, haemolytic anaemia, serum sickness

♥ **CVS** infective endocarditis, atrial myxoma, Dressler's syndrome, pericarditis, thrombophlebitis

♠ **E&M** thyroiditis, thyrotoxicosis, phaeochromocytoma

♦ **RS** sarcoidosis, Wegener's granulomatosis, lymphomatoid granulomatosis, pulmonary embolism

♣ **GIT** inflammatory bowel disease, Whipple's disease, pancreatitis, alcoholic hepatitis, granulomatous hepatitis, granulomatous peritonitis

♥ **CNS** meningitis (bacterial, tuberculous, carcinomatous)

♠ **LMS** rheumatic fever, polymyalgia rheumatica, temporal arteritis, polyarteritis nodosa, Still's disease, Behcet's syndrome

- ♦ **KUS** retroperitoneal fibrosis
- ♣ **IS** erythema multiforme, Fabry's disease

Very High Temperatures

Very high temperatures usually reflect disorders of thermoregulation where compensatory mechanisms fail. The causes include conditions affecting the:

- ♥ **CNS** pontine lesions, encephalitis, meningitis
- ♠ **Drugs** anaesthetic agents, neuroleptic malignant syndrome
- ♦ **Heat stroke** where thermoregulatory mechanisms fail after prolonged exposure to heat

Hypothermia

Hypothermia may be due to:

- ♣ **E&M disorders** hypothyroidism, hypopituitarism
- ♥ **Exposure** which refers to accidental exposure in the country
- ♠ **Urban Hypothermia**. This is multifactorial and occurs in the elderly, patients with co-existent disease and in association with drug and alcohol use

Rate

The rate of rise of body temperature is not usually useful. However, seeing the paroxysmal, rapid rise in temperature in association with severe chills in a patient from the tropics usually makes the diagnosis of malaria obvious.

Rhythm

The rhythm displayed by the fever is important. Fevers quite often display rhythms that may be of diagnostic value.

- ♦ **Continued Fever**

  Continued fever is a fever that does not fluctuate more than 1.5 degrees Celsius and at no time reaches the baseline temperature

- ♣ **Remittent Fever**

  Remittent fever is a fever that fluctuates more than 2 degrees Celsius within a 24-hour period but at no time reaches the baseline.

  A high swinging fever is characteristically seen in patients who have a localised collection of pus.

- ♥ **Intermittent Fever**

  Intermittent fever refers to a fever that reaches the baseline thus providing fever free intervals. This type of fever is classically seen in malaria where the fever may recur every 48 hours, tertian malaria, in infestation by *Plasmodium vivax, ovale, falciparum* or every 72 hours, quartan malaria, in infestation by *Plasmodium malariae*

Pel-Ebstein Fever

Pel-Ebstein fever is an intermittent fever that lasts from hours to days and is followed by afebrile periods lasting from days to weeks. It occurs in Hodgkin's disease.

Associated Features

The associated features of fever that give clues to aetiology are:

♣ **Chills and rigors**

Chills and rigors would suggest malaria, kidney infections

♦ **Break-bone fevers**

Severe pain (break-bone pain) would suggest dengue fever

♣ **Tachycardia**

The hypermetabolic state represented by a fever is usually reflected in the cardiovascular system by an accompanying tachycardia. A degree rise in temperature is usually associated with an increase in heart rate of ten beats per minute.

♥ **Lack of Tachycardia**

The association of tachycardia with fever may be lost in:

Infections typhoid fever, brucellosis

CNS lack of tachycardia may reflect an increase in intracranial pressure in central nervous system infections

Drugs such as beta-blockers that reduce the heart rate result in loss of the associated tachycardia

Regional Examination

The abnormalities that one may detect on regional examination are as follows:

Head

Abnormalities may be noted of the following:

♣ Mental state

♥ Dimensions

Mental State (The Cortex)

The abnormalities that one may detect are as follows:

Level of Consciousness

A decreased level of consciousness may occur in disorders of:

♣ **Temperature Control**

High fever or hypothermia

♦ **Thyroid disorders**

Hypothyroidism

♣ **Glucose Homeostasis**

Hyperglycaemia in association with:

Hyperosmolar non-ketotic coma, ketotic coma

Hypoglycaemia, which may be due to:

Treatment of diabetes mellitus either insulin or oral hypoglycaemic agents, insulinoma

Hypoglycaemia may also be due to:

Glucocorticoid deficiency (adrenal failure, panhypopituitarism), hepatic failure, mesothelial tumours of the thorax or retroperitoneum

Orientation

The patient may not be orientated in place, time and person and may even be frankly psychotic in:

♥ **Adrenal disorders**: Cushing's syndrome

♠ **Thyroid disorders**: hypothyroidism

♦ **Pancreatic disorders**: irritability and confusion would be features of hypoglycaemia.

Mood

Variations in mood that may be encountered are:

♣ Hypomania

♥ Depression

Hypomania

Hypomania may occur in:

♠ Thyrotoxicosis

Depression

Depression may occur in:

♦ **Thyroid disorders**: hypothyroidism, apathetic thyrotoxicosis

♣ **Adrenal disorders**: Cushing's syndrome, Addison's disease

Dimensions

On assessing the dimensions of the head one may note abnormalities of:

♥ Size

♠ Shape

Size

When assessing size one may detect abnormalities of:

♦ Length

♣ Bi-parietal circumference

♥ Overall size

Length

Abnormalities that one may detect in the length of the head are:

♥ A long face or dolicocephaly is seen in rare syndromes for example Soto's syndrome (cerebral gigantism) and Marfan's syndrome.

♠ A short face or brachycephaly is seen in Down's syndrome

Bi-Parietal Circumference

This is an important measurement in paediatric practice. The bi-parietal circumference would be increased in hydrocephalus. The bi-parietal circumference would be decreased in microcephaly.

Overall Size

The overall size of the head may be greater than normal. This increase in size may be due to an increase in bone, lean tissue, fat, fluid or due to an accumulation of pathological tissue.

♦ **Bone and Lean Tissue**

An increase in growth of bone and lean tissue will lead to the characteristic increase in size seen in acromegaly.

♣ **Fat**

An increase in size may occur due to excess fat, which causes the rounded or moon face of Cushing's syndrome. Excess fat may also be due to simple obesity.

♥ **Mucopolysaccharide**

An accumulation of mucopolysaccharide in the subcutaneous tissues may give an apparent increase in size in hypothyroidism.

♠ **Congestion**

Congestion of the head would occur in obstruction of the superior vena cava.

Shape

As with changes in size, a change in shape may be due to changes in the quantity and distribution of bone, lean tissue, fat, fluid or pathological tissue. One may note:

♦ Exaggerated features

♣ Rounded appearance

♥ Skeletal appearance

Exaggerated Features

A combination of an increase in bone and lean tissue gives the characteristic changes seen in:

♠ Acromegaly

Rounded Appearance

A rounded appearance may be due to:

♣ **Fat**

Fat deposition will result in the moon face of Cushing's syndrome.

♥ **Mucopolysaccharide**

Deposition of mucopolysac-charide and fluid will cause the rounded appearance of hypothy-roidism.

♠ **Congestion**

Venous congestion will cause a rounded appearance. This occurs in obstruction of the superior vena cava, which may occur as a complication of a retrosternal goitre.

Skeletal Appearance

Changes in shape may also occur due to a decrease in fat and lean tissue. A skeletal appearance may be observed in:

♦ Nutritional failure

♣ Cachexia consequent on chronic disease or malignancy

♥ Lipoatrophic diabetes, which is a rare syndrome that consists of non-ketotic insulin resistance, generalised atrophy of adipose tissue, acanthosis nigricans (in one form of the condition) hepatosplenomegaly and severe hyperlipidaemia.

♠ Partial lipodystrophy

♦ Thyrotoxicosis

Nose

When examining the nose one may note changes in:

♣ Size

♥ Colour

♠ Surface

♦ Circulation

♣ Function

Size

The nose would be enlarged in:

♣ Acromegaly

Colour

Changes in the colour of the skin over the nose could be:

♥ Brown pigmentation of the skin of the nose may occur in pregnancy and in treatment with the oral contraceptive pill. This is called chloasma.

Surface

Abnormalities that one may note are:

♠ The surface of the skin may be oily and affected by acne in Cushing's syndrome

Circulation

Changes that one may observe in the circulation are:

♦ Telangiectasia may occur in Cushing's syndrome

♣ The nose may be plethoric in Cushing's syndrome

Function

On examination of the functions of the nose one may note:

♥ Anosmia as a feature of Kallman's syndrome

♠ In diabetic ketoacidosis, one may note the smell of ketones in the breath of the patient

Eyes

On examination of the eyes one may note abnormalities of the following:

Visual Acuity

Visual acuity may be decreased because of pathology in the following:

♥ Cornea

♠ Anterior chamber

♦ Lens

♣ Vitreous

♥ Retina

♠ Optic nerve

Cornea

Abnormalities in the cornea that result in decreased visual acuity are:

♦ Involvement of the cornea by keratitis in ophthalmic Grave's disease may decrease visual acuity.

♣ Keratomalacia with resultant ulceration of the cornea, perforation and secondary endophthalmitis may occur in vitamin A deficiency and thus lead to blindness.

Anterior Chamber

Lesions that occur in the anterior chamber are:

♥ Rubeosis iridis in diabetes mellitus. This interferes with the drainage of aqueous humour and may result in glaucoma and blindness

Lens

Lesions that occur in the lens are:

♠ The lens may become opaque due to cataract and this would reduce visual acuity. (Causes of cataract are discussed later)

Vitreous

Lesions that may occur in the vitreous are:

♦ Haemorrhage into the vitreous in diabetic retinopathy will result in decreased visual acuity.

Retina

Retinal lesions that result in decreased visual acuity are:

♣ The retina may be damaged in diabetic retinopathy.

♥ Night blindness may occur in vitamin A deficiency

Optic Nerve

Lesions that could occur in the optic nerve are:

♠ The optic nerve could be involved in Grave's ophthalmopathy and this could result in decreased visual acuity.

♦ The optic nerve may be compressed by pituitary lesions

Visual Fields

Abnormalities that one may note on examination of the visual fields are:

♣ **Bitemporal Hemianopia**

The characteristic field defect seen in endocrine disease is bitemporal hemianopia. This feature is due to compression of the optic chiasma by pituitary enlargement

♥ **Homonymous Hemianopia**

Strokes consequent on diabetes mellitus may result in these visual field defects.

Eyeball

On examination of the eyeball one may note changes in the:

Site

The abnormality that may occur is:

♠ **Proptosis**

The eyeball may be displaced forward by the accumulation of an inflammatory infiltrate within the orbit and within the extra-ocular muscles. This forward displacement of the eyeball in relation to the orbit is known as proptosis. This is a feature of ophthalmic Grave's disease. The proptosis is usually bilateral. It may rarely be unilateral and this occurs in ophthalmic Grave's disease in which there is no associated hyperthyroidism. The asymmetry seen in this condition is usually mild and if severe other causes of unilateral proptosis should be considered.

Unilateral Proptosis

Unilateral proptosis may be due to:

♦ Orbital Tumour

♣ Orbital cellulitis

♥ Granuloma

Eyelids

On examination of the eyelids one may note changes in:

♣ Size

♥ Shape

♠ Margins

♦ Colour

♣ Surface

♥ Consistency

Size

Abnormalities in the size of the eyelids are:

♣ The size of the eyelids may change due to deposition of mucopolysaccharide in hypothyroidism. This will cause thickening of the eyelids and if severe may also result in periorbital oedema.

Shape

The shape of the palpebral fissure is dependent on racial origin.

♦ In oriental races there is an upward slope from medial to lateral. The presence of this shape in a patient who is from a different ethnic background signifies an abnormality. This may be associated with an epicanthic fold and these features are seen in Down's syndrome.

♣ The reverse where the slant is downwards from medial to lateral is seen in rare conditions such as Soto's syndrome.

Margins

Changes in the margins of the eyelids are:

♥ The margin may be irregular due to the presence of neuromas in MEN type II B

Colour

Changes in the colour of the eyelids will reflect the generalised changes in colour of the skin due to the underlying conditions that have already been described.

Surface

Abnormalities that may occur on the surface of the eyelids are:

♠ **Xanthelasma**

The smooth surface of the eyelids may be broken by the presence of xanthelasma. These are yellow, sharply demarcated papules or plaques seen on the surface of the eyelids. They indicate hyperlipidaemia and occur in diabetes mellitus, hypothyroidism and familial hypercholesterolaemia.

Consistency

Changes in the consistency of the eyelids are:

♦ Deposition of mucopolysaccharide in hypothyroidism causes the consistency to change in addition to a change in the size of the eyelids. This may also cause peri-orbital oedema.

Conjunctiva

On examination of the conjunctiva one may note changes in the:

♠ Surface

♥ Consistency

Surface

The surface may differ from normal in being:

♣ **Moist**

The surface may be more moist than normal in chemosis.

♥ **Dry**

The surface may be dry. This may be due to destruction of the lacrimal glandular tissue if there is associated Sjogren's syndrome or due to failure of secretory function in vitamin A deficiency.

♠ **Conjunctivitis**

The conjunctiva may be inflamed in severe ophthalmic Grave's disease. This is because the combination of proptosis, lid retraction and exophthalmos causes the palpebral fissure to widen to such an extent that protection of the eyeball is not possible. This results in exposure keratoconjunctivitis

The conjunctiva may also be inflamed due to infection as a result of a dry conjunctiva.

♦ **Bitot's spots**

Bitot's spots refer to dry foamy spots that occur on the conjunctiva in vitamin A deficiency.

Consistency

Changes in the consistency of the conjunctiva are:

♣ **Chemosis**

The conjunctiva may be thickened due to oedema. This is called chemosis and may occur in thyroid ophthalmopathy.

Cornea

On examination of the cornea one may note changes in:

♠ Colour

♦ Surface

♣ Consistency

Colour

The colour of the cornea may alter in certain metabolic conditions.

♥ **Greenish-Brown Pigmentation**

A Kayser-Fleischer ring, a ring of greenish-brown pigmentation, is seen in Wilson's disease

♠ **White Ring**

Arcus senilis, a white ring at the edge of the cornea, may be seen in hyperlipidaemia.

♦ **Band Keratopathy**

Band keratopathy refers to ectopic calcification in the conjunctiva or the lateral margins of the cornea as a result of hypercalcaemia

Surface

Changes that may occur on the surface of the cornea are:

♣ **Keratitis**

The surface may be inflamed due to exposure keratitis in ophthalmic Grave's disease.

Consistency

Variations in the consistency of the cornea could be:

♥ Keratomalacia (softening of the cornea), which occurs in vitamin A deficiency

Anterior Chamber

Abnormalities that one may note in the anterior chamber are:

♠ **Hyphaema**

Hyphaema refers to blood in the anterior chamber. This may occur as a consequence of rubeosis iridis complicating diabetes mellitus.

Iris

On examination of the iris one may note abnormalities of:

♦ Site

♣ Shape

♥ Circulation

Site

Abnormalities of site would be:

♦ **Synechiae**

The free border of the iris may be attached either to the back of the cornea, anterior synechiae, or to the anterior aspect of the lens, posterior synechiae. This may occur as a consequence of either inflammation or haemorrhage.

Shape

Abnormalities of shape could be:

♣ The shape of the iris may be irregular due to synechiae

Circulation

Changes that one may note in the circulation in the iris are:

♥ **Rubeosis Iridis**

New blood vessels may grow on the anterior aspect of the iris. This

is known as rubeosis iridis and occurs in diabetes mellitus. It may result in glaucoma.

Lens

On examination of the lens one may note a cataract. Cataract refers to any opacity in the lens of the eye that results in blurred vision.

Cataract

Cataract may occur in:

♠ **Pancreatic disorders**: diabetes mellitus

♦ **Parathyroid disorders**: hypoparathyroidism

♣ **Adrenal disorders**: steroid therapy causes cataract but it is uncommon in Cushing's syndrome

Posterior Chamber

Abnormalities that may occur in the posterior chamber are:

♦ **Vitreous Haemorrhage**

The main abnormality that could occur in the posterior chamber would be vitreous haemorrhage as a consequence of diabetic retinopathy.

Optic Fundus

On examination of the fundus one may note:

♣ Diabetic Retinopathy

♥ Papilloedema

♠ Optic Atrophy

Diabetic Retinopathy

The types of diabetic retinopathy are:

79

- Background Retinopathy
- Diabetic Maculopathy
- Preproliferative Retinopathy
- Proliferative Retinopathy

Background Retinopathy

In background retinopathy one would see capillary microaneurysms (dot haemorrhages), leakage of blood into the deeper layers of the retina (blot haemorrhages) and hard exudates

Diabetic Maculopathy

In diabetic maculopathy there is loss of vision and exudates and haemorrhages may be seen in the macula.

Preproliferative Retinopathy

In preproliferative retinopathy, in addition to the background changes, cotton wool spots (soft exudates), venous beading and venous loops would be observed.

Proliferative Retinopathy

Proliferative retinopathy is characterised by new vessel formation in addition to the above changes.

In advanced retinopathy vitreous haemorrhages and scarring would be observed. In addition laser burns may be seen.

Papilloedema

Papilloedema may occur in:

- Hypoparathyroidism

Optic Atrophy

Optic atrophy may be seen in the:

- DIDMOAD syndrome. In this syndrome a combination of Diabetes Insipidus, Diabetes Mellitus, Optic Atrophy and Deafness occur.

Eye Movements

In endocrine disease abnormalities of eye movements are usually caused by:

- Thyroid ophthalmopathy
- A pituitary tumour may rarely be large enough to involve the relevant cranial nerves as they travel along the wall of the cavernous sinus.
- Diabetes mellitus may affect the nerves by causing mononeuritis multiplex.

Position of the Eyes at Rest

On examination one may note abnormalities of the position of the:

- Eyelids
- Eyeballs

Eyelids

Abnormalities in the position of the eyelids would be:

- **Lid Retraction**

  The upper eyelid usually covers the upper part of the iris. The upper eyelid may be retracted revealing a rim of sclera between the iris and the lower border of the upper eyelid. This is called lid retraction. It is a feature of the eye disease associated with thyrotoxicosis, Grave's ophthalmopathy.

It is not a specific sign of Grave's ophthalmopathy and may reflect sympathetic overactivity.

♠ **Exophthalmos**

Where the lower eyelid is concerned, normally its upper border is in line with the lower margin of the iris. The lower eyelid may be retracted downwards thus exposing a rim of sclera between the lower eyelid and the iris. This is known as exophthalmos and is a feature of Grave's ophthalmopathy.

♦ **Lagophthalmos**

Lagophthalmos refers to a wide palpebral fissure caused by proptosis, exophthalmos and lid retraction. This may result in an inability to shut the eyes.

♣ **Ptosis**

Ptosis will be seen if there is a third nerve lesion or Horner's syndrome.

Eyeballs

Variations in the position of the eyeballs are:

♥ Strabismus may be observed in lesions affecting the 3rd, 4th or 6th cranial nerves. These lesions may be due to mononeuritis multiplex consequent on diabetes mellitus or due to compression by a pituitary tumour.

Eye Movements

When examining eye movements one may note abnormal movements of the:

♠ Eyelids

♦ Eyeballs

Eyelids

Abnormal movement of the eyelids are:

♠ **Lid Lag**

When eye movements are tested, on asking the patient to follow the examiner's finger in a downward direction the rate of movement of the upper eyelid would be slower than that of the eyeball. This would result in a gradually increasing rim of sclera becoming visible as the eye moves downward. This delay in movement of the upper eyelid is known as lid lag and is a feature of thyroid ophthalmopathy.

Eyeball

Abnormal movement of the eyeball would occur due to weakness of the extraocular muscles.

Weakness of Extraocular Muscles

Weakness of the eye muscles results in a decreased range of movements and may result in diplopia.

Weakness of the extraocular muscles may be due to:

♦ **Muscle involvement**

In Grave's ophthalmopathy

♣ **Neuromuscular junction involvement**

Involvement of the neuromuscular junction may occur due to associated myasthenia gravis

♥ **Cranial nerve involvement**

Cranial nerve involvement may be due to mononeuritis multiplex or compression by enlargement of the pituitary gland

Pupil

Lesions that may affect the pupil are the following:

- ♠ Afferent Pupillary Defect
- ♦ 3rd Nerve Lesion
- ♣ Horner's Syndrome

Afferent Pupillary Defect

An afferent pupillary defect may be due to:

- ♠ Optic neuropathy as a result of ophthalmic Grave's disease

3rd Nerve Lesion

A 3rd nerve lesion could be due to:

- ♦ Compression by a large pituitary tumour
- ♣ Mononeuritis multiplex

Horner's Syndrome

Horner's syndrome may occur in:

- ♣ Diabetes mellitus

Face

On examination of the face one may note abnormalities of the following:

Scalp

On examination of the scalp one may note abnormalities of scalp hair. The abnormalities could be variations in the:

- ♥ Quantity
- ♠ Colour
- ♦ Surface

- ♣ Consistency
- ♥ Connections

Quantity of Hair

Abnormalities that one may detect would be in relation to:

- ♠ Hair loss
- ♦ Pattern of hair loss

Hair Loss

Hair loss occurs in conditions affecting the:

- ♥ **E&M** hypothyroidism, hyperthyroidism, hypopituitarism, excess androgens
- ♠ **GIT** protein-energy malnutrition, iron deficiency

Pattern of Hair Loss

The pattern of hair loss could be:

- ♦ **Diffuse Loss of Hair**

  Diffuse loss of hair occurs in protein-energy malnutrition, iron deficiency, hypothyroidism, hyperthyroidism and hypopituitarism.

- ♣ **Frontal Balding**

  Frontal balding occurs in androgen excess

Colour of Hair

The colour of the patient's hair depends on genetic and racial influences. These influences would determine the melanin content, which determines the colour of the hair. Melanin is a protein and the production of this protein is dependent on a normal state of nutrition.

♥ Protein-energy malnutrition would result in loss of colour of the hair.

♠ Pernicious anaemia also results in white hair.

♦ White patches (leucotrichia) occur in autoimmune disease

Surface of Hair

The surface of the hair normally has a sheen, which is a result of the production of sebum.

♣ In hypothyroidism this sheen is lost and the hair looks dull and lacklustre

Consistency

The consistency of the hair depends on the state of nutrition and hormonal balance. It would be:

♥ Brittle in protein-energy malnutrition

♠ Brittle in hypothyroidism

♦ Coarse in hypothyroidism

Connections

Abnormalities of the connections of the hair may be:

♣ The attachment of the hair root would not be firm in protein-energy malnutrition and this would result in easy pluckability.

Forehead

Abnormalities that one may note in the forehead are:

♥ Thickened skin folds may occur in acromegaly.

Eyebrows

When examining the eyebrows one may note the following:

♠ Prominent supra orbital ridges are a feature of acromegaly.

♦ The outer third of the eyebrows may be lost in hypothyroidism

♣ Leucotrichia may occur in autoimmune disease.

Malar Region

On examination of the malar region one may note abnormalities of:

♥ Colour

♠ Surface

♦ Consistency

♣ Circulation

Colour

Changes in colour that one may observe are:

♥ Pigmentation in chloasma

♠ A peaches and cream appearance may be seen in hypothyroidism. This is due to a yellow tinge occurring as a result of carotenaemia together with pallor.

Surface

The surface of the skin in the malar region may be:

♦ Oily and affected by acne in Cushing's syndrome

♣ Dry in hypothyroidism

♦ Acne would be a feature of hyperandrogenisation

Consistency

Changes that may occur in the consistency of the skin in the malar region are:

♠ The skin would be thickened in myxoedema

Circulation

Changes that may occur in the blood vessels of the skin in the malar region are:

♦ Telangiectases may occur and the skin would be plethoric in Cushing's syndrome

Chin

Abnormalities that one may note in the chin are:

Males

Reduced growth of hair on the chin occurs in disorders of the:

♥ **Pituitary**: hypopituitarism, gonadotrophin deficiency

♠ **Gonads**: testicular failure

♦ **Systemic Conditions**

Conditions affecting the:

GIT cirrhosis of the liver

Females

Growth of hair on the chin may indicate the presence of disorders of the:

♣ **Ovary**: polycystic ovarian syndrome, ovarian tumours

♥ **Adrenal**: Cushing's syndrome, congenital adrenal hyperplasia, virilising tumour

♠ **Pituitary**: acromegaly

♦ **Systemic Factors**

Conditions affecting the:

E&M porphyria cutanea tarda

Facial Nerve

On testing function of the facial muscles one may note:

♣ **Chvostek's Sign**. Tap over the facial nerve at the point where it leaves the parotid gland. Twitching of the lips and drawing up of the angle of the mouth is considered a positive sign and this indicates hypocalcaemia.

Mouth

When examining the mouth one may note abnormalities of the following:

Jaw

One may note changes in:

♣ Size

♥ Shape

♠ Temperomandibular joint

Size

The size of the jaw may be:

♣ Increased in acromegaly.

♥ Decreased in Turner's syndrome

Shape

Variations that one may note in the shape of the jaw are:

♠ **Prognathos**

Protrusion of the jaw may occur in acromegaly and in Soto's syndrome

Temperomandibular Joint

Lesions that may occur in the temperomandibular joint are:

- Arthritis in acromegaly

Lips

On examination of the lips one may note changes in:

- Size
- Surface

Size

The lips may be:

- Large in acromegaly

Surface

The surface of the lips may show:

- Reddening and cracking of the angles (angular stomatitis or angular cheilosis) in nutritional deficiencies (pyridoxine, riboflavin, folate, B_{12})
- Mucosal neurofibroma may be seen in MEN type 2B

Teeth

One may note abnormalities in:

Position

The teeth may be widely separated in:

- Acromegaly. Malocclusion may also be a feature as the lower teeth may overbite the upper due to prognathism.

Gums

Abnormalities that may occur in the gums are:

- Scurvy may result in bleeding gums.

Buccal Mucosa

When examining the buccal mucosa one may note changes in:

- Colour
- Surface

Colour

Changes that may occur in the colour of the buccal mucosa are:

- Pigmentation of the buccal mucosa may occur in haemochromatosis and in Addison's disease

Surface

Changes that may occur on the surface of the buccal mucosa are:

- Candidiasis would be a feature of uncontrolled diabetes mellitus.

Tongue

On examination of the tongue one may note changes in:

- Size
- Colour
- Surface

Size

Changes that may occur in the size of the tongue are:

- **Macroglossia**

  The tongue may be larger than normal in hypothyroidism, acromegaly. Other causes of a large tongue are Down's syndrome and amyloidosis

Colour

Changes that may occur in the colour of the tongue are:

♣ **Red Beefy Tongue**

Initially nutritional deficiency would result in glossitis due to atrophy of the papillae. This would allow the red colour of the underlying blood vessels to become more obvious.

♥ **Shiny and Pale Tongue**

In the later stages of nutritional deficiency, as anaemia supervenes the tongue would become shiny and pale

Surface

Changes that may occur on the surface of the tongue are:

♠ **Glossitis**

The surface may be smooth due to loss of the papillae. This occurs in nutritional deficiencies such as vitamin B_{12}, folate, niacin, pyridoxine, thiamine, riboflavin and iron.

♦ **Furring**

Furring of the tongue would occur in mouth breathers and in fevers

Salivary Glands

Abnormalities that may occur in the parotid glands are:

♣ Parotid enlargement may occur in diabetes mellitus.

Functions of the Mouth

One of the functions of the mouth is the production of speech. This would have been assessed at the time of history taking but it would be wise to formally document it.

Speech

When listening to the patient's speech one may note:

♣ **Slow Speech**

The rate at which speech is produced would be reduced and speech becomes slow in hypothyroidism.

♥ **Dysarthria**

The rhythm may be disrupted in the hypothyroid patient and dysarthria may occur.

♠ **Aphonia**

In recurrent laryngeal palsy the volume may decrease resulting in aphonia

♦ **Dysphonia**

The character may change and the patient's voice may be hoarse in hypothyroidism

Ears

On examination of the ears one may note abnormalities of:

♠ Size

♦ Shape

♣ Hearing

Size

The size of the ears may be:

♥ Increased in acromegaly

Surface

The surface of the ears may be:

♠ Irregular due to the presence of gouty tophi

Hearing

On testing hearing one may note:

♦ **Deafness**

Deafness may occur in hypothyroidism. The character of deafness in hypothyroidism is a sensorineural deafness. This occurs in a familial type of hypothyroidism where there is a genetic defect in the production of thyroxine. Patients develop hypothyroidism and goitre. This is known as Pendred's syndrome.

Upper Limbs

When examining the upper limbs in general one may note changes in the:

♠ Dimensions

♦ Integument

Dimensions

One may note changes in the:

♣ Length

♥ Circumference

Length

The length of the upper limbs should be in proportion to the length of the body.

♣ Disproportion may occur in relation to tall statue and short stature and these conditions have already been discussed

Circumference

The circumference of the upper limbs should be proportional to the circumference of the torso.

♥ A discrepancy occurs in Cushing's syndrome where an obese body is seen in relation to thin, "matchstick", arms and legs

Integument

The causes of changes in the colour and the surface of the integument have already been discussed. Changes may also occur in:

♠ Consistency

♦ Circulation

Consistency

Variations in the consistency of the skin are:

♠ Thickened skin occurs in hypothyroidism.

♦ Localised areas of myxoedema may occur in thyrotoxicosis. This is more common in the lower limb, but may occur in the upper limb rarely. It is called thyroid acropachy

♣ Thin atrophic skin occurs in Cushing's syndrome

Circulation

Changes that may occur in the circulation of the skin are:

♣ Telangiectases occur in Cushing's syndrome

♥ Ecchymoses are common in hyperadrenocorticism

Hands

On examination of the hands one may note changes in the following:

Dimensions

Changes in the dimensions could affect:

♠ Size

♦ Length

♣ Shape

Size

Variations in the size of the hands could be:

♠ The overall size of the hands may be increased in acromegaly, obesity, hypothyroidism, primary amyloidsosis and in people engaged in heavy manual work

Length

Changes in the length of the hands could be:

♦ The length of the fingers may be increased in Marfan's syndrome giving rise to spider-like fingers or arachnodactyly.

♣ The length may be decreased in pseudohypoparathyroidism.
Short fourth or fifth fingers may be seen. This arises as a result of metacarpal shortening giving the appearance of a short fourth and or fifth finger. The abnormality is more apparent when a fist is made

Shape

The shape of the hands would differ from normal due to the changes in size that occur in the above conditions.

Nails

When examining the nails one may note changes in:

♥ Shape

♠ Colour

♦ Consistency

♣ Surface

♥ Connections

♠ Circulation

Shape

Changes that may be observed in the shape of the nails are:

♥ **Clubbing**

Clubbing may be seen in thyrotoxicosis. This is known as thyroid acropachy and is almost always seen in association with ophthalmopathy and localised myxoedema.

♠ **Pseudoclubbing**

Pseudoclubbing is seen in hyperparathyroidism. This is due to resorption of the terminal phalanges causing the nail to slope towards the palmar aspect resulting in an appearance that may be mistaken for clubbing.

♦ **Koilonychia**

Koilonychia refers to spoon shaped nails (concavity of the upper surface). This is seen in iron deficiency anaemia

Colour

Changes in the colour of the nails could be:

♠ Yellow Nails Syndrome

This is a condition in which the nails appear yellow in colour. It is associated with chronic lymphoedema of the skin, pleural effusions and thyroid disease.

♥ Blue Discolouration

Blue discolouration of the lunulae may occur in Wilson's disease.

♠ White Nails

Leuconychia occurs in hypoalbuminaemia.

♦ White Bands

White bands that lie parallel to the lunulae are seen in hypoalbuminaemia (Muehrke's lines). They occur in the nail plate and not the nail bed. They resolve when the hypoalbuminaemia is corrected.

♣ Terry's Nails

Terry's nails are white proximally with distal reddening. They may occur in non-insulin dependent diabetes mellitus

Consistency

Changes in the consistency of the nails could be:

♥ Brittle Nails

Nails in which the borders are irregular, frayed and torn are seen in thyrotoxicosis, malnutrition, calcium deficiency, iron deficiency

Surface

Changes that may occur on the surface of the nails are:

- ♠ A transverse groove may occur in the nail, Beau's line. This indicates growth arrest due to severe illness such as fever, cachexia and malnutrition.

- ♦ Multiple horizontal grooves may occur due to secondary nail plate damage in paronychia

Connections

The connections of the nails may be disrupted due to:

- ♣ Onycholysis, which refers to separation of the nail from its bed. This may occur in thyrotoxicosis

Circulation

Changes that one may observe in the nail bed circulation are:

- ♥ Splinter haemorrhages may give a clue to the cause of a fever.

Nail Fold

Abnormalities that one may observe in the nail fold are:

- ♠ Chronic paronychia

  In chronic paronychia the nail fold is decreased in size, the shape changes, the margins become ragged and the surface is irregular. Chronic paronychia may occur in hypoparathyroidism, multiple endocrine deficiencies and in chronic iron deficiency.

Skin

The main changes that may be seen in the skin are changes in colour, surface and consistency. Changes in colour, consistency and surface changes have already been described. Other abnormalities that may occur are:

♦ Pigmented skin creases are a feature of Addison's disease.

♣ Yellow skin is seen in carotenaemia. This would be most noticeable over the palms. Carotenaemia occurs due to excessive consumption of food containing carotene, hypothyroidism, diabetes mellitus, anorexia nervosa

♥ Palmar erythema occurs in thyrotoxicosis and pregnancy

♠ Palmar xanthomata, a yellowish-orange discolouration of the palms and skin creases is seen in hyperlipidaemia

♦ Granuloma annulare may be associated with insulin dependent diabetes mellitus

Locomotor System

Most abnormalities usually picked up on examination of the bones and joints would have already become obvious as one performed assessment of size and shape. That is the changes seen in acromegaly or pseudohypopararthyroidism. Other abnormalities that may occur are those affecting the:

Joints

Abnormalities that one may note in the joints of the hands are:

♣ The second and third metacarpophalangeal joints may be involved in the arthropathy complicating haemochromatosis

Tendons

In the tendons one may note the following abnormalities:

♥ Tendon xanthomata occur in familial hypercholesterolaemia.

♠ Dupuytren's contracture may occur in insulin dependent diabetes mellitus.

Peripheral Circulation

When palpating the hands one may note:

♦ Warm, moist hands in thyrotoxicosis

♣ Cold, dry skin in hypothyroidism

Radial Pulse

On examination of the radial pulse one may note abnormalities of:

♥ Rate

♠ Rhythm

♦ Volume

♣ Character

Rate

Changes in rate could be:

♥ Tachycardia in thyrotoxicosis, fever

♠ Bradycardia in hypothyroidism

Rhythm

Changes in rhythm are:

♦ Atrial fibrillation in thyrotoxicosis

♣ Varying degrees of heart block may occur in hypothyroidism

Volume

Changes that may occur in the volume of the pulse are:

- ♥ A large volume pulse may occur in thyrotoxicosis, fever.
- ♠ The pulse may be of small volume in hypothyroidism

Character

Changes in the character of the pulse are:

- ♦ A collapsing pulse may occur in thyrotoxicosis and in fevers.

Function of the Hands

The function of the hands is movement. This is dependent on the structural and functional integrity of the locomotor system, the nervous system and the integument. These systems may be involved in diseases of the endocrine and metabolic system and thereby function of the hands may be compromised. This would result in abnormalities of active and or passive movement and in abnormal movement.

Involuntary Movements

The involuntary movements one may note are:

- ♣ Physiological tremor is exaggerated in thyrotoxicosis.
- ♥ Choreoathetosis may occur in thyrotoxicosis

Decreased Movement

Restricted movements of the hand may be caused by development of the:

- ♠ Diabetic stiff hand syndrome. In this condition thickened, waxy skin occurs on the dorsum of the hands and this is associated with joint stiffness. This is called diabetic cheiroarthropathy and is best demonstrated by showing that the patient is unable to place the hands together as if in prayer (Prayer sign). The patient would not be able to oppose the metacarpophalangeal joints and the interphalangeal joints.

Neuropathies

Neuropathies that may occur in relation to the endocrine and metabolic system are the following:

- ♦ **Entrapment Neuropathy**

  Carpal tunnel syndrome is seen in hypothyroidism and in acromegaly. This results in wasting and weakness of the muscles of the lateral part of the thenar eminence, sensory loss in the distribution of the median nerve and Tinel's sign and Phalen's sign may become positive.

- ♣ **Mononeuritis Multiplex**

  Mononeuritis multiplex may occur in diabetes mellitus.

- ♥ **Peripheral Neuropathy**

  Peripheral neuropathy may occur in diabetes mellitus.

Forearms

This is not an area that gives a lot of information on clinical examination. Most of the features seen in disease would have already become evident during the course of the examination conducted up to now. These features would be in relation to the dimensions and the cover.

Function of the Forearms

Grip Strength

The assessment that is performed in relation to the metabolic and endocrine system is determination of grip strength which is dependent on the forearm muscle mass. This is an excellent functional assessment in nutritional deficiency. The test is performed using a dynamometer and is mentioned here for the sake of completeness.

Elbows

Most of the features are the same as those that may be detected on regional examination elsewhere. A few features of particular relevance to the elbow will be mentioned. They are in relation to:

♣ Dimensions

♥ Integument

Dimensions

Shape

Carrying Angle

When the arms are held out straight by the sides of the body, a slight angulation is evident between the upper arms and forearms. This angulation is known as the carrying angle. It is normally greater in females than in males. The carrying angle is increased in:

♠ Turner's syndrome

Skin (Cover)

In the skin over the elbow one may note changes in:

Colour

Increased pigmentation may be seen in the crease of the elbow in:

♥ Addison's disease

Surface

The surface of the skin over the elbows may show:

♣ Eruptive xanthomata. This is a yellow, papular eruption that may be observed in severe hyper-triglyceridaemia

Upper Arms

Abnormalities that one may note are the following:

Size

The size of the upper arms is of importance in the assessment of the nutritional state of the patient and ideally measurements should be made. They are given here for the sake of completeness.

Mid Arm Circumference

This is the circumference of the upper arm at a point mid way between the acromial and olecranon processes. The measurement should be >23 cms in a male and > 22 cms in a female. Readings less than this indicate malnourishment.

Triceps Skin Fold

The skin over the triceps is pinched between thumb and middle finger and measured using callipers.

Mid Arm Muscle Circumference

This is the mid arm circumference minus π x triceps skin fold thickness

MAMC = MAC- (πx TSF)

This value should be over 19 cms in males and over 17 cms in females.

Blood Pressure

Variations that one may note are the following:

♥ The blood pressure would be high in Cushing's syndrome, Conn's syndrome, phaeochromocytoma and acromegaly.

♠ The blood pressure would be low in Addison's disease, salt and water depletion. The earliest sign is a postural drop in blood pressure of more than twenty millimetres of mercury.

♦ Postural hypotension may be a feature of diabetic autonomic neuropathy

Trousseau's sign

To demonstrate Trousseau's sign, occlude the arterial pulse for five minutes by inflating a blood pressure cuff to above systolic blood pressure. In hypocalcaemia this will cause carpal spasm. The fingers will flex at the metacarpophalangeal joints and extend at the interphalangeal joints. The thumb will adduct. This resembles an obstetrician's hand when performing manual removal of the placenta and is thus known as *main d' accoucheur.*

Shoulders and Axillae

When examining the shoulders and axillae one may note abnormalities of the:

Dimensions

When assessing the dimensions of the shoulders one may note changes in size and shape.

Size

The size of the supraclavicular and suprascapular regions may be abnormal due to the following:

♣ The size may be increased due to deposition of excess fat in Cushing's syndrome.

♥ Wasting would occur in malnutrition.

♠ Muscle wasting may be a feature of the metabolic myopathy, which can occur in acromegaly, hyperthyroidism, hypothyroidism, Cushing's syndrome, osteomalacia

Shape

The shape of the shoulders may vary from normal:

♦ In Cushing's syndrome excess deposition of fat would result in the typical "Buffalo Hump" appearance.

♣ Wasting of tissue in malnutrition would result in a squared appearance.

Integument (Cover)

Changes that one may observe in the skin are:

♥ Increased pigmentation would be seen in the axillae in acanthosis nigricans where the skin would be thickened, have a velvety texture and there may be skin tags. It occurs in diabetes mellitus, Cushing's syndrome and acromegaly

Function

When examining power of the shoulder muscles one may note:

♠ Weakness of the muscles of the shoulder girdle due to a metabolic myopathy

Neck

On examination of the neck one may note changes in the:

Dimensions

On examination of the dimensions one may note abnormalities of size and shape.

Size

The size of the neck may be:

♦ Increased in obesity, Cushing's syndrome and hypothyroidism. It would also be increased in thoracic inlet obstruction due to a retrosternal goitre.

♣ Decreased in cachexia

Shape

Variations in shape are:

♥ A webbed neck occurs in Turner's syndrome

Integument (Cover)

When examining the skin over the neck one may note:

♣ A scar indicating previous thyroid surgery

♥ A scar due to previous parathyroid surgery

Consistency

The consistency of the tissues of the neck may vary due to:

♥ Increased fat in Cushing's syndrome, simple obesity

♠ Congestion in thoracic inlet obstruction

Thyroid Gland

When examining the thyroid gland one may note changes in its:

♦ Position
♣ Size
♥ Shape
♠ Margins
♦ Surface
♣ Consistency
♥ Tenderness
♠ Mobility
♦ Circulation
♣ Pemberton's sign

Position

The gland is normally situated in the neck with its isthmus below the cricoid cartilage and the two lateral lobes on either side of the trachea. Less commonly:

♦ The whole or part of the gland may be situated in a retrosternal position

Size

The normal gland is usually not visible nor is it palpable.

♣ Enlargement of the gland, goitre, may vary from minimal diffuse enlargement to massive multinodular goitres

Shape

Small goitres maintain their normal shape but as the gland enlarges the normal shape is lost and it becomes globular

Margins

The margins are usually easily palpable. It is important to define the inferior margin, as inability to palpate this could indicate retrosternal extension

Surface

The surface of the gland is usually smooth.

♣ Nodularity may become apparent as the gland enlarges

Consistency

The consistency of the thyroid gland is important.

♥ Normally the gland is soft.

♠ It may be firm in a simple goitre.

♦ It would be rubbery in consistency in Hashimoto's thyroiditis.

♣ It may be hard in carcinoma, if there is calcification or if it is fibrotic. Rarely, a hard consistency

would be indicative of Riedl's thyroiditis.

♥ A cyst may occur in the gland and this may be transilluminated

Tenderness

The presence of tenderness in the thyroid gland could indicate:

♠ Thyroiditis

♦ Bleeding

Mobility

The thyroid gland moves with swallowing.

♣ Decreased mobility could indicate malignancy.

Circulation

Abnormalities that one may note are:

♥ The carotid arteries may be involved by malignant infiltration. This would be indicated by loss of pulsation.

♠ Increased vascularity of the gland may result in a palpable thrill and a bruit

Pemberton's Sign

Pemberton's sign would be positive if there is:

♦ A retrosternal goitre

Findings

The abnormalities that one may detect on examination of the thyroid gland are summarized in table 2.1.

Table 2.1

Diffuse enlargement	Simple goitre.
Diffuse enlargement	Thyrotoxicosis. In this case the gland may have a bosselated surface, an associated thrill and bruit may also occur. Signs of thyrotoxicosis may be present. There may be evidence of thyroid ophthalmopathy or dermopathy (localised myxoedema, thyroid acropachy)
Diffuse enlargement with a rubbery consistency	This indicates Hashimoto's thyroiditis. It may be associated with features of hypothyroidism.
Diffuse enlargement with associated pain and tenderness	This is seen in de Quervain's thyroiditis, a viral condition that may produce transient hyperthyroidism
Nodular goitre	Multinodular goitre is the commonest cause of thyroid enlargement
Solitary nodule	Usually a single or first nodule of a multinodular goitre. More rarely carcinoma or adenoma may cause a solitary nodule. Rapid enlargement, pain or lymphadenopathy would suggest cancer. A toxic nodule may rarely occur. This is known by the eponym Plummer's syndrome. A cyst may present as a solitary nodule. This may be transilluminated.
Hard gland	A hard gland may occur in carcinoma and may be associated with decreased mobility and involvement of the adjacent structures. A hard, irregular gland may also occur in Riedl's thyroiditis, which causes fibrosis of the gland and is associated with other forms of midline fibrosis.

Thyroid Cancer

Thyroid cancer may be of the following types:

♣ Papillary (younger patients, lymph node spread)

♥ Follicular (older patients, blood borne spread)

♠ Anaplastic (elderly patients, aggressive tumours)

♦ Medullary (younger patients, secretes calcitonin sometimes ACTH, may be part of MEN)

♣ Lymphoma (usually arises in the thyroid of a patient with Hashimoto's thyroiditis)

Sternocleidomastoid Muscle

Abnormalities that one may note in the sternocleidomastoid muscle are:

The muscle may be infiltrated in thyroid malignancy

Jugular Venous Pressure

When examining the jugular venous pressure one may observe:

♠ An elevated jugular venous pressure occurs in retrosternal extension of the thyroid causing obstruction of the superior vena cava in which case it will be a non-pulsatile elevation.

♦ The JVP may be elevated due to pericardial effusion or heart failure consequent on endocrine disease and in atrio-ventricular block due to hypothyroidism

Carotids

On examination of the carotids one may note:

♣ In thyroid malignancies the carotids may undergo local invasion.

Trachea

Abnormalities that may occur in relation to the trachea are:

♥ The trachea may be deviated by a large gland

♠ Stridor could occur due to narrowing of the trachea by a large thyroid gland or due to damage to the recurrent laryngeal nerve

Lymph Nodes

The cervical lymph nodes may be:

♦ Enlarged in thyrotoxicosis.

♣ Lymphadenopathy may occur in thyroid cancer

Chest Wall

When examining the chest wall one may note changes in:

♥ Dimensions

♠ Integument

♦ Breasts

Dimensions

Size

The size of the chest may be:

♥ Increased in obesity, especially the central type, in Cushing's syndrome, hypothyroidism

♠ Decreased in malnutrition, cachexia

Integument

The colour and surface characteristics would reflect changes that have been dealt with earlier. Other changes that may occur are:

♦ Hair distribution in the male would represent individual and ethnic differences. Body hair loss occurs in hypogonadism.

♣ Spider naevi may occur in thyrotoxicosis.

♥ Skin elasticity may be decreased in diabetes mellitus and in Addison's disease.

Breasts

When examining breast tissue one may note:

♠ Gynaecomastia

♦ Breast atrophy

♣ Galactorrhoea

Gynaecomastia

The endocrine causes of gynaeco-mastia are:

- ♠ **Pituitary disorders**: hypogo-nadotrophic hypogonadism
- ♦ **Thyroid disorders**: thyrotoxi-cosis
- ♣ **Adrenal disorders**: congenital adrenal hyperplasia, adrenal cancer, Addison's disease

Breast Atrophy

Breast atrophy may occur in:

- ♥ Hypopituitarism

Galactorrhoea

The function of the breast is the production of milk, lactation. This is physiological after childbirth but at any other time it is pathological and is known as galactorrhoea.

The causes of galactorrhoea are:

- ♠ **Pituitary disorders**: hyperpro-lactinaemia, acromegaly
- ♦ **Adrenal disorders**: Cushing's syndrome
- ♣ **Thyroid disease**
- ♥ **Drugs**: oral contraceptives, phenothiazines, tricyclic antide-pressants, methyldopa

Heart

In the heart the abnormalities that may be noted are:

- ♠ Cardiomegaly may be evident in acromegaly
- ♦ A gallop rhythm may occur in thyrotoxicosis

- ♣ Valvular lesions may occur in the carcinoid syndrome:

  Right-sided lesions in gastroin-testinal, hepatic or ovarian carcinoid

  Left-sided lesions in bronchial carcinoid

- ♥ Pericardial effusion may occur in hypothyroidism
- ♠ Coronary artery disease may occur in diabetes mellitus and in hypothyroidism

Lungs

Abnormalities that may occur in the lungs are:

- ♦ Kussmaul's respiration occurs in metabolic acidosis
- ♣ Wheezing may occur in the carcinoid syndrome
- ♠ Pleural effusions may occur in hypothyroidism

Abdominal Wall

On examination of the abdominal wall one may note changes in the following:

- ♠ Dimensions
- ♦ Integument

Dimensions

On examination of the dimensions one may note abnormalities of:

Size

The size of the abdomen may be increased because of:

- ♠ Deposition of fat in obesity

◆ Ascites in hypothyroidism

Shape

The shape of the abdomen may change:

♣ A distended abdomen could be due to fat or fluid.

♥ The abdomen may be scaphoid in malnutrition

Integument

The colour and surface characteristic may change as described earlier.

♠ There may be striae in Cushing's syndrome

◆ An adrenalectomy scar may be seen in Nelson's syndrome

Liver and Spleen

Abnormalities that may be noted are:

♣ Hepatomegaly and splenomegaly may occur in thyrotoxicosis, rarely.

♥ Hepatomegaly and splenomegaly may also occur in acromegaly

Bladder

The bladder may be:

♠ Distended in autonomic neuropathy consequent on diabetes mellitus

Ascites

Ascites may occur in:

◆ Myxoedema

Bruits

A bruit may be heard in:

♣ Renal artery stenosis, complicating diabetes mellitus

Male External Genitalia

In the context of the endocrine and metabolic systems one would concentrate mainly on the dimensions and the cover

Dimensions

When examining the dimensions one may note changes in size and shape.

Size

The size of the testes may be:

♥ Increased in precocious puberty.

♠ The testes would be enlarged in Soto's syndrome.

◆ The size of the testes would be decreased in hypogonadism, acromegaly and hypopituitarism.

> Soto's syndrome or cerebral gigantism is probably of autosomal dominant inheritance and is characterised by mental retardation, gigantism, slight downslant of the eyes, characteristic facies and scoliosis.

Shape

Variations in the shape of the genitalia are:

♣ Hypospadias may be associated with decreased exposure to sex hormones in the developing foetus

Integument (Cover)

When examining the skin over the genitalia one may note:

♥ The amount of pubic hair would be decreased in hypogonadism

Female External Genitalia

On examination of the female genitalia one may note:

♠ Changes in size may occur and an enlarged clitoris may be evident in masculinising syndromes.

♦ Decreased pubic hair would be a feature of hypogonadism

Lower Limbs

When examining the lower limbs one may note abnormalities of:

♣ Length

♥ Circumference

♠ Integument

Length

Variations in the length of the limbs could be:

♣ Increased length in relation to the torso occurs in the eunuchoidal types of tall stature

Circumference

Changes that may occur in the circumference of the limbs are:

♥ Reduced circumference in relation to the torso (matchstick limbs) occurs in Cushing's syndrome. Reduced circumference would also occur in malnutrition.

♠ Localised variations in the amount of fat would be seen in diabetic lipodystrophy

Integument

The surface characteristics may show the changes that have been dealt with earlier. In addition features that are most likely to be seen in the lower limb are:

♦ Necrobiosis lipoidicum diabeticorum

♣ Pretibial myxoedema

Pelvic Girdle and Hips

On examination of the pelvic girdle and hips one may note changes in the:

Dimensions

One may note changes in size and shape.

Size

The size of the hips would be:

♥ Increased in obesity of the peripheral type.

♠ Decreased in malnutrition

Shape

The shape of the hips would vary according to the type of obesity.

♦ The hips would be wide in the female peripheral type of obesity

Hip Joints

Abnormalities that may occur at the hip joints are:

- ♠ Osteoarthrosis may occur in acromegaly

Function

When testing power of the muscles of the pelvic girdle one may note:

- ♦ Proximal myopathy, which may occur in Cushing's syndrome, thyrotoxicosis, acromegaly, and osteomalacia
- ♣ Periodic paralysis may occur in thyrotoxicosis.

Thighs

When examining the thighs one may note changes in the following:

Shape

Variations in the shape of the thighs could be:

- ♥ Lipodystrophy in insulin dependent diabetics. This causes localised fat atrophy

Integument

One may note:

- ♠ Candidiasis in the groin (intertrigo) in diabetics

Function

When examining power of the quadriceps one may note:

- ♦ In diabetic amyotrophy, weakness and wasting of the quadriceps would occur.

Knees

Lesions that may occur at the knees are:

Skin

The skin over the knee may be affected by:

- ♣ Eruptive xanthoma

Joints

Abnormalities that may occur at the knee joint are:

- ♥ Pyrophosphate arthropathy, which may complicate haemochromatosis, commonly affects the knees
- ♠ Osteoarthrosis can occur in acromegaly

Tendons

The tendons of the knee joint may be affected by:

- ♦ Tendon xanthomata which may occur in hyperlipidaemia

Lower Legs

When examining the lower legs one may note changes in:

Shape

Abnormalities that may occur are:

- ♣ Bowed legs may occur in acromegaly

Integument

Abnormalities that may occur in the skin over the lower legs are:

♥ Necrobiosis lipoidica diabeticorum is commonly seen over the shins. These are well-demarcated plaques, which may coalesce. The surface is shiny and atrophic. The centre is yellow and waxy. The edge is brownish-red. There may be telangiectasia on the surface.

♠ In diabetic dermopathy patches of atrophy and pigmentation may occur.

♦ Pre-tibial myxoedema may be seen in thyrotoxicosis. It is a shiny, red, non-tender infiltration on the front of the shins. When it becomes chronic it has the appearance of localised elephantiasis

Ankle

Lesions that may occur at the ankle are those affecting the:

Joints

Lesions that may affect the ankle joint are:

♣ Charcot's joints may occur in diabetes mellitus

Tendons

The tendons may be affected by:

♥ Tendon xanthomata

Function

When testing the ankle jerks one may demonstrate the following abnormalities:

♠ Increased ankle jerk relaxation time may occur in hypothyroidism. Ideally one should demonstrate this by asking the patient to kneel on a chair or bed with the feet hanging over the edge of it.

♦ Reduced ankle jerks would indicate the development of neuropathy in diabetes mellitus.

Feet

The changes seen here are similar to those occurring in the hand.

Shape

One may observe the following changes in shape:

♣ Loss of the transverse arch along the metatarsal heads may occur in diabetes mellitus

♥ Short fourth and fifth toes may be noted due to shortening of the metatarsals in pseudohypoparathyroidism

Integument

When examining the skin one may note:

♠ Ulceration, which may occur in diabetes mellitus. This would indicate peripheral vascular disease or neuropathy.

♦ Callus formation may occur over pressure points in diabetes mellitus

Pulses

On examination of the arterial pulses of the foot one may note the following:

♣ Absent foot pulses due to peripheral vascular disease. This may occur in diabetes mellitus and in hypothyroidism

Neuropathy

Neuropathies that may develop are:

- ♥ Peripheral neuropathy may present with absent touch, pain, temperature and vibration sense. Peripheral neuropathy occurs in diabetes mellitus.
- ♠ Foot drop could occur due to common peroneal lesions consequent on mononeuritis multiplex or it could be the result of loss of the protective fat pad in severe wasting.

Buttocks

Conditions that may be observed are:

- ♦ A migratory, necrolytic, erythematous eruption may be seen in glucagonoma.

Spine

Size and Shape

One may note changes in the dimensions such as:

- ♣ Decreased length of the spine and kyphosis may occur in osteoporosis and in hyperparathyroidism.

Gait

On assessing gait, the abnormalities that may be detected are:

- ♥ Cerebellar ataxia in hypothyroidism
- ♠ A stamping gait may occur due to peripheral neuropathy.
- ♦ A rolling gait may occur in acromegaly.

Trendelenburg Test

The Trendelenburg test may be positive in:

- ♣ Proximal (metabolic) myopathy

Standing from a Seated or Squatting Position

The patient may have difficulty standing from a seated or squatting position if there is:

- ♣ Proximal (metabolic) myopathy

103

Chapter 9

The Integumental System (the skin and its appendages)

The study of the integumental system deals with diseases that affect the skin and its appendages. However, one should bear in mind that of equal importance is the fact that the skin and its appendages often reflect manifestations of systemic disease. The structures that should be assessed are the skin together with the mucosa that is easily accessible and the appendages of the skin; the hair and the nails.

History Taking

One should enquire about:

- ♥ Rash
- ♠ Sweating
- ♦ Dry Skin
- ♣ Pigmentation
- ♥ Itching
- ♠ Hair
- ♦ Nails

A review of systems is extremely important, as this would give clues to any systemic illness that manifests as a skin disorder.

Physical Examination

Physical examination is of crucial importance in the evaluation of disorders of the integument. As with examination of any system one should commence with a general examination where one should note the position of the patient, assess the state of growth and development and the metabolic state. Any striking changes in the integument should be noted and the body temperature should be ascertained. (Position, Height and Proportions, Weight and Shape, Integument, Body Temperature)

This should be followed by examination of the anatomical regions of the body.

Examination of the integument follows the same principles as examination of any other system. One should examine structure and evaluate function.

Skin and Mucosa

Structure of the Skin

Inspect the skin paying attention to the features of structure. The dimensions should be assessed. Size would be reflected by contraction of the skin or conversely the skin being redundant. The shape would be a reflection of the state of the underlying tissue together with either contraction or redundancy of the skin. Note the colour of the skin.

When examining the surface the most important feature is the evaluation of a rash and this will be discussed in detail later. The other features of importance when evaluating the surface are the presence of and quantity of sweat and sebum.

The blood vessel pattern is of importance and should be noted.

Palpate the skin noting the characteristics of the surface (rash, sweat, sebum), the consistency of the skin, the temperature of the skin and the presence of any tender areas. Note the degree of skin elasticity and the mobility of the skin over underlying structures, Check capillary refill if required.

Percussion and auscultation would not be required.

Function of the Skin

The skin has many functions. They are:

♣ Protection

♥ Production of sebum

♠ Production of sweat

♦ Temperature control

Protective Function

The protective function of the skin is dependent upon its structural integrity and this has been assessed when examining structure.

Sebum and Sweat

The production of sebum and sweat has already been noted during the course of examination of structure.

Temperature Control

Temperature control is an important function of the skin. Changes in temperature may be:

♣ Generalised changes

♥ Localised changes

Generalised Changes

Generalised changes in skin temperature reflect efforts to maintain body temperature or reflect changes in the cutaneous circulation either due to systemic disturbances or due to generalised cutaneous disease.

Localised Changes

Localised changes in skin temperature reflect inflammation or vascular insufficiency.

Hair

Hair may be categorised as scalp hair and hair on the body.

Body hair is comprised of facial hair, hair in the axillae, pubic hair, hair on the torso and limbs. Body hair represents secondary sexual characteristics and reflects sexual maturation. Hence, the quantity and distribution of body hair would be dependent on the sex hormone environment. In addition, one should bear in mind that in scalp hair loss, the pattern of loss would be dependent on the sex hormone environment.

In examination of the hair inspection is the most important modality of examination.

One should define the site of examination and then define the quantity of hair and the pattern of distribution.

The shape and colour of the hair should be defined. This should be followed by an evaluation of surface characteristics such as the sheen of the hair and the presence of foreign bodies notably lice or their ova.

Palpation is of limited value but rarely one may define easy pluckability or that the hair is brittle.

Percussion and auscultation are obviously of no importance.

Nails

Remember to look at the nail fold and cuticle as well as the nail itself.

Define the site being examined. Note the size and shape of the nail and note the condition of the margins.

Note the colour of the nail and look at the surface carefully.

Look carefully at the attachment of the nail to the underlying nail bed. Observe the underlying network of blood vessels and the blood vessels in the nail fold.

Palpation is useful to look for fluctuation in early clubbing. It will also determine any tender areas. Use palpation to elicit capillary pulsations in aortic regurgitation and to detect capillary refill time in vascular insufficiency.

Elicit capillary refill by exerting pressure on the nail to blanche the nail bed. Release pressure and see how long it takes for the blanched area to refill with blood.

The method of performing Quincke's test is described in the chapter on the cardiovascular system.

Obviously percussion and auscultation are of no value here.

Skin Rashes

An important aspect of examination of the skin is the definition and analysis of skin rashes. This is a subject that should be studied in depth.

When describing skin lesions one should define the type of lesion seen. Next, if multiple lesions are evident their arrangement in relation to one another should be defined. Finally, the distribution of lesions over the surface of the body should be defined. Thus one should define:

♣ **T**ype

♥ **A**rrangement

♠ **D**istribution

Aide Memoire

*This will give an acronym that should hopefully make it a **TAD** easier to remember.*

Types of Lesions

The types of lesions may be classified as:

♦ Primary Lesions

♣ Secondary Lesions

Primary Lesions

Primary lesions may in turn be classified as:

♥ Flat Lesions

♠ Raised Lesions

♦ Depressed Lesions

Flat (non-palpable) Lesions

Macules

Macules are flat non-palpable lesions that differ from the surrounding normal skin in being:

♣ Pigmented

♥ Depigmented

♠ Erythematous

♦ Haemorrhagic

Large macules (more than 1 cm) are sometimes referred to as patches.

> Depending on the size of the haemorrhage into the skin, haemorrhagic lesions are further subdivided into petechiae, purpura and ecchymoses. (Petechiae refers to lesions less than 3 mm in size, ecchymoses are large lesions)

Raised (palpable) Lesions

Raised (palpable) lesions may be subdivided into:

♣ Solid lesions

♥ Fluid filled lesions

Solid Raised Lesions

Solid raised lesions may be:

♠ Papules

♦ Milia

♣ Comedones

♥ Plaques

♠ Nodules

♦ Weals

♣ Burrows

Papules

Papules are raised, solid skin lesions that are smaller than 1 cm at their greatest diameter

Milia

Milia refers to small, firm, white papules filled with keratin

Comedones (Blackheads)

Comedones are hair follicles plugged by keratin. They occur in acne

Plaques

Plaques are raised, palpable lesions that are greater than 1 cm in diameter. They are superficial and flat-topped.

Nodules

Nodules are raised, palpable lesions greater than 1 cm in diameter. They are either deep seated or project outwards

Weals

A weal refers to oedema of the skin. Weals usually occur due to insect bites or allergic reactions. They are raised, flat-topped lesions with ill-defined margins.

Burrows

Burrows are linear elevations of the epidermis that occur due to infestation by parasites

Raised Fluid Filled Lesions

Raised fluid filled lesions may be:

- ♥ Vesicles
- ♠ Bullae
- ♦ Whiteheads
- ♣ Pustules
- ♥ Target lesions
- ♠ Cysts

Vesicles

Vesicles are fluid-filled lesions less than 5 mm in diameter

Bullae

Bullae are larger, fluid-filled lesions. They are greater than 5 mm in diameter

> **Nikolsky's sign**
>
> Nikolsky's sign refers to fluid moving from a bulla into the surrounding skin when pressure is applied with the examining finger. This is due to separation of cells that are not closely adherent. This sign allows differentiation of pemphigus from pemphigoid

Whiteheads

Whiteheads are distended sebaceous glands. They are seen in acne.

Pustules

Pustules are vesicles filled with pus

Target Lesions

Target lesions are lesions consisting of three concentric zones of skin change. They are a central, dark area or blister surrounded by a pale, oedematous zone, which in turn is surrounded by an area of erythema.

Cysts

Cysts are large fluid-filled lesions. They are usually surrounded by a well-defined capsule.

Depressed Lesions

Depressed lesions may be:

- ♦ Erosions
- ♣ Ulcers
- ♥ Fissures
- ♠ Atrophy

Erosions

An erosion refers to a breach in the continuity of the epithelium resulting in a depressed lesion involving only the epidermis

Ulcer

An ulcer is a breach in the continuity of the epithelium resulting in a depressed lesion involving the whole or part of the dermis

Fissure

A fissure is a linear depressed lesion

Atrophy

Atrophy of the skin gives rise to areas that are paler than normal, more shiny, thinner than normal and have

loss of skin markings and appendages

Secondary Lesions

Secondary lesions are:

- ♦ Scales
- ♣ Crusts
- ♥ Excoriations
- ♠ Lichenification
- ♦ Dyschromia
- ♣ Scars

Scales

Scales refer to flaking of the epidermis resulting in clumps of epidermal cells.

Crusts

Crusts refer to dried exudate.

Excoriations

Excoriations refer to marks caused by scratching

Lichenification

Lichenification refers to thickening of the skin caused by chronic irritation and scratching

Dyschromia

Dyschromia refers to a change in the colour of the skin as a result of chronic inflammation

Scar

A scar refers to tissue resulting from healing of an injured area. A scar is usually flat or depressed but it may be hypertrophic and then it is referred to as keloid.

Complex Lesions

Lesions are not always uniform but are quite commonly complex with different types of lesion featured.

Arrangement

This refers to the way in which lesions are arranged in respect to one another. This is important. Lesions may be arranged in a linear fashion, in clusters, in an annular fashion, a reticular arrangement or a gyrate fashion. They may be confluent or discrete.

Arrangement of Lesions

- ♥ Linear
- ♠ Cluster
- ♦ Annular
- ♣ Reticular
- ♥ Gyrate

Linear

Linear refers to lesions arranged along a line

Cluster

A cluster refers to lesions grouped together

Annular

Annular refers to a ring-like arrangement

Reticular

Reticular refers to a net-like arrangement

Gyrate

Gyrate refers to a snake-like (winding) arrangement

Confluent or Discrete

When grouped together lesions may coalesce or remain discrete.

Distribution

The distribution of lesions across the body should be carefully noted and defined. The distribution may be:

- ♠ Generalised
- ♦ Localised

Lesions of the Integument

Lesions of the integument may be due to:

- ♣ External agents
- ♥ Primary disease of the integument
- ♠ Systemic disease with manifestations in the integument

External Agents

External agents that result in lesions of the integument are:

- ♦ **Chemical Agents**

  Cosmetics, detergents, nickel, agents used in industry and agriculture

- ♣ **Physical Agents**

  Heat, sunlight, radiation, trauma

- ♥ **Biological Agents**

  Parasites, bacteria, fungi, viruses

Primary Disease of the Integument

Primary disease of the integument may be:

- ♠ **Developmental Lesions**

  Genetic abnormalities

- ♦ **Inflammatory Lesions**

  These may be acute or chronic and are usually autoimmune in aetiology

- ♣ **Tumours**

  Primary tumours of the skin are melanoma, basal cell carcinoma and squamous carcinoma.

Systemic Disease

Systemic diseases that have manifestations in the integument are conditions affecting the:

- ♥ **HS** these are usually neoplastic disorders such as lymphoma, leukaemia, polycythaemia rubra vera. Haemolytic anaemia may also have skin manifestations.

- ♠ **RAG** diseases of the RAG system such as the sexually transmitted diseases like syphilis, AIDS have skin manifestations.

  Disorders of sexual development would also have skin manifestations.

- ♦ **GIT** disorders of the GIT that have skin manifestations are usually the inflammatory disorders of the liver and gastrointestinal tract and neoplasms of the upper gastrointestinal tract. Examples are:

Inflammatory bowel diseases: Crohn's disease, ulcerative colitis, coeliac disease, Whipple's disease

Liver disease: cirrhosis of the liver, primary biliary cirrhosis

Stomach and pancreatic cancer also result in skin manifestations.

- ♣ **RS** the diseases that have skin manifestations are inflammatory conditions such as tuberculosis and sarcoidosis and neoplasms.
- ♥ **CNS** the phakomatoses
- ♠ **LMS** systemic lupus erythematosus, rheumatoid arthritis
- ♦ **E&M** disorders of the endocrine and metabolic system that have skin manifestations are those affecting the:

Pituitary: hypopituitarism, Nelson's syndrome, acromegaly

Thyroid: thyrotoxicosis, hypothyroidism

Adrenal: Cushing's syndrome, Addison's disease

Pancreas: diabetes mellitus, glucagonoma

- ♣ **CVS** infective endocarditis, rheumatic fever, vasculitis, Raynaud's phenomenon
- ♥ **KUS** chronic renal failure

Findings on History

The findings that one may obtain on taking a history are as follows:

Itch (Pruritus)

Itch may be caused by:

- ♠ External agents

- ♦ Primary skin disease
- ♣ Systemic causes

External Agents

External agents that cause itch are:

- ♥ Water (Aquagenic pruritus)
- ♠ Parasites such as scabies, onchocerciasis, trichinella, schistosomiasis
- ♦ Insect bites

Primary Skin Disease

Itch may be due to primary skin disease:

- ♣ Dryness and desiccation, which is common in the elderly
- ♥ Lichen simplex or neurodermatitis
- ♠ Dermatitis herpetiformis

Systemic Causes

The systemic causes of itch are lesions of the:

- ♦ **GIT** obstructive jaundice where bile salts rather than bilirubin cause itch
- ♣ **HS** polycythaemia rubra vera, lymphatic leukaemia, Hodgkin's disease, iron deficiency
- ♥ **KUS** itch is a feature of chronic renal failure but not acute renal failure. It is relieved if the patient undergoes parathyroidectomy.
- ♠ **E&M** itch may occur in diabetes mellitus, hyperthyroidism and hypothyroidism

Itch may also occur in internal malignancy particularly carcinoma of the bronchus.

Findings on Physical Examination

Abnormalities that may be detected in relation to the skin, hair and nails will be discussed initially and this will be followed by a discussion of the findings on regional examination.

Skin

When examining the skin one may note abnormalities of the following:

- ◆ Dimensions
- ♣ Colour
- ♥ Surface
- ♠ Consistency
- ◆ Temperature
- ♣ Tenderness
- ♥ Mobility
- ♠ Circulation

Dimensions

On examination of the dimensions one may note changes in size and shape.

Size

The size of the skin may be:

- ◆ Reduced in scleroderma.
- ♣ Increased in size and redundant in pseudoxanthoma elasticum, Ehlers-Danlos syndrome and cutis laxa.

Cutis laxa may be inherited or occur following episodes of urticaria and angioedema, it can also occur in complement deficiency, lupus erythematosus, sarcoidosis, syphilis, multiple myeloma.

Shape

The shape of the skin reflects the shape of the underlying tissue:

- ♥ In scleroderma; the nose would become smaller and beak like. The mouth would be smaller and appear more rounded. The fingers would also demonstrate a change in shape, becoming more pointed. The skin would definitely appear smaller and more taut

Colour of the Skin

The colour of the skin may vary and present in disease states as:

- ♣ Hypopigmentation
- ♥ Hyperpigmentation
- ♠ Yellow Discolouration
- ◆ Purple Discolouration
- ♣ Pallor
- ♥ Flush
- ♠ Cyanosis
- ◆ Muddy Discolouration

Hypopigmentation

Hypopigmentation of the skin may be:

- ♣ Diffuse
- ♥ Localised

113

Diffuse Hypopigmentation

Diffuse hypopigmentation of the skin may occur in:

♠ **Primary Skin Disease**

Albinism. This refers to a group of genetic syndromes, characterised by the failure to synthesise melanin (the enzyme tyrosinase is defective). This affects the skin, the eye and the cochlea.

Partial albinism causes piebaldism and albinoidism. Albinoidism is where pale skin occurs without eye changes.

Complete albinism can be categorised as oculocutaneous albinism or ocular albinism. In ocular albinism skin changes are not seen but deafness may occur.

♦ **Systemic Conditions**

Phenylketonuria, hypopituitarism

Localised Hypopigmentation

Leucoderma refers to whiteness of the skin and may range from mild hypopigmentation to complete loss of pigment.

Localised hypopigmentation may occur in:

♣ **Primary Skin Disease**

Piebaldism (partial albinism) where a congenital white forelock occurs in association with symmetrical patches of depigmentation

Halo naevus where a hypopigmented halo surrounds a naevus (it is a common early sign of vitiligo)

Pityriasis verscicolor, leprosy

As a complication of lichen planus, lichen simplex, atopic dermatitis, discoid lupus erythematosus

♥ **Systemic Disease**

Systemic diseases that cause localised hypopigmentation are:

Vitiligo

Vitiligo refers to depigmented macules. They may occur in association with autoimmune diseases such as:

E&M thyrotoxicosis, hypothyroidism, Addison's disease, diabetes mellitus

HS pernicious anaemia

IS alopecia areata

RAG premature ovarian failure

KUS renal tubular acidosis

GIT primary biliary cirrhosis, autoimmune hepatitis

Other systemic diseases that may be associated with localised hypopigmentation are:

CNS ash leaf macules occur in tuberose sclerosis

RAG syphilis

Hyperpigmentation

Hyperpigmentation may be:

♦ Brown

♣ Grey

Brown

Due to increased melanin in epidermal cells

Grey

Due to increase melanin in the dermis

Hyperpigmentation of the skin may be:

- ♠ Diffuse
- ♦ Localised

Diffuse Hyperpigmentation

The causes of diffuse hyperpigmentation of the skin are:

- ♣ **External Causes**

  Sunburn

- ♥ **Primary Disease of the Skin**

  Scleroderma

- ♠ **Systemic Disease**

  Systemic diseases that manifest as diffuse hyperpigmentation of the skin are conditions affecting the

  E&M

  Endocrine: Addison's disease, Nelson's syndrome, Cushing's disease, ectopic ACTH secretion

  Metabolic: porphyria cutanea tarda, haemochromatosis, vitamin B_{12} deficiency, folate deficiency, pellagra, cachexia

  GIT primary biliary cirrhosis, malabsorption

  Toxins silver (argyria), arsenic

  Drugs amiodarone, phenothiazines, minocycline, busulphan

Localised Hyperpigmentation

Localised hyperpigmentation may be classified as conditions in which the:

- ♦ **Epidermis is Altered**

The epidermis is altered in:

Acanthosis nigricans, seborrheic keratosis, pigmented actinic keratosis

- ♣ **Proliferation of Melanocytes**

  Proliferation of melanocytes occurs in:

  Lentigo, naevus, melanoma

- ♥ **Increased Pigment Production**

  Increased pigment production occurs in:

  Freckles (ephelides), café au lait spots

Systemic Conditions associated with Localised Hyperpigmentation

Systemic conditions associated with localised hyperpigmentation are the following:

- ♠ Acanthosis nigricans is associated with metabolic disturbances, internal malignancy.

- ♦ Lentigo is associated with Peutz-Jeghers syndrome.

- ♣ The LEOPARD syndrome is Lentiginosis, ECG abnormalities, Ocular hypertelorism, Pulmonary stenosis, Abnormal genitalia, Retardation of growth, Deafness.

- ♥ Café au lait spots. The presence of more than 5 spots is associated with neurofibromatosis.

Yellow Discolouration

Yellow discolouration of the skin may be seen in:

- ♠ Jaundice
- ♦ Carotenaemia
- ♦ Lycopenaemia

115

Jaundice

Jaundice may be haemolytic, hepato-cellular or obstructive

Carotenaemia

Carotenaemia causes yellow pigmentation of the skin as a result of high carotene levels in the blood. The yellow pigmentation is enhanced by artificial light. It is increased in the palms, soles of the feet and the naso-labial folds as carotene is excreted by the sebaceous glands. The causes of carotenaemia are:

♥ Increased dietary consumption, hypothyroidism, diabetes mellitus, anorexia nervosa, liver disease, renal disease, familial

Lycopenaemia

Lycopenaemia causes an orange-yellow pigmentation of the skin. It is due to ingestion of large amounts of tomatoes, which contain lycopenes.

Purple Discolouration

A purplish (heliotrope) discoloration of the skin occurs in:

♣ Dermatomyositis.

Pallor

Pallor of the skin may be due to anaemia or vasoconstriction.

♥ Vasoconstriction may be gener-alised due to cardiovascular collapse or localised due to areas of diminished blood flow.

♠ Pallor, if caused by anaemia, indicates significant anaemia. It is more easily seen in the mucous membranes of the mouth and eyelids.

Flush

A flushed appearance may be due to:

♦ **Primary Skin Disease**

Vasodilatation in erythroderma

♣ **Systemic Disease**

Systemic diseases that result in flushing are those that affect the:

E&M fevers, carcinoid syndrome

RS carbon dioxide narcosis, carbon monoxide poisoning

HS polycythaemia rubra vera

Cyanosis

Cyanosis occurs if the concentration of reduced haemoglobin in the blood is more than 5 g/dl. Cyanosis may be peripheral or central in origin.

♥ **Peripheral Cyanosis**

Peripheral cyanosis may be due to:

Low cardiac output, peripheral vascular disease, cold weather, increased tissue oxygen extraction.

Localised cyanosis may be a feature of Raynaud's phenomenon

♠ **Central Cyanosis**

Central cyanosis may be due to conditions affecting the:

RS acute and chronic lung disease, pulmonary embolism, hypoventilation

HS polycythaemia (this may be cause or effect)

CVS right to left shunt

Methhaemoglobin

Methhaemoglobin occurs as a result of oxidation of haemoglobin. It is similar to cyanosis and causes a bluish or leaden appearance. Methaemoglobinaemia may be due to:

- Genetic causes
- Acquired causes

Genetic causes

Genetic causes of methaemoglobinaemia are:

- Defect in the red cell (NADH diaphorase deficiency)
- An abnormality in haemoglobin known as haemoglobin M of which there are many types

Acquired causes

Acquired causes of methaemoglobinaemia are:

- **Chemicals**: nitrites
- **Drugs**: primaquine, sulphonamides, phenacetin, dapsone

Sulphaemoglobinaemia

Sulphaemoglobinaemia is very rare. It is produced by the action of hydrogen sulphide on haemoglobin. It causes a similar appearance to methaemoglobinaemia. It may be caused by:

- **Drugs** sulphonylureas, phenacetin
- **GIT** it may also be seen in malabsorption and chronic constipation.

Muddy Discolouration

A muddy colour of the skin occurs in:

- Chronic renal failure.

Surface of the Skin

When assessing the surface of the skin, the commonest manifestation of a skin disorder that may be observed would be the presence of a rash. This will be dealt with in depth later. The other abnormalities that may occur on the surface are:

- Dry Skin
- Greasy Skin
- Increased Sweating (Hyperhidrosis)
- Lack of Sweating (Hypohidrosis)
- Striae or Stretch Marks
- Pitting
- Calcium Deposition

Dry Skin

Dry skin could be due to:

- **Primary Skin Conditions**

  Anhidrotic ectodermal dysplasia, a genetically determined condition in which ectodermal structures are not developed

  Xerosis, which is a dry, flaky condition of the skin that occurs in the elderly

- **Systemic Conditions**

  Systemic conditions that cause dry skin are those involving the:

  E&M hypothyroidism, vitamin A deficiency, zinc deficiency

  KUS chronic renal failure

117

GIT liver failure, malabsorption

RAG AIDS

Greasy Skin

Greasy skin may be due to:

♥ **Primary Skin Conditions**

Senile sebaceous hyperplasia

♠ **Systemic Conditions**

Systemic conditions that cause greasy skin are:

E&M acromegaly, Cushing's syndrome

CNS Parkinsonism

Increased Sweating (Hyperhidrosis)

The causes of increased sweating are:

♦ **Primary Skin Conditions**

Idiopathic hyperhidrosis. This can cause a problem to patients especially teenagers

♣ **Systemic Conditions**

Systemic conditions that cause increased sweating are those involving the:

E&M thyrotoxicosis, acromegaly, diabetes mellitus, hypoglycaemia, phaeochromocytoma, fevers

GIT nausea, gustatory sweating

Toxins alcoholic intoxication

HS lymphoma

CNS lesions of the sympathetic nervous system, cortical lesions, lesions of the basal ganglia and the spinal cord

Other causes like cancer should be considered.

Lack of Sweating (Hypohidrosis)

Hypohidrosis may be:

♦ Generalised

♣ Localised

Generalised Hypohidrosis

Generalised hypohidrosis could be due to:

♥ **Primary Skin Conditions**

Hypohidrotic ectodermal dysplasia, severe exfoliative dermatitis, erythroderma. Miliaria crystallina, a condition in which there is blockage of the sweat ducts resulting in clear vesicles

♣ **Systemic Conditions**

Systemic conditions that cause hypohidrosis are those affecting the:

E&M hypothyroidism

CNS chronic autonomic nervous system failure. This would result in sudomotor failure, which causes lack of sweating and heat intolerance

Ectodermal Dysplasia

Ectodermal dysplasias are congenital conditions in which abnormalities of the skin, hair, nails, teeth and sweat glands occur.

♠ **Hidrotic Ectodermal Dysplasia**

An autosomal dominant condition which is characterised by:

Nails: dystrophy with thick, short, slow-growing, discoloured nails

Hair: sparse, pale, fine and brittle (scalp, eyebrows, body)

Skin: palmoplantar keratoderma (variable)

♦ **Hypohidrotic Ectodermal Dysplasia**

This is an X-linked recessive form that has the following features:

Sweat: absent or reduced sweating

Teeth: abnormal teeth (conical)

Face: saddle nose, sunken cheeks

Hair: sparse, dry, fine

Localised Hypohidrosis

Localised hypohidrosis may be due to:

♥ Tuberculoid leprosy, syringomyelia, diabetes mellitus

Striae or Stretch Marks

Striae may occur in conditions involving the:

♠ **E&M** Cushing's syndrome, in obesity and following growth spurts in childhood and adolescence.

♦ **RAG** they are common in pregnancy

Pitting

Pitting may be seen in localised areas of oedema. This would result in an orange peel or *peau d'orange* appearance. It may be due to:

♣ **Local Factors**

Lymphatic obstruction, which is usually due to malignancies such as breast cancer or infestations such as filariasis

♥ **Systemic Factors**

Conditions affecting the:

E&M pretibial myxoedema in thyrotoxicosis

Calcium Deposition

Calcium deposition may be due to:

♠ **Primary Skin Conditions**

Scleroderma, dermatomyositis

♦ **Systemic Conditions**

Conditions affecting the:

E&M hypoparathyroidism (subcutaneous calcification)

Consistency of the Skin

Changes in the consistency of the skin could be:

♣ Lax Skin

119

- ♥ Taut Skin
- ♠ Thick Skin
- ♦ Thin Skin

Lax Skin

Lax skin may be due to:

- ♣ **Primary Skin Conditions**

  Age related laxity in the elderly, pseudoxanthoma elasticum, Ehlers-Danlos syndrome, cutis laxa

- ♥ **Systemic Conditions**

  Salt and water loss

Taut Skin

Taut skin occurs in:

- ♠ **Primary Skin Conditions**

  Scleroderma

- ♦ **Systemic Conditions**

  Conditions affecting the:

  E&M diabetic dermopathy

Thick Skin

Thick skin may be due to:

- ♣ **Primary Skin Conditions**

  Localised Scleroderma. In scleroderma localised induration with formation of poorly defined plaques may occur. This is known as morphoea. The lesion begins as a bluish-red plaque but later it becomes pale and may atrophy.

  Cutaneous amyloid

- ♥ **Local (External) Factors**

  Lymphatic obstruction due to filariasis, malignancy

- ♠ **Systemic Conditions**

  Conditions involving the:

E&M acromegaly, thyroid acropachy, myxoedema, diabetes mellitus

Thin Skin

Thin skin may be due to:

- ♦ **Primary Skin Conditions**

  Ageing, poikiloderma

- ♣ **Systemic Conditions**

  Conditions involving the:

  E&M Cushing's syndrome, diabetes mellitus

Skin Temperature

The temperature of the skin will reflect body temperature and changes in local blood flow. The changes that may occur are:

- ♥ Generalised Warm Skin
- ♠ Localised Warm Skin
- ♦ Generalised Cold Skin
- ♣ Localised Cold Skin

Generalised Warm Skin

Generalised warmth of the skin could occur in:

- ♥ **Primary Skin Conditions**

  Erythroderma

- ♠ **Systemic Conditions**

  Fever, thyrotoxicosis

Localised Warm Skin

Localised warmth of the skin could occur in:

- ♦ Erysipelas
- ♣ Cellulitis

Generalised Cold Skin

Generalised cold skin could occur in:

- ♥ Hypothermia
- ♠ Cardiovascular collapse

Localised Cold Skin

Localised cold skin would reflect diminished regional blood flow. This may occur as a consequence of:

- ♦ Peripheral vascular disease
- ♣ Raynaud's phenomenon

Tenderness

The presence of tenderness would indicate inflammation as in:

- ♥ Cellulitis

Mobility of the Skin

Changes in mobility could be:

- ♠ The skin would be taut and less mobile in systemic sclerosis.
- ♦ Reduced mobility may reflect an underlying infiltrating lesion.

Blood Vessels

Assessment of the blood vessels of the skin may show important changes. They are changes in:

- ♣ Structure
- ♥ Function

Structure

Structural changes are:

- ♣ Telangiectasia
- ♥ Haemangioma

Telangiectasia

Telangiectasia refers to permanently dilated, visible vessels in the dermis. They may be due to:

- ♠ **External Factors**

  Radiation dermatitis

- ♦ **Primary Skin Conditions**

  Rosacea, discoid lupus erythematosus, Fabry's disease

- ♣ **Systemic Conditions**

  Conditions involving the:

  CVS hereditary haemorrhagic telangiectasia

  GIT chronic liver disease

  RAG pregnancy

  E&M Cushing's syndrome, carcinoid syndrome, mastocytosis

  CNS ataxia telangiectasia

  LMS scleroderma, lupus erythematosus, dermatomyositis

Haemangioma

Cutaneous haemangioma may present as:

- ♥ **Port-Wine Stain** which occurs in the distribution of the trigeminal nerve in the Sturge-Weber syndrome
- ♠ **Campbell di Morgan spots** are small, bright-red angioma on the upper trunk. They are of no significance.

Function

Changes in function of the blood vessels are those affecting:

- ♦ Blood Flow
- ♣ Haemoglobin concentration

121

Blood Flow

In pathological states, blood flow in the cutaneous vessels may be altered. The changes that may result are as follows:

- ♥ Increased blood flow
- ♠ Decreased blood flow
- ♦ Livedo reticularis
- ♣ Delayed capillary refill time

Increased Blood Flow (Flushing)

Increased blood flow to the skin, which manifests as flushing and warmth of the skin, may be due to:

- ♥ **Primary Skin Conditions**

  Erythroderma, mastocytosis

  Localised increase in blood flow and warmth of the skin may occur in inflammation due to cellulitis or erysipelas.

- ♠ **Systemic Conditions**

  E&M Cushing's syndrome, phaeochromocytoma, carcinoid syndrome, fever

  RS carbon dioxide narcosis

  HS polycythaemia rubra vera

Decreased Blood Flow

Decreased blood flow may be:

- ♦ Localised
- ♣ Generalised

Localised Decrease in Blood flow

A localised decrease in blood flow, which manifests as pallor and cold skin with decreased capillary refill time, could occur in:

- ♦ **Primary Skin Conditions**

  Scleroderma

- ♣ **Systemic Conditions**

  CVS peripheral vascular disease, Raynaud's phenomenon

Generalised Decrease in Blood Flow

A generalised decrease in blood flow, which manifests as pallor and cold skin, would occur in states of:

- ♥ Cardiovascular collapse

Livedo Reticularis

Livedo reticularis refers to a reticular or chicken wire pattern of blood vessels caused by decreased blood flow resulting in deoxygenation of blood in the vessels. It may be due to:

- ♠ **External factors**

  Cold environment

- ♦ **Primary Skin Conditions**

  Cutis marmorata telangectatica. This occurs in infants

- ♣ **Systemic Conditions**

  Conditions affecting the:

  LMS polyarteritis nodosa, antiphospholipid syndrome

  HS cryoglobulinaemia, cryofibrinogenaemia, macroglobulinaemia, polycythaemia, sickle cell disease

  CVS emboli from subacute bacterial endocarditis, left atrial myxoma, atheromatous emboli

  E&M cholesterol emboli, blockage of vessels by oxalate or calcium

Capillary Refill Time

Capillary refill time would indicate adequacy of regional blood flow. It would be increased in:

- ♥ Peripheral vascular disease

♠ Raynaud's phenomenon

It would also be increased in:

♦ States of cardiovascular collapse

Quantity of Haemoglobin

A rough assessment may be made of the quantity of haemoglobin within the blood vessels

♦ **Pallor** would indicate anaemia

♣ **Suffusion** would indicate polycythaemia

Poikiloderma

Poikiloderma refers to a combination of mottled pigmentation, skin atrophy and telangiectasia. It may be due to:

♥ **External Factors**

Radiation damage, actinic damage

♠ **Primary Skin Conditions**

Genodermatoses (genetically determined skin disorders), discoid lupus erythematosus, dermatomyositis. Poikiloderma of Civatte is a common form of pigmentary disturbance seen on the neck of women.

♦ **Systemic Conditions**

HS graft versus host disease

Smell

The sense of smell is not used that often in clinical medicine but in certain conditions of the skin a characteristic odour may emanate. They are:

♣ Darier's disease

♥ Fish odour syndrome. This is an autosomal recessive condition.

The smell is the result of the inability of the body to break down trimethylamine a product that is formed in the intestine by bacterial action on substances such as choline. Trimethylamine is excreted in the sweat, urine and breath.

Hair

The characteristics of hair will depend on the site considered that is, scalp or body. One should consider changes in:

♣ Quantity

♥ Shape

♠ Colour

♦ Surface

♣ Consistency

♥ Connections

Quantity (Size)

The quantity of hair present depends on a variety of factors. They are genetic and racial factors, the state of nutrition and the presence of local or systemic disease. The variations that may occur are the following:

♣ Loss of Hair (Alopecia)

♥ Male Pattern Balding

♠ Feminisation

♦ Localised Loss of Hair

♣ Hypertrichosis

♥ Lanugo Hair

♠ Hirsutism

Loss of Hair (Alopecia)

Alopecia may be due to:

- **Primary Skin Conditions**

  Alopecia areata (refers to a patchy loss of scalp hair), alopecia totalis (refers to loss of hair over the entire scalp), alopecia universalis (refers to loss of hair over the whole body), tinea capitis, scleroderma, lichen planus

- **External Factors**

  Trauma, trichotillomania

- **Systemic Conditions**

  Those affecting the:

  E&M hypothyroidism, hyperthyroidism, deficiency of iron, biotin, zinc

  RAG secondary syphilis, HIV infection, telogen effluvium following pregnancy

  LMS lupus erythematosus

  RS sarcoidosis

  Telogen effluvium, which occurs after any severe illness, is a transient increase in the number of hairs in the resting phase of the growth cycle

  Anagen effluvium refers to the hair loss that occurs after cancer chemotherapy, radiotherapy to the scalp and following administration of drugs such as colchicine

Male Pattern Balding

The male pattern of balding in a female would suggest:

- Hyperandrogenisation

Feminisation

Feminisation is characterised by loss of body hair and decreased facial hair in a male and occurs in:

- Hypopituitarism
- Hypogonadism

Localised Loss of Hair

Localised loss of hair would be seen as a result of:

- Decreased blood flow in peripheral vascular disease

Hypertrichosis

Hypertrichosis refers to excess body hair in a distribution that is not influenced by the sex hormones. It may be due to:

- **External Factors**

  Plaster casts, chronic irritation

- **Primary Skin Conditions**

  Becker naevus

- **Systemic Conditions**

  E&M porphyria, mucopolysaccharidoses

  CNS spina bifida

  Drugs cyclosporin, minoxidil

  Neoplasia it could be due to an underlying neoplasm

Lanugo Hair

In adults, lanugo hair occurs in:

- Anorexia nervosa

Hirsutism

Hirsutism refers to the male pattern of body and facial hair distribution with associated baldness. It would be obvious in females and in pre-pubertal children. The causes are:

- **Primary Skin Conditions**

  Familial or a racial tendency

♦ **Systemic Conditions**

RAG virilising syndromes such as polycystic ovarian syndrome, arrhenoblastoma

E&M

Adrenal lesions: adrenal tumours, Cushing's syndrome, congenital adrenal hyperplasia

Pituitary disorders: acromegaly, prolactinoma

Drugs androgens, anabolic steroids

Shape

The shape of the hair depends on ethnic origin and genetics. Variations that may occur in disease are:

♣ Corkscrew hair in vitamin C deficiency

Colour

The colour of the hair depends on ethnic origin and genetic make up.

Decreased Colour of Hair

Decreased colour of the hair may be due to:

♥ **External Factors**

Bleaching or dyeing

♠ **Primary Disease of Hair**

Poliosis is a localised area of white hair that may occur as part of Waardenburg's syndrome (heterochromia iridis, confluent eyebrows and deafness)

Piebaldism, over areas of vitiligo, after regrowth of alopecia areata

♦ **Systemic Conditions**

GIT malnutrition

Drugs chloroquine, mephenesin

Surface of Hair

The surface of the hair is usually smooth due to the presence of sebum.

♣ Reduced production of sebum results in a lack of lustre. This occurs in endocrine disease and malnutrition.

♥ Parasites such as head and pubic lice may be seen on the surface in infestations.

Consistency of Hair

The consistency of the hair may change and hair could be brittle in:

♠ Malnutrition

Connections

The connections of the hair may become loose and hair may be easily plucked out in:

♦ Malnutrition

Nails

When examining the nails one may detect abnormalities in relation to the following:

♣ Dimensions

♥ Colour

♠ Surface

♦ Consistency

♣ Connections

♥ Circulation

125

Dimensions

On examination of the dimensions of the nails one may note abnormalities of:

- ♣ Size
- ♥ Shape
- ♠ Margins

Size

Variations in the size of the nails could be:

- ♣ Small Nails
- ♥ Absent Nails
- ♠ Brachyonychia (Short Nails)
- ♦ Dolichonychia (Long nails)

Small Nails

Small nails may be seen in the:

- ♣ Nail patella syndrome where deformed small nails and absence of the patella occurs

Absent Nails

Loss of nails may be due to:

- ♥ **External Factors**

   Trauma, nail bed infections
- ♠ **Primary Skin Disease**

   Lichen planus, Stevens-Johnson syndrome
- ♦ **Systemic Disease**

   HS chronic graft versus host disease, amyloidosis

Brachyonychia (Short Nails)

Brachyonychia refers to a condition where the width of the nail is greater than its length. It may be seen where

resorption of the terminal phalanx occurs. The causes are:

- ♣ Hyperparathyroidism
- ♥ Psoriatic arthropathy

Dolichonychia (Long nails)

Dolichonychia or long nails occurs in conditions affecting the:

- ♠ **LMS** Marfan's syndrome
- ♦ **IS** Ehlers-Danlos syndrome
- ♣ **E&M** hypopituitarism
- ♥ **RAG** eunuchs

Shape of the Nails

The shape of the nails is extremely important as it gives clues to systemic disease. The variations that may occur are:

- ♠ Clubbing
- ♦ Pseudoclubbing
- ♣ Koilonychia

Clubbing

Clubbing is caused by soft tissue deposition resulting in elevation of the nail base. It results in the following characteristic features:

- ♣ A change in the angle between the nail and the nail fold, Lovibond's angle. This is normally less than 180 degrees. In clubbing, initially, this angle is lost and it becomes a straight line. When clubbing is more severe the angle becomes greater than 180 degrees.
- ♥ The nail bed becomes ballotable. If the nail fold is palpated with two digits the base of the nail is ballotable.

♠ Distal phalangeal depth becomes greater than interphalangeal depth. The depth of the finger at the level of the nail fold becomes greater than the depth at the distal interphalangeal joint.

♦ Schamroth's sign. If the terminal phalanges of opposite fingers are held together with their nails touching each other, a diamond shaped space is apparent between them. Loss of this space is indicative of clubbing.

Five Stages of Clubbing

Five stages of clubbing are described. They are:

1. Increased nail bed fluctuation

2. Loss of the nail bed angle

3. Increased curvature of the long axis of the nail

4. Soft tissue swelling of the ends of the fingers giving a drum stick appearance

5. Hypertrophic pulmonary osteoarthropathy

Causes of Clubbing

Clubbing may be due to:

♣ **Primary Nail Disorders**

Congenital clubbing

♥ **Systemic Conditions**

CVS brachial arterio-venous fistula, which causes unilateral clubbing. Clubbing also occurs in subacute infective endocarditis, left atrial myxoma.

RS lung abscess, bronchial carcinoma, bronchiectasis, pulmonary fibrosis, fibrosing alveolitis, asbestosis, mesothelioma, empyema

GIT cirrhosis of the liver, Crohn's disease, coeliac disease

E&M thyrotoxicosis

HS dysproteinaemia (especially light chain disease)

KUS pyelonephritis

RAG syphilis, pregnancy

Pseudoclubbing

Pseudoclubbing occurs due to resorption of the terminal phalanges causing the nail to slope towards the palmar aspect resulting in an appearance that may be mistaken for clubbing. Pseudoclubbing is seen in:

♥ Hyperparathyroidism

Koilonychia

Koilonychia refers to flat or spoon shaped nails. It is seen in:

♠ Iron deficiency anaemia

Margins of the Nail

The margins may become irregular and frayed or even torn in conditions in which the nails become brittle.

Colour of the Nails

The changes that may occur in the colour of the nails are:

♦ White Colour

♣ Yellow Nails

♥ Blue Nails

♠ Red Colour

♦ Localised Pigmentation

White Colour

White discolouration of the nails could present as:

* ♣ **White Nails (leuconychia)** are seen in liver disease

* ♥ **Muehrcke's Lines** refer to two white lines parallel to the nail fold. This indicates hypoalbuminaemia.

* ♠ **Mee's Lines** are multiple white lines parallel to the nail fold. This is seen in chemotherapy for cancer, cardiac or renal failure, Hodgkin's disease. It is also seen in poisoning by arsenic and thallium.

Yellow Nails

Yellow discolouration of the nails occurs in:

* ♦ Yellow nails syndrome. Here the presence of yellow nails is associated with lymphoedema of the lower limbs and sterile pleural effusions.

Blue Nails

Blue discolouration would be seen in the following conditions:

* ♣ Blue lunulae are seen in Wilson's disease

* ♥ Blue nails are seen in argyria, which is caused by deposition of silver absorbed as a result of industrial skin contact or ingestion.

Red Colour

Red discolouration of the nails would occur in the following conditions:

* ♠ **Lindsay's Nails** are nails in which the proximal half of the nail is white and the distal half brown or pink or red. This is seen in chronic renal failure

* ♦ **Terry's Nails** are nails in which the proximal part of the nail is white with a peripheral red rim. This is seen in cirrhosis of the liver, type 2 diabetes mellitus, heart failure.

* ♣ **Red Lunulae** are seen in heart failure

Localised Pigmentation

Localised pigmentation may be due to a:

* ♥ Subungual melanoma

Surface of the Nails

Changes that may occur on the surface of the nails are:

* ♠ **Pitting** of the surface is seen in psoriasis, alopecia areata

* ♦ **Grooves** in the nail, parallel to the nail fold, occur in any severe illness that results in temporary restriction of growth of the nail. These are called Beau's lines.

* ♣ **Ridging**: longitudinal ridging of the nails occurs in lichen planus

Consistency of the Nails

Variations in the consistency of the nails are:

* ♥ **Brittle Nails** may occur due to dystrophy of the nails and this is a feature of thyrotoxicosis, malnutrition, iron deficiency, calcium deficiency

- ♠ **Onychomycosis** refers to dystrophy and destruction of the nails due to fungal infection
- ♦ **Onychogryphosis** refers to hypertrophy and thickening of the nail. It is often due to trauma but may be a consequence of ischaemia or neglect.

Connections of the Nails

The connection of the nail to the nail bed may be lost in:

- ♣ **Onycholysis**. In onycholysis the attachment of the nail to the underlying nail bed is lost. This results in a nail that is lifted off its base. Onycholysis is seen in thyrotoxicosis, psoriasis, fungal infections

Blood Vessels of the Nails

Abnormalities that may be observed in the blood vessels of the nail bed are:

- ♥ **Splinter Haemorrhages** are small, linear, subungual haemorrhages. They are an important sign in bacterial endocarditis. They may also occur as a result of trauma.
- ♠ **Pulsations** of the blood vessels in the nail base may be observed in severe aortic regurgitation. This is known as Quincke's sign.

Nail Fold and Cuticle

When examining the nail fold and cuticle one may note abnormalities of:

- ♦ Site
- ♣ Size
- ♥ Shape
- ♠ Margins
- ♦ Colour
- ♣ Surface
- ♥ Consistency
- ♠ Temperature
- ♦ Tenderness
- ♣ Connection
- ♥ Blood vessels

Site

The site of attachment of the cuticle may be abnormal.

- ♦ The cuticle may be pushed back in paronychia. This may be either cause or effect.

Size

The size of the nail fold and cuticle would be:

- ♣ Decreased in chronic paronychia.
- ♥ In acute paronychia the nail fold would be swollen.

Shape

The shape of the cuticle would be:

- ♠ Lost in both acute and chronic paronychia

Margins

The margins of the nail fold and cuticle would be:

- ♦ Irregular in paronychia.
- ♣ The margins would be ragged in dermatomyositis

Colour

The colour of the nail fold would change and the area would be:

- ♥ Reddened in acute paronychia
- ♠ A reddish or purplish discolouration occurs in dermatomyositis

Surface

The surface of the nail fold may be abnormal and one may observe:

- ♦ Nodules around the nails, periungual fibroma, in tuberose sclerosis.
- ♣ The surface would be irregular in inflammation (acute or chronic paronychia)

Consistency

The consistency may change and there may be:

- ♥ A boggy feel in inflammation

Temperature

The temperature may change and the nail fold may be:

- ♠ Warm in acute paronychia

Tenderness

The nail fold would be tender in:

- ♦ Acute paronychia

Connections

Attachments of the cuticle may be lost in:

- ♣ Chronic paronychia

Blood Vessels

Abnormalities that may occur in the blood vessels of the nail fold are:

- ♥ **Telangiectases** may be seen in scleroderma, systemic lupus erythematosus, dermatomyositis
- ♠ **Haemorrhages** may occur in dermatomyositis

Chronic Paronychia

Chronic paronychia occurs in:

- ♦ Hypoparathyroidism
- ♣ Multiple endocrine deficiencies
- ♥ Chronic iron deficiency

Rashes

Next, a more detailed analysis of rashes will be undertaken. The analysis will be of the:

- ♠ Types of rashes
- ♦ Arrangement of rashes
- ♣ Distribution of rashes

Types of Rashes

The types of rashes that will be analysed are the following:

Flat (non-palpable) Lesions

Macules

Macules may be:

- ♥ **Pigmented Macules** the causes of pigmented macules have been dealt with earlier.
- ♠ **Depigmented Macules** the causes of depigmented macules have been dealt with earlier.

- **Erythematous Macules** occur in drug reactions, viral infections such as measles, rubella and infectious mononucleosis. Usually these lesions are maculopapular rather than solely macular.

- **Purple Macules** could be port wine stains or Kaposi's sarcoma

- **Reddish-Brown Macules** are seen in urticaria pigmentosa (cutaneous mastocytosis). The lesions become itchy and urticated if they are rubbed. This is known as Darier's sign.

  In systemic mastocytosis bones may be involved and hepatosplenomegaly can occur.

Haemorrhages into the Skin

Haemorrhages into the skin are characterised by the fact that they do not blanch on pressure. They may be classified according to size as:

- Petechiae
- Purpura
- Ecchymoses

Petechiae

Petechiae are small macules less than 3 mm in size. They occur in:

- Thrombocytopaenia
- Thrombasthenia

Purpura

Purpura are larger than petechiae. The causes of purpura are as follows:

- Vasculitis. This results in palpable purpura. This may be caused by conditions affecting the:

LMS rheumatoid arthritis, systemic lupus erythematosus

IS Henoch-Schonlein purpura

RS Churg-Strauss syndrome, Wegener's granulomatosis

GIT hepatitis B and C

Drugs penicillin, sulphonamides

CVS subacute bacterial endocarditis, polyarteritis nodosa

Other causes of purpura are:

- Viral haemorrhagic fevers
- Meningococcal septicaemia
- Amyloidosis which causes periorbital purpura

Ecchymoses

Ecchymoses are larger lesions. They may be due to:

- **Primary Skin Conditions**

  Age related fragility of the skin and blood vessels, hyperelasticity of the skin as in Ehlers-Danlos syndrome. In Ehlers-Danlos syndrome when the haematomas heal they may form nodules or pseudotumours.

- **Systemic Conditions**

  E&M scurvy, Cushing's syndrome

  Drugs warfarin

  HS haemophilia, Christmas disease

Raised (Palpable) Lesions

Raised palpable lesions may be:

- Solid lesions
- Fluid filled lesions

131

Raised Solid Lesions

Raised solid lesions could be:

- ♠ Papules
- ♦ Milia
- ♣ Comedones
- ♥ Plaques
- ♠ Nodules
- ♦ Weals
- ♣ Burrows

Papules

Papules are elevated solid lesions less than 0.5 cms in diameter. They could be:

- ♦ **Flesh Coloured Papules**: neurofibromata, adenoma sebaceum
- ♣ **Erythematous Papules**: drug reactions, viral infections
- ♥ **Red Papules**: angioma
- ♠ **White Papules**: calcinosis, molluscum contagiosum
- ♦ **Yellow Papules**: xanthoma, sebaceous hyperplasia
- ♣ **Translucent Papules**: basal cell carcinoma
- ♥ **Purple Papules**: Kaposi's sarcoma
- ♠ **Haemorrhagic Papules**: vasculitis
- ♦ **Brown Papules**: naevus, malignant melanoma
- ♣ **Reddish-Brown Papules**: urticaria pigmentosa
- ♥ **Violaceous Papules**: lichen planus, lupus pernio

Urticaria Pigmentosa

Urticaria pigmentosa is caused by nests of mast cells in the skin. They present as reddish-brown, pigmented macules and papules. If they are rubbed they become red, itchy and urticated (Darier's sign). Rarely there may be systemic involvement with infiltration of the liver, spleen and bone marrow. A leukaemic variety is recognised.

Plaques

Plaques may be:

- ♠ **Inflammatory Plaques**: eczema, psoriasis, lichen planus, discoid lupus erythematosus, granuloma annulare, morphoea

Lichen planus has a violaceous appearance and demonstrates Wickham's striae, which are fine white streaks on the surface. The Koebner phenomenon may be observed, that is, lesions appearing in a linear arrangement along a scratch mark

- ♦ **Neoplastic Plaques**: mycosis fungoides, Bowen's disease, Paget's disease, Kaposi's sarcoma
- ♣ **Degenerative**: lichen sclerosis et atrophicus
- ♥ **Metabolic**: xanthelasma
- ♠ **Traumatic**: lichen simplex chronicus (neurodermatitis)

Nodules

Nodules are elevated solid lesions greater than 0.5 cms in diameter.

They may be due to:

♦ **Primary Skin Conditions**

Neurofibromatosis, lipoma, mycosis fungoides, healed haematomas in Ehlers-Danlos syndrome, malignant melanoma

♣ **Systemic Conditions**

Erythema nodosum, rheumatoid nodules, metastatic cancer

Weals

Weals occur in urticaria, which may be due to:

♥ **External Factors**

Cold, sunlight, heat, insect bites

♠ **Primary Skin Conditions**

Cholinergic urticaria where heat, exercise or anger causes urticaria

Dermographism where immediate pressure causes urticaria

♦ **Systemic Conditions**

HS

Serum sickness, which is a delayed reaction to blood products

Urticaria pigmentosa where mast cell hyperplasia occurs in the skin

LMS lupus erythematosus

Drugs may cause weals by non-allergic mechanisms. Examples are salicylates, codeine, morphine, ACE inhibitors and antibiotics such as ciprofloxacin, vancomycin, rifampicin.

Allergies to food, drugs, radiological contrast media, insect bites, helminths

Angioedema

Angioedema affects the subcutaneous tissues and is less well demarcated than weals. It is not itchy. An inherited form occurs due to C_1 esterase inhibitor deficiency.

Burrows

Burrows occur in:

♥ Scabies, which is caused by the mite *Sarcoptes scabiei*

♠ Cutaneous larva migrans (cutaneous lesions caused by migrating helminth larvae, more commonly animal helminths)

Raised Fluid Filled Lesions

Raised fluid filled lesions could be:

♥ Vesicles

♠ Bullae

♦ Whiteheads

♣ Pustules

♥ Target lesions

♠ Cysts

Vesicles

Vesicles are fluid filled lesions less than 5 mm in diameter formed by accumulation of fluid in the skin and associated with disintegration of cells in the affected area. They occur in:

♦ Herpes simplex

♣ Herpes zoster

133

♥ Dermatitis herpetiformis

Bullae

Bullae are fluid filled lesions more than 0.5 cms in diameter. Bullae occur in the following conditions:

♠ Pemphigus vulgaris

♦ Pemphigoid

♣ Epidermolysis bullosa

♥ Bullous impetigo

♠ Porphyria cutanea tarda

♦ Benign familial pemphigus or Hailey Hailey disease

♣ Dermatitis herpetiformis

Pemphigus vulgaris

Pemphigus vulgaris results in thin-roofed blisters, which rupture easily leaving a red area that exudes. Blisters commonly occur in the mouth but they could be missed as they rupture easily leaving erosions. In the skin Nikolsky's sign may be demonstrated.

Pemphigus vulgaris is an autoimmune disease. It may be associated with the use of penicillamine, captopril and rifampicin.

Pemphigus vegetans

Pemphigus vegetans refers to hypertrophy of the repairing epidermis and granulomatous change in the dermis resulting in vegetations.

Pemphigus foliaceous

Pemphigus foliaceous refers to a more benign condition in which the blisters are more superficial. The face and upper trunk are most commonly affected. Oral lesions are not common and it is associated with systemic lupus erythematosus and myasthenia gravis.

Pemphigoid

Pemphigoid results in tense blisters with erythematous patches around and separate from them.

Epidermolysis Bullosa

Epidermolysis bullosa may be:

♥ Congenital

♠ Acquired.

The acquired type of epidermolysis bullosa is associated with inflammatory bowel disease, internal malignancy and amyloidosis.

Bullous Impetigo

Impetigo is a highly infectious skin disease that is most common in children. The commonest causative organism is *Staphylococcus aureus* although group A *Streptococcus* may also be responsible. It is spread by direct contact.

Porphyria Cutanea Tarda

Porphyria cutanea tarda has a genetic predisposition and presents with a bullous eruption on exposure to sunlight. The aetiological agents are alcohol, hepatitis C, iron overload, HIV.

Benign Familial Pemphigus (Hailey-Hailey disease)

Hailey-Hailey disease is inherited as an autosomal dominant trait and results in blistering and erosions at the flexures

Dermatitis Herpetiformis

Dermatitis herpetiformis is a blistering disorder that is associated with gluten-sensitive enteropathy. It presents with small, itchy blisters that are most common over the extensor surfaces of the elbows, forearms, buttocks and scalp. The blisters are usually scratched off and presentation is with crusted lesions.

Pustules

Pustules occur in:

- ♦ Varicella
- ♣ Folliculitis
- ♥ Impetigo
- ♠ Acne
- ♦ Pustular psoriasis

Target Lesions

Target lesions consist of three concentric zones of skin change. They are a central dark area or blister surrounded by a pale, oedematous zone, which is in turn surrounded by an area of erythema. They occur in erythema multiforme.

Erythema Multiforme

The causes of erythema multiforme are conditions affecting the:

- ♣ **HS** multiple myeloma, lymphoma
- ♥ **LMS** systemic lupus erythematosus, dermatomyositis, polyarteritis nodosa, rheumatoid arthritis
- ♠ **GIT** ulcerative colitis
- ♦ **Drugs** sulphonamides, salicylates, penicillin, barbiturates, antimalarials
- ♣ **Infections** streptococci, mycoplasma, herpes simplex, AIDS

- ♥ **Malignancy**
- ♠ **Idiopathic**

Stevens-Johnson Syndrome

Stevens-Johnson syndrome refers to erythema multiforme with severe blistering and mucosal lesions.

Cysts

Cysts are seen in:

- ♦ Acne
- ♣ Sebaceous cysts

Depressed Lesions

Depressed lesions could be:

- ♦ Erosions
- ♣ Ulcers
- ♥ Fissures
- ♠ Atrophy

Erosions

Erosions refer to superficial skin loss limited to the epidermis. Erosions occur in:

- ♥ Pemphigus
- ♠ Pemphigoid
- ♦ Stevens-Johnson syndrome

Ulcer

An ulcer refers to loss of the epidermis and the whole or part of the dermis. Ulcers may be due to:

- ♣ **Primary Skin Disease**

  Ulcers may be due to primary skin disease caused by:

  Infections such as syphilis, tuberculosis, other bacteria, malignant ulcers

♥ Systemic Conditions

Systemic conditions that result in ulcers are those affecting the:

GIT pyoderma gangrenosum

LMS pyoderma gangrenosum

CVS vascular ulcers due to venous congestion, peripheral vascular disease, vasculitis

CNS neuropathic ulcers

HS sickle cell anaemia, cryoglobulinaemia

E&M diabetes mellitus

Fissure

A fissure refers to a deep, narrow, crack in the skin. Fissures occur in:

- ♠ Chronic eczema
- ♦ Intertrigo
- ♣ Psoriasis (occasionally)

Atrophy

Atrophy of the skin may be:

- ♥ Post-inflammatory atrophy
- ♠ Due to necrobiosis lipoidica

Secondary Lesions

Secondary lesions are the following:

- ♦ Scales
- ♣ Crusts
- ♥ Excoriations
- ♠ Lichenification
- ♦ Dyschromia
- ♣ Scars

Scales

Scales are dry plates of desquamated cells. They may be:

- ♥ Psoriasiform
- ♠ Icthyotic
- ♦ Localised Fine Scales
- ♣ Generalised Fine Scales
- ♥ Greasy Adherent Scales

Psoriasiform (Thick silvery scales)

Thick silvery scales occur in:

- ♠ Psoriasis
- ♦ Secondary syphilis
- ♣ Lupus erythematosus

Icthyotic (Fish scale appearance)

Icthyosis or a fish scale appearance may be:

- ♥ Inherited
- ♠ Acquired

Inherited Icthyosis

Inherited icthyosis may be:

- ♦ Icthyosis vulgaris (autosomal dominant)
- ♣ X-linked recessive icthyosis
- ♥ Rare forms such as: epidermolytic hyperkeratosis (autosomal dominant), icthyosis bullosa of Siemans, Netherton's syndrome, Sjorgen-Larsson syndrome
- ♠ Refsum's disease (autosomal recessive) in which there are associated neurological lesions

Acquired Icthyosis

Acquired icthyosis occurs in conditions affecting the:

- ♦ **E&M** malnutrition
- ♠ **HS** lymphoma, multiple myeloma
- ♥ **RAG** breast cancer

Localised Fine Scales (Pityriasiform scales)

Localised fine scales may be due to:

- ♠ Xerosis or dry skin
- ♦ Atopic eczema
- ♣ Pityriasis rosea
- ♥ Pityriasis verscicolor
- ♠ Fungal infections

Generalised Fine Scales

Generalised fine scales are seen in:

- ♦ Exfoliative dermatitis

Greasy Adherent Scales

Greasy adherent scales occur in:

- ♣ Seborrheic dermatitis
- ♥ Darier's disease which is an autosomal dominant disease in which there are brown papules covered with scales

Crusts

Crusts refer to dried exudate. The antecedent lesions may be:

- ♠ Bullae
- ♦ Vesicles
- ♣ Pustules
- ♥ Eczema
- ♠ Pyogenic granuloma
- ♦ Bowen's disease
- ♣ Squamous cell carcinoma

Excoriations

Excoriations refer to skin damage caused by scratching. They occur in:

- ♥ Eczema
- ♠ Fungal infections

- ♦ Dermatitis herpetiformis
- ♣ Lichen planus
- ♥ Any cause of generalised pruritus.

Lichenification

Lichenification refers to thickening of the skin. This may occur in:

- ♠ Acanthosis nigricans
- ♦ Lichen planus
- ♣ Lichen simplex

Dyschromia

Dyschromia or discolouration of the skin is usually post-inflammatory, it may occur in:

- ♥ Lichen planus
- ♠ Fixed drug eruptions
- ♦ Atopic eczema

Scars

Scarring occurs as a result of dermal damage.

- ♣ **Hypertrophic Scars**

    Hypertrophic scars occur in keloid

- ♥ **Tissue Paper Scars**

    Tissue paper scars occur in Ehlers-Danlos syndrome

Dermatitis (Eczema)

Dermatitis refers to an inflammatory reaction of the skin to endogenous or exogenous factors. The clinical features of these conditions are caused by dermal and epidermal components, which give rise to a heterogeneous pattern of involvement. The result is a mixture

137

of papules, vesicles, excoriations, weeping, crusts, scales, lichenification and dyschromia.

Dermatitis could be:

♠ Exogenous Dermatitis

♦ Endogenous Dermatitis

Exogenous Dermatitis

Exogenous dermatitis refers to an inflammatory response of the skin to exogenous factors. The types of exogenous dermatitis are:

♣ Irritant contact dermatitis

♥ Allergic contact dermatitis

♠ Phototoxic dermatitis

♦ Photoallergic dermatitis

Irritant Contact Dermatitis

Irritant contact dermatitis is caused by regular exposure to the causative agent with resultant wear and tear.

Allergic Contact Dermatitis

Allergic contact dermatitis is caused by an immune reaction.

Phototoxic Dermatitis

Phototoxic dermatitis refers to dermatitis due to the direct toxic effect of sunlight

Photoallergic Dermatitis

Photoallergic dermatitis refers to dermatitis caused by the effect of sunlight following prior sensitisation with agents, which are commonly drugs, certain plants

Irritants and Sensitisers

The irritants and sensitisers that could cause dermatitis are cosmetics, clothing, textiles, food, plastics, rubber, resins, plants, wood, medications, metals, employment as in hairdressing, baking, builders and agriculture

Endogenous Dermatitis

Endogenous dermatitis may be of the following types:

♣ Atopic eczema

♥ Nummular eczema

♠ Asteatotic eczema

♦ Hand/Foot Eczema

♣ Seborrheic Dermatitis

♥ Pityriasis alba

♠ Venous Eczema

Atopic Eczema

Atopic eczema is caused by a defect in immunity. It results in a heterogenous pattern of involvement as described earlier.

Nummular Eczema

Nummular eczema causes discoid lesions, which are vesicular and itchy

Asteatotic Eczema

Asteatotic eczema is caused by drying of the skin. It is common in the elderly and in malnutrition.

Hand/Foot Eczema

Hand/Foot eczema refers to eczema confined to the hands and feet. It may present as vesicles (pompholyx), diffuse erythematous scaling and peeling or scaling and peeling at the fingertips.

Seborrheic Dermatitis

Seborrheic dermatitis affects the areas of sebaceous activity. It is common in Parkinsonism and AIDS

Pityriasis Alba

Pityriasis alba is seen in children. It is a low-grade, dry eczema with loss of pigment.

Venous Eczema (gravitational eczema, varicose eczema)

Venous eczema occurs in the lower legs and is due to chronic venous hypertension.

Arrangement of Rashes

Skin lesions may be arranged in:

♠ Clusters

Or the arrangement may be:

♦ Linear

♣ Annular

♥ Reticular

♠ Gyrate

Clusters

Clusters are seen in:

♥ Dermatitis herpetiformis

♠ Herpes simplex

Linear

A linear arrangement may be due to lesions arising in relation to:

♥ Blood Vessels

♠ Lymphatics

♦ Nerves

♣ Developmental Lines

Blood Vessels

Lesions that arise in relation to blood vessels are:

♥ Thrombophlebitis, temporal arteritis

Lymphatics

Lesions that arise in relation to lymphatics are:

♠ Lymphangitis, fish tank granuloma, sporotrichosis

Nerves

Lesions that arise in relation to nerves are conditions such as:

♦ Leprosy

Developmental Lines

Lesions that arise in relation to developmental lines are:

♣ Linear lichen planus, linear psoriasis, lichen striatus

Koebner phenomenon

The Koebner phenomenon refers to new lesions developing in areas of trauma and irritation. It occurs in:

♥ Psoriasis

♠ Lichen planus

♦ Lichen nitidus

♣ Vitiligo

Annular

An annular arrangement results from spreading infiltration or a healing centre. Examples are:

- ♥ Impetigo
- ♠ Dermatophytosis
- ♦ Lupus vulgaris
- ♣ Granuloma annulare

Reticular

A reticular arrangement of skin lesions is seen in:

- ♥ Erythema ab igne
- ♠ Livedo reticularis

Gyrate

A gyrate arrangement is seen in:

- ♣ Erythema gyratum repens. This presents as repeated concentric rings of erythema with desquamation. The rings are irregular and wavy and are most common on the neck, trunk and extremities. It is associated with internal malignancy.

Distribution of Rashes

The distribution of a rash may be:

- ♥ Generalised
- ♠ Localised

Generalised Rashes

Generalised rashes occur in:

- ♦ Chicken pox
- ♣ Measles
- ♥ Exfoliative dermatitis
- ♠ Erythroderma

- ♦ Stevens-Johnson syndrome

- ♣ In exfoliative dermatitis the entire skin is reddened and scaly.
- ♥ In erythroderma the entire skin is red but not scaly.

Localised Rashes

Rashes may be localised to the:

- ♠ Extensor Aspects
- ♦ Creases
- ♣ Dermatomes
- ♥ Sunlight Exposed Areas
- ♠ Areas of Contact
- ♦ Dependent Areas (Gravitational)
- ♣ Symmetrical Sites
- ♥ Asymmetrical Sites
- ♠ Accessible Areas

Extensor Aspects

Rashes distributed over the extensor aspects occur in:

- ♦ Psoriasis
- ♣ Henoch-Schonlein purpura (limbs and buttocks)
- ♥ Dermatitis herpetiformis

Creases

Rashes in the skin creases are seen in:

- ♠ Scabies

Dermatomes

Rashes localised to the dermatomes occur in:

- ♦ Herpes zoster

Sunlight Exposed Areas

Rashes in areas of sunlight exposure occur in:

♣ Photosensitivity

Areas of Contact

Rashes in areas of contact with extraneous substances occur in:

♥ Contact dermatitis

Dependent Areas

Rashes in dependent areas are due to:

♦ Venous stasis

Symmetrical

Symmetrical rashes occur in:

♣ Endogenous causes of rashes; psoriasis, atopic eczema, viral exanthema, vitiligo

Asymmetrical

Asymmetrical rashes occur in:

♥ Exogenous causes such as infection

Accessible Areas

A rash in accessible areas may be due to:

♦ Dermatitis artefeacta. This refers to self-induced injury to the skin. It may take many forms but is restricted to accessible areas of the skin.

A discussion of the findings that may be obtained on general and regional examination follows:

General Examination

On general examination one may detect abnormalities of the following:

Dimensions

Weight

The state of nutrition would be important.

♣ **Decreased Weight**

Malnutrition would give rise to changes in the integument due to protein calorie deficiency and vitamin deficiency.

♦ **Increased Weight**

Obesity may be associated with hormonal imbalances and changes in lipid and carbohydrate metabolism that may result in changes in the integument.

Regional Examination

On regional examination one may detect abnormalities of the following:

Head

Dimensions

Changes that one may note in the dimensions of the head are:

♣ The head may appear fuller and more rounded in hypothyroidism and in Cushing's syndrome.

♥ The head may appear larger and the features would be more prominent in acromegaly.

Nose

On examination of the nose one may note abnormalities of:

- ♠ Size
- ♦ Shape
- ♣ Surface
- ♥ Smell

Size

The size of the nose may be:

- ♣ Enlarged in acromegaly, rhinophyma
- ♥ The nose may appear smaller in scleroderma

Shape

The shape of the nose may differ from normal. The abnormal shapes may be:

- ♠ A flat nasal bridge occurs in Ehlers-Danlos syndrome
- ♦ A beak like nose occurs in scleroderma
- ♣ Destruction of cartilage may occur in secondary syphilis, Wegener's granulomatosis, lupus vulgaris, relapsing polychondritis.
- ♥ A leonine facies occurs in leprosy. This due to thickening of the skin over the nose.
- ♠ A bulbous nose is seen in rhinophyma

Surface of the Nose

Rash

A rash may occur over the nose in:

- ♦ Lupus pernio which causes a bluish-red infiltrate
- ♣ Rosacea
- ♥ Lupus erythematosus

Rosacea presents with flushing, telangiectasia, acneiform papules and pustules. The skin becomes thickened and the hair follicles appear enlarged. Later rhinophyma occurs

Smell

Abnormalities that may occur are:

- ♠ In the fish odour syndrome, there may be the smell of fish on the patient's breath.

Eyes

On examination of the eyes one may detect abnormalities of the following:

Vision

Visual problems may occur in the following:

- ♠ Myopia occurs in Ehlers-Danlos syndrome
- ♦ Photophobia occurs in albinism

Eyelids

When examining the eyelids one may note changes in the following:

Shape

Abnormalities that may occur in the shape of the eyelids are:

♣ An epicanthic fold may be seen in Ehlers-Danlos syndrome.

Colour

One may note change in the colour of the eyelids in the following conditions:

♥ A purple (heliotrope) discoloration occurs in dermatomyositis.

♠ Periocular purpura may be a feature of amyloidosis.

Surface

The surface of the eyelids may be abnormal in the following conditions:

♦ Plaques of xanthelasma may be observed in hyperlipidaemia

♣ Contact dermatitis may occur in the eyelids

Consistency

Changes that could occur in the consistency of the eyelids are:

♥ Angioneurotic oedema may be observed in the eyelids.

Conjunctiva

When examining the conjunctiva one may note:

♠ Cicatrical pemphigoid (benign mucosal pemphigoid), which causes scarring and adhesions and may lead to blindness.

♦ Conjunctivitis may be infective, allergic or part of the Stevens-Johnson syndrome.

Sclera

On examination of the sclera one may note:

♣ The sclera may be blue in Ehlers-Danlos syndrome, pseudoxanthoma elasticum

Cornea

When examining the cornea one may note:

♥ Keratoconus or bulging of the apex of the cornea occurs in atopic eczema.

Iris

Lesions that may occur in the iris are:

♣ Lisch nodules are small, circular, pigmented hamartoma that occur in neurofibromatosis.

Fundus

The lesions that may occur in the fundus are:

♦ Angioid streaks occur in pseudoxanthoma elasticum

♣ Capillary malformations occur in the Sturge-Weber syndrome

♥ Potato like tumours occur in tuberose sclerosis

♣ Retinal hamartoma occur in neurofibromatosis

♦ Retinal detachment occurs in Ehlers-Danlos syndrome

Eye Movements

Abnormalities that may be noted when examining eye movements are:

♣ Nystagmus and strabismus may occur in albinism.

Face

When examining the face one may note abnormalities of the following:

Scalp

Disorders of hair have already been dealt with. Other conditions of note are:

♥ Alopecia areata causes localised patches of hair loss. At the edges of the lesions there are short, stubby hairs, which are referred to as exclamation mark hairs. Coalescence of hair loss may result in total scalp alopecia or universal body alopecia. Alopecia areata may be associated with:

Autoimmune diseases (such as thyrotoxicosis, Addison's disease, pernicious anaemia), hypogammaglobulinaemia, Down's syndrome

♠ Exclamation mark hairs occur in systemic lupus erythematosus

♦ Dermatitis occurring in the scalp may be seborrheic or due to fungal infections such as tinea capitis

♣ Kerion is a mass of inflammatory tissue of fungal aetiology

♥ The rash of psoriasis is common in the scalp

♠ *En coup de sabre* refers to linear scleroderma occurring in the scalp or face. It results in a depressed, ivory appearance reminiscent of the scar caused by a sabre wound (to those who have seen a sabre wound!)

Forehead

Changes that may occur in the forehead are:

♦ Hypertrichosis

♣ Seborrheic dermatitis

♥ Herpes zoster

♠ Haemangioma occur in the Sturge-Weber syndrome

Eyebrows

The eyebrows do not always give a lot of clinical information. Changes that may be noted are:

♦ Loss of the outer one third of the eyebrows may be noted in hypothyroidism

♣ The area may be thickened in leprosy

♥ Greasy scales would be seen in seborrheic dermatitis

Malar Region

When examining the malar region one may note changes in:

Colour

Changes in the colour of the skin in the malar region may be:

♠ Chloasma or increased pigmentation in the malar region may occur in pregnancy or it may be due to the oral contraceptive pill or due to exposure to sunlight.

Surface

Rash

Rashes that may occur in the malar region are as follows:

♦ **Erythema**

Erythema may be due to:

Erysipelas, rosacea, Sjogren's syndrome may be associated with an annular, non-itching oedematous, erythematous lesion

♣ **Papules**

Papules may occur in:

Acne vulgaris

Angiofibromata occur in tuberose sclerosis (they are salmon-coloured and glisten)

Acne vulgaris presents with comedones (blackheads), white-heads, papules, pustules, cysts, greasy skin and scarring

♥ **Plaques**

Plaques may be seen in:

Lupus vulgaris, which results in red-brown plaques with an irregular edge. The surface has fine scales. Lupus pernio may occur in the malar region. Butterfly rash occurs in systemic lupus erythematosus

♠ **Blistering**

Blistering may be seen in:

Porphyria cutanea tarda

♦ **Dermatitis**

Dermatitis may be due to:

Tinea facie, which causes an annular plaque with a raised edge and central clearing. Itching and scaling may occur but this is variable.

Contact dermatitis

Seborrheic dermatitis, which occurs in the flexures and the naso-labial fold and causes scaliness of the eyebrows (it is associated with Parkinsonism and AIDS)

Circulation

Abnormalities that may be noted in the circulation in the malar region are:

♣ Capilllary haemangioma occur in the Sturge-Weber syndrome (port-wine stain)

♥ Telangiectasia occur in systemic sclerosis

Chin

Abnormalities that one may note over the chin are:

♠ In males reduced beard growth would occur with loss of secondary sexual characteristics in hypogonadism and liver disease.

♦ Fungal infection may occur in the beard (tinea barbae)

♣ In females growth of hair would occur in virilising syndromes

Mouth

On examination of the mouth one may note abnormalities of the:

145

Dimensions

Size

The mouth would be:

♥ Small in scleroderma

Lips

On examination of the lips one may note abnormalities of the:

♠ Dimensions

♦ Colour

♣ Surface

♥ Circulation

Dimensions

Size

Variations that may occur in the size of the lips are:

♠ Swelling. This may be due to contact allergy, angioedema or oro-facial granulomatosis, which may be associated with Crohn's disease or sarcoidosis.

Colour

Lesions that result in a change in the colour of the lips are:

♦ Peutz-Jeghers syndrome where localised hyperpigmentation would occur (multiple pigmented macules)

♣ Malignant melanoma

Surface

Abnormalities that may occur on the surface of the lips are:

♥ Inflammation. The causes of inflammation of the lip are:

Peri-oral dermatitis, which is an erythematous, papular eruption seen around the mouth in young women

Cheilitis may be caused by contact, atopy, it may be granulomatous (toothpaste allergy, candida, Crohn's disease), actinic or due to discoid lupus erythematosus

Stomatitis may be due to vitamin B deficiency, debilitation

Herpes simplex

♠ Peri-oral furrowing (pseudorhagades) occurs in systemic sclerosis

♦ Molluscum sebaceum (keratoacanthoma) presents as a nodule with a central crater. It heals spontaneously,

♣ Squamous cell carcinoma may present as a nodule or an ulcer.

Circulation

Lesions that may be seen in relation to the blood vessels of the lips are:

♥ Telangiectasia in Osler-Rendu-Weber syndrome (Hereditary Haemorrhagic Telangiectasia)

Teeth

On examination of the teeth one may note changes in:

♠ Dimensions

♦ Colour

♣ Surface

Dimensions

Shape

The teeth may be abnormal in shape in:

♠ Ectodermal dysplasia, congenital syphilis

Colour

Changes in the colour of the teeth could be:

♦ An abnormal colour occurs following treatment with tetracycline in childhood

Surface

Changes that may occur on the surface of the teeth are:

♣ Lack of enamel occurs in dystrophic epidermolysis bullosa

Gums

Abnormalities that may be seen in the gums are:

♥ Gingival hyperplasia occurs in patients treated with drugs such as phenytoin, calcium channel blockers, cyclosporin

♠ Bleeding occurs in scurvy

Tongue

When examining the tongue one may note changes in the following:

Dimensions

Size

Changes in the size of the tongue are:

♦ A large tongue occurs in amyloidosis

Surface

On examination of the surface of the tongue one may note the following:

♣ A dry tongue occurs in Sjogren's syndrome, scleroderma

♥ Glossitis occurs in iron deficiency, B_{12} deficiency, malabsorption

♠ Hairy leukoplakia presents as a corrugated white patch. It is caused by the Epstein Barr virus and occurs in immunodeficiency especially HIV

♦ A geographical tongue refers to a map like pattern on the tongue. It is of no consequence.

♣ Acute atrophic candidiasis (antibiotic sore tongue) results in a smooth, erythematous tongue

Buccal Mucosa

When examining the buccal mucosa one may note abnormalities of the following:

Colour

Pigmentation occurs in:

♥ Addison's disease

Surface

Abnormalities that one may note on the surface of the buccal mucosa are:

♠ Pseudomembranes

♦ Plaques

♣ Blisters

♥ Ulcers

Pseudomembranes

Pseudomembranes may be seen in:

♠ Candidiasis

Plaques

The causes of plaques on the buccal mucosa are:

♦ Lichen planus. This presents as a white, lacy pattern

♣ Leukoplakia are white patches or plaques on the buccal mucosa caused by chronic irritation. They are pre-malignant and may transform into squamous cell carcinoma.

Blisters

Blistering of the buccal mucosa may be due to:

♥ Erythema multiforme

♠ Pemphigus vulgaris (large blisters or erosions)

Ulcers

Ulceration of the buccal mucosa may be due to:

♦ Aphthous ulcers, which occur in coeliac disease, Behcet's disease, Crohn's disease

♣ Mouth ulcers may occur in neutropaenia

♥ Snail track ulcers occur in syphilis

Fauces

On examination of the fauces one may note:

♠ Lymphadenopathy in infectious mononucleosis, lymphoma

Ears

When examining the ears one may note abnormalities on the:

Surface

Lesions that one may note on the surface of the ears are:

♦ Tophi occur in gout

♣ Discoid lupus erythematosus may occur here

♥ Ramsay-Hunt syndrome is characterised by a vesicular rash on the ear. It is due to herpes zoster of the geniculate ganglion.

♠ Lupus pernio refers to a bluish-red or violaceous swelling that occurs in sarcoidosis

Inflammation

Inflammation of the ear may be due to:

♦ Atopic eczema

♣ Seborrheic dermatitis

Upper Limb

General

On general examination of the upper limbs one may note abnormalities of the:

Dimensions

One may note:

♥ The upper limbs would be thin in comparison to the torso in Cushing's syndrome.

Hands

When examining the hands one may note abnormalities of the:

Dimensions

When examining the dimensions of the hands one may note:

- ♠ The hands would be apparently smaller in sclerodactyly

Dorsum of Hand

On examination of the dorsum of the hands one may note abnormalities of the following:

Nails

In addition to the nail changes that have already been described notable lesions are:

- ♦ Atrophic nails occur in scleroderma
- ♣ Pitting occurs in psoriasis, alopecia areata
- ♥ Longitudinal ridging of the nails is seen in lichen planus
- ♠ In Darier's disease there is a longitudinal ridge which ends in a V shaped notch at the free border of the nail
- ♦ In the yellow nails syndrome the nails are slow growing, the curvature is increased, they are yellow and thickened and have loss of cuticles and lunulae. They are associated with pleural effusions, bronchiectasis, sinusitis and peripheral oedema.
- ♣ Fibroma occur in tuberose sclerosis

- ♥ Nail fold telangiectasia occur in dermatomyositis
- ♠ Nail fold and nail edge infarcts occur in vasculitis

Skin

Lesions that occur in the skin over the back of the hand may affect:

Colour

Changes that may occur are:

- ♦ Dermatomyositis causes a purple rash over the back of the hands.

Surface

Rash

Rashes that occur on the back of the hand are:

Papules

Papules that occur on the back of the hands are:

- ♣ Gottron's papules, which occur over the knuckles in dermatomyositis. They are violaceous, flat-topped papules
- ♥ Granuloma annulare may occur over the back of the hands. It is seen as a ring of papules with a healing centre and centrifugal spread. It is commoner in diabetics.

Plaques

The causes of plaques on the back of the hands are:

- ♠ Psoriasis
- ♦ Systemic lupus erythematosus

Bullae

Bullae may be seen on the backs of the hands in:

♣ Porphyria cutanea tarda. This results in bullae, fragile skin, photosensitivity, milia

Papules and Burrows

Papules and burrows may be seen in:

♥ Scabies. This causes papules and burrows over the finger webs and wrists

Inflammation

Inflammation may be due to:

♠ Dermatitis which may be contact dermatitis, photosensitivity dermatitis

Consistency

Changes in the consistency of the skin over the back of the hands are:

♦ Loose skin occurs in Ehlers-Danlos syndrome, pseudoxanthoma elasticum, cutis laxa

♣ Tight skin occurs in scleroderma

♥ Fragile skin occurs in porphyria cutanea tarda

Palms

Abnormalities may be detected in:

Colour

Changes in the colour of the palms are:

♠ Palmar erythema occurs in liver disease, rheumatoid arthritis, systemic lupus erythematosus, pregnancy

♦ Plane xanthoma would be seen as orange-yellow macules over the palmar creases.

Surface

Abnormalities that occur on the surface of the palms are:

Rash

Rashes are uncommon on the palm. Those that may occur are:

♦ Secondary syphilis causes a pinkish-brown maculopapular rash with fine scaling

♣ Pustular psoriasis

♥ Systemic lupus erythematosus

♠ Erythema multiforme

♦ Acrodermatitis

♣ Hand, foot and mouth disease results in small, greyish vesicles with a faint, pink rim. It is due to coxsackie virus or enterovirus infection.

Dermatitis

Dermatitis occurring on the palm may be:

♠ Contact dermatitis

♦ Tinea

♣ Pellagra

♥ Hand Eczema

Calcinosis

Calcinosis refers to multiple spots of calcification in the soft tissues.

♠ Calcinosis occurs in scleroderma

Consistency

Changes in the consistency of the skin on the palms may be:

- ♦ Thick skin (keratoderma) occurs in arsenic poisoning

- ♣ Tylosis is hyperkeratosis of the palms and soles of the feet. It presents as a diffuse, yellow thickening of the skin. It is associated with internal malignancy (carcinoma of the oesophagus). It is familial.

- ♥ Inherited keratodermas are characterised by thickened skin on the palms and soles of the feet. Many types have been described.

Circulation

Raynaud's phenomenon is discussed in the chapter on the locomotor system.

LMS

Abnormalities that affect the locomotor system of the hands are:

- ♠ Joint changes occur in psoriatic arthropathy

- ♦ Joint changes may be seen in gout

- ♣ Hyperextensible joints are seen in Ehlers-Danlos syndrome

- ♥ Tendon xanthomata occur in hyperlipidaemia. They present as firm, localised, swellings of the tendons.

Psoriatic Arthritis

Psoriatic arthritis may be of five types:

- ♠ Distal interphalangeal

- ♦ Arthritis mutilans

- ♣ Symmetrical (rheumatoid like)

- ♥ Pauciarticular

- ♠ Spinal

Forearms

Lesions that may occur on the forearms are:

- ♦ Loose skin occurs in pseudoxanthoma elasticum

- ♣ Lichen planus may be seen over the anterior aspect of the wrist and the forearms

Elbows

Lesions that may occur at the elbows are:

- ♥ Dermatitis herpetiformis would present as itchy papules and vesicles with excoriations.

- ♠ Eruptive xanthoma would present as orange or yellow papules. They occur in hyperlipidaemia.

- ♦ Tuberose xanthoma present as firm orange or yellow nodules or plaques over the extensor surfaces. They occur in hyperlipidaemia.

- ♣ Pseudotumours are organised, calcified haematomas which are seen in Ehlers-Danlos syndrome

151

♥ Poor healing of wounds, thin scars occur in Ehlers-Danlos syndrome

♠ Hyperextension of the elbows occurs in Ehlers-Danlos syndrome

♦ Loose skin would be seen over the antecubital fossa in pseudoxanthoma elasticum.

Upper Arm

In the upper arm one may note abnormalities of the blood pressure. Elevated blood pressure may be due to:

♣ Renal involvement in scleroderma, pseudoxanthoma elasticum

♥ Phaeochromocytoma may be associated with neurofibromatosis.

Shoulders

Abnormalities that one may note at the shoulders are:

♥ Recurrent dislocation of the shoulder occurs in Ehlers-Danlos syndrome

♠ Proximal muscle weakness and tenderness occur in dermatomyositis

Axillae

Lesions that may occur in the axillae are:

♦ Axillary freckling occurs in neurofibromatosis

♣ Hidradenitis suppuritiva. This is caused by blockage of the apocrine glands with secondary anaerobic infection

♥ Dermatitis may occur in the axilla. This may be either contact or seborrheic

♠ Candidiasis may occur in the axilla

♦ Darier's disease

♣ Benign familial pemphigus (Hailey Hailey disease)

♥ Acanthosis nigricans presents as pigmented, velvety thickening of the skin with skin tags. Associated conditions are:

E&M acromegaly, hypothyroidism, hyperthyroidism, Cushing's syndrome, diabetes mellitus

RAG polycystic ovaries

GIT cancer of the stomach

♠ Loose skin occurs in pseudoxanthoma elasticum

Neck

Lesions that may occur in the neck are:

♦ Tight skin occurs in scleroderma

♣ Loose skin with a chicken-skin appearance would be seen in pseudoxanthoma elasticum

Trunk

Lesions that may occur on the trunk are:

♥ Café au lait spots occur in neurofibromatosis

♠ Shagreen patches occur in tuberose sclerosis. They are

leathery, firm, flesh-coloured plaques.

- Ash leaf macules are leaf-like hypopigmented macules that occur in tuberose sclerosis

- Bowen's disease presents as a scaly, red macule or plaque. It is an intraepidermal carcinoma-in-situ

- Rash

  Rashes that are likely to occur over the trunk are:

  Urticaria, pustular psoriasis, systemic lupus erythematosus, dermatomyositis, systemic sclerosis, acne, mycosis fungoides, pemphigus, dermatitis herpetiformis, tinea corporis, pityriasis verscicolor

- Contact dermatitis may occur over the trunk

- Atopic eczema may occur over the trunk

- Anderson-Fabry's disease or angiokeratoma corporis diffusum presents with multiple, small, red, raised, vascular skin lesions (angiokeratoma). These patients also have acoparasthesiae, autonomic dysfunction, cardiac hypertrophy and suffer from strokes (due to disease of the capillaries and medium sized vessels) and renal failure (due to impaired capillary circulation). They may also have high-tone hearing loss.

Breasts

Lesions that may occur are:

- Paget's disease of the breast

- Contact Dermatitis
- Nummular eczema
- Candidiasis

Chest Wall

Lesions that may occur on the chest wall are:

- Herpes zoster

Heart

Lesions that may occur in the cardio-vascular system are the following:

- Pericardial effusion, pulmonary hypertension occur in scleroderma

- Dissecting aneurysm, mitral valve prolapse, rupture of the large arteries occur in Ehlers-Danlos syndrome

- Mitral regurgitation, coronary artery disease occur in pseudoxanthoma elasticum

Lungs

Lesions that may occur in the respiratory system are:

- Pleural effusion, pulmonary fibrosis, overspill pneumonitis occur in scleroderma

- Pneumothorax occurs in Ehlers-Danlos syndrome

- Pulmonary arteriovenous fistulae occur in Osler-Rendu-Weber syndrome

Back

Lesions that may occur over the back are:

- ♣ Shagreen patch occurs in tuberose sclerosis
- ♥ The initial lesions of lichen planus may occur in the lumbar region

Abdomen

Lesions that may occur in the abdomen are:

- ♠ Herpes zoster
- ♦ Striae occur in Cushing's syndrome, pregnancy, obesity, growth spurt
- ♣ Erythema ab igne (reticular erythema or pigmentation) occurs due to application of heat. This would indicate pain due to underlying chronic pancreatitis or intra-abdominal malignancy
- ♥ Hepatosplenomegaly may occur in systemic mastocytosis

Groin

Lesions that may occur in the groin are:

- ♠ Infestation by *Pediculosis pubis*
- ♦ Infestation by *Phthyrus pubis*
- ♣ Scabies
- ♥ Tinea cruris presents as a well-defined erythematous plaque, which may spread into the thighs. Scaling is seen in the periphery with central clearing.
- ♠ Candidiasis
- ♦ Contact dermatitis

- ♣ Acanthosis nigricans
- ♥ Pseudoxanthoma elasticum

Genitals

Lesions that may occur are:

- ♠ Lichen planus may be seen on the penis
- ♦ Behcet's disease causes genital ulcers
- ♣ Circinate balanitis occurs in Reiter's syndrome
- ♥ Chancre occurs in primary syphilis
- ♠ Chancroid. This is a sexually transmitted infection caused by *Haemophilus ducreyi*

Lower Limbs

On examination of the lower limbs in general one may note abnormalities of the:

Dimensions

Size

One may observe:

- ♦ Discrepancy between the size of limbs and the torso is seen in Cushing's syndrome

Hips

Abnormalities that may occur are:

- ♣ Weakness and tenderness of the proximal muscles occurs in dermatomyositis

Thighs

Lesions that may occur over the thighs are:

♥ Erythema marginatum occurs in rheumatic fever. This begins as a faint, red macule, which spreads outwards whilst the centre returns to normal. The margins are irregular and adjacent lesions may coalesce. The rash usually fades in about a day but may recur.

♠ Livedo reticularis

Knees

Lesions that may occur at the knees are:

♦ Genu recurvatum and recurrent dislocation occur in Ehlers-Danlos syndrome

♣ Dermatitis herpetiformis

Legs

Lesions that may occur on the legs are:

♥ Corkscrew hairs with perifollicular haemorrhage in scurvy

♠ Pretibial myxoedema presents as a shiny, red, non-tender infiltration on the front of the shins. Chronic forms may look like localised elephantiasis.

♦ Necrobiosis lipoidica diabeticorum presents as well-defined plaques, which may coalesce. They have yellowish centres with raised, brownish-red edges (the lesion may be red at first). The surface is shiny and appears atrophic.

♣ Diabetic dermopathy presents as pigmented macules

♥ Erythema nodosum presents as tender, red swellings on the front of the shins. It may occur in conditions affecting the:

IS leprosy

RS tuberculosis, sarcoidosis, streptococcal infection

LMS rheumatoid arthritis, rheumatic fever, Behcet's disease

GIT inflammatory bowel disease, systemic fungal infections, *Yersina enterocolitica*

HS lymphoma, leukaemia

RAG syphilis, lymphogranuloma venereum, pregnancy

Drugs oral contraceptive pill, sulphonamides, penicillin

♠ Pyoderma gangrenosum begins as a tender, red or blue nodule that breaks down into a necrotic ulcer. It occurs in conditions affecting the:

GIT inflammatory bowel disease, autoimmune hepatitis

LMS rheumatoid arthritis, seronegative arthritis

HS leukaemia, polycythaemia rubra vera, multiple myeloma, Ig A monoclonal gammopathy

RS Wegener's granulomatosis

♦ Henoch-Schonlein purpura may occur over the legs

♣ Erythema ab igne may be seen in elderly patients. It is caused by sitting in front of fireplaces for prolonged periods.

155

♥ Eczema over the legs may be discoid, stasis, asteatotic, atopic

♠ Venous ulcer occurs around the medial malleolus. The ulcer is surrounded by an area of pigmentation

♦ Lichen planus may occur over the ankles

Feet

Lesions that occur in the feet are similar to those that occur on the hand. Other notable lesions that may present are:

Dimensions

Shape

One may note the following:

♣ Flat feet occur in Ehlers-Danlos syndrome

Dorsum of the Feet

Lesions that occur on the dorsum of the feet are:

♥ Dermatitis

♠ Tinea pedis. In tinea pedis the skin between the toes becomes moist and macerated with fine scaling.

♦ Psoriasis

♣ Gouty tophi

♥ Onychomycosis, which is due to infection by fungi, causes the nail to become thickened and friable

Soles of the Feet

Lesions that may occur on the soles of the feet are:

♠ Pustular psoriasis

♦ Keratoderma blenorrhagica in Reiter's syndrome

♣ Arterial ulcers usually occur on the plantar surface

♥ Kaposi's sarcoma presents as well demarcated red-brown vascular lesions

Buttocks

Lesions that may occur on the buttocks are:

♠ Migratory necrolytic erythema in glucagonoma

♦ Dermatitis herpetiformis

♣ Eruptive xanthoma may occur over the buttocks

♥ Tuberose xanthoma

Spine

Abnormalities that may be noted in the spine are:

♠ Kyphoscoliosis occurs in Ehlers-Danlos syndrome, neurofibromatosis

♦ Spondyloarthropathy may occur in psoriasis

Gait

Abnormalities of gait that may be relevant are:

♣ Proximal myopathy occurs in Cushing's syndrome and results in a waddling gait

♥ Proximal muscle weakness occurs in dermatomyositis and this may result in a waddling gait

Chapter 10

The Cardiovascular System

In the cardiovascular system one will study the heart, the blood vessels and the associated features of cardiovascular disease. The clinical features that result from the causes and effects of diseases that involve the cardiovascular system but are reflected in other systems will also be studied.

History Taking

In taking a history, one should ask about symptoms that relate to the heart, the arterial side of the circulation and the venous side of the circulation. Symptoms that relate to the heart are chiefly chest pain and palpitations. Arterial insufficiency would result in pain in the extremities and rarely visceral pain, cold peripheries and cyanosis, fatigue and syncope. Venous congestion would result in dyspnoea and swelling. A review of systems would evaluate the effects of cardiovascular dysfunction on other organ systems and seek evidence of causes of cardiovascular disease reflected in other systems.

Cardiovascular History

One should ask about:

- ♥ Chest pain
- ♠ Palpitations
- ♦ Dyspnoea (with effort or at rest and associated orthopnoea or paroxysmal nocturnal dyspnoea)
- ♣ Swelling (of the ankles, the abdomen and the genitalia)
- ♥ Claudication
- ♠ Cold extremities
- ♦ Cyanosis
- ♣ Fatigue
- ♥ Syncope

This should be followed by a review of systems.

Physical Examination

On physical examination one should assess the structure and function of the heart, the arteries and veins and the peripheral circulation. In addition one should evaluate the associated features of cardiovascular disease.

General Examination

Begin by examining the posture of the patient, the state of growth and development and the metabolic state of the patient. Note any gross changes in the integument. Note the body temperature. (Position, Height and Proportions, Weight and Shape, Integument, Body Temperature)

Regional Examination

Next, proceed to examine the regions of the body.

Head

Examine the head. In practice one would begin by noting cerebral cortical function if this has not been done already. In a professional examination this would not be done. Perform a general examination of the head, noting the dimensions, the integument and movement. Then examine the regions of the head; the nose, the eyes, the face (scalp, forehead, eyebrows, malar region, chin), the mouth (jaw, lips, teeth, gums, buccal mucosa, tongue, palate, fauces, salivary glands) and the ears.

Upper Limbs

Perform a general examination of the upper limbs and then focus on the hands.

Hands

First, assess the dimensions of the hands. Next, examine the dorsum of the hands. Examine the nails and skin, the bones, joints, tendons and muscles. Ask the patient to turn the hands over palms upwards. Repeat inspection of the skin, the bones, joints, tendons and muscles. Palpate the hands and assess the state of the peripheral circulation. Look for Quincke's sign and check capillary refill. Evaluate the radial pulse

Radial Pulse

Palpate the radial pulse with three fingers, the second, third and fourth. One may use the right or left hand for palpation. However, use of one's left hand will allow the use of the right hand to simultaneously palpate the opposite radial pulse and the right femoral pulse. Note the following characteristics of the pulse:

- ♥ Condition of the Vessel Wall
- ♠ Transmission
- ♦ Rate
- ♣ Rhythm
- ♥ Volume
- ♠ Character

Condition of the Vessel Wall

Note the condition of the vessel wall. This is strictly speaking examination of structure of the blood vessel but it is traditionally included in examination of function of the radial pulse. Occlude the radial pulse with the second and fourth fingers and palpate the vessel wall with the third.

Transmission

Check whether transmission of the pulse wave occurs in a normal fashion. To do this whilst palpating the radial pulse with the fingers of the left hand simultaneously examine the opposite radial pulse with the fingers of the right hand and then examine the femoral pulse with the fingers of the right hand. Note whether these pulses are palpable and whether there is any radio-radial or radio-femoral delay.

Rate

Count the rate. Ideally for one minute. More than one hundred is a tachycardia, less than sixty a bradycardia.

Rhythm

Note the rhythm of the pulse and whether the rhythm varies with respiration

Volume

Note the volume of the pulse and whether there is a variation in volume between beats and any variation with respiration.

Character

The normal character of the pulse consists of an initial sharp upstroke, the percussion wave, which is followed by a second slower upstroke called the tidal wave. The pulse wave then subsides but as it subsides it is interrupted by another upstroke called the dicrotic notch, which represents aortic valve closure. These characteristics are not discernible by the palpating fingers but by plethysmography.

However, one should carefully evaluate the upstroke of the pulse noting its height and the rate of ascent. Evaluate the downstroke noting the rate of descent, which is of importance. The intervening segment should also be evaluated.

Collapsing Pulse

To check for a collapsing pulse, first ask the patient whether they experience any pain in the arms or shoulder. Then hold the patients right wrist with one's right hand so that the palmar surface of the examining hand overlies the palmar surface of the patient's wrist. The heads of the metacarpals of the examining hand should overlie the radial pulse. Do not exert pressure. The radial pulse should not be palpable. Now hold the patient's right hand with one's left hand and raise the patient's hand up to about head height. If the pulse, which was not palpable, now becomes palpable this indicates a collapsing pulse. Move the patient's hand back to the starting position and note whether the pulse is now impalpable. This cross check will ensure that excess pressure was not used during the manoeuvre.

Another method that is described is to raise the patient's arm and use the palmar aspect of the fingers of the left hand to palpate the radial pulse whilst the right hand is used to simultaneously palpate the more proximal vessels. This method may be used if one wishes.

To complete examination of the hands look for involuntary movements. Ask the patient to stretch his or her arms out in front of him or her and look for a fine tremor. Then ask the patient to extend the wrists and spread the fingers apart and look for a flapping tremor. Examine the nervous system and function of the locomotor system of the hands in more detail if required.

Forearms and Upper Arms

Perform a quick examination of the structure of the forearms and upper arms and then examine the brachial artery.

Brachial Artery

Examine the brachial artery by performing:

♥ Inspection

♠ Palpation

♦ Auscultation

Inspection

A thickened tortuous brachial artery may be observed. This is called locomotor brachialis and indicates severe arteriosclerosis.

Palpation

Feel the brachial pulse. The character of the pulse is better determined here. Look for brachio-radial delay. This is done by palpating the brachial artery with the thumb or fingers of the right hand whilst simultaneously palpating the radial artery with the fingers of the left hand.

Auscultation

The blood pressure should be measured in both upper arms. In a professional examination this would not be required but it should be mentioned for the sake of completeness.

Shoulders and Axillae

Make a quick note of any abnormality of the shoulders and axillae. Examine in detail only if required.

Next move on to examine the neck.

Neck

Note the dimensions of the neck. Note the state of the integument. Look for any enlargement of the thyroid gland and examine in detail if required. Inspect the sternocleidomastoid muscle and then examine the jugular venous pressure.

Jugular Venous Pressure (JVP)

To examine the jugular venous pressure, position the patient so that he or she is in a reclining position with the torso making an angle of 45 degrees with the bed or couch. The patient's head should be supported so that the sternocleidomastoid muscle is relaxed. Observe pulsations of the internal jugular vein. It is preferable to observe pulsations in the right internal jugular vein rather than the left. The pulsations are best seen by leaning across the patient and observing the pulsations in silhouette from the left hand side of the patient.

An alternative method is to shine the beam of a torch tangentially across the right hand side of the patient's neck so that the shadow of the neck is thrown onto the bedclothes. Now observe the shadow for pulsations.

Note the following characteristics of the JVP:

♥ Height

♠ Character

♦ Transmission

♣ Modifying Factors

Height

Assess the height of the jugular venous wave in relation to the manubriosternal angle. The simplest method is to place one's clenched right fist on the chest with the ulnar surface of one's hand over the angle of Louis (manubriosternal angle). Read off the height of the venous wave as the number of fingers reached by the upper limit of the wave. It would be best to measure one's fingers beforehand so that one may improve the accuracy of this method. The normal is less than 3 cms of water.

The heights of the waves vary with respiration; decreasing with inspiration as reduced intrathoracic pressure sucks blood into the thorax and increasing with expiration when increased intrathoracic pressure impedes venous return. Carefully note this.

Apply gentle pressure at the root of the neck with the ulnar border of one's right hand and note that the jugular venous pulse may be obliterated by this manoeuvre.

Character

Note the character of the venous waves. The normal jugular venous pulse exhibits three upward waves (the a, c, v waves) and two downward troughs (the x and y descents). The **a** wave coincides with atrial contraction. This is followed by the **c** wave, which is caused by ventricular contraction making the atrioventricular valves bulge into the atrium. Following this one would observe the first trough, the **x** descent, which is caused by right ventricular emptying drawing the tricuspid valve away from the right atrium thus reducing right atrial pressure and sucking blood into the right atrium. The **x** descent ends with a rise in pressure, the **v** wave, which is due to venous return causing a build up of pressure within the atrium whilst the tricuspid valve remains closed. With opening of the atrioventricular valves in diastole the second trough, the **y** descent, occurs as blood rushes from the right atrium into the right ventricle.

Timing

The timing of the venous waves is determined by simultaneous palpation of the left carotid pulse or the apex beat. If one experiences difficulty in timing, one may repeat this assessment whilst listening to the heart sounds. Time the waves in relation to the heart sounds.

Transmission

Place one's right hand over the patient's right hypochondrium and gently exert pressure. Note transmission. Pressure over the liver increases the venous return to the right atrium thus increasing the jugular venous pressure. This is known as hepatojugular reflux.

Modifying Factors

Note the modifying factors. The JVP varies with posture and respiration and it is obliterated by pressure at the root of the neck.

When examining the jugular venous pressure one must always remember to elicit all the signs that differentiate pulsations in the neck. In other words the signs that differentiate whether a pulsation seen in the neck is carotid or jugular venous. This may seem obvious at first but when faced with a patient who has a very high jugular venous pressure as a result of severe pulmonary hypertension and tricuspid regurgitation, the importance of this will be realised.

Differentiating Signs

The signs that differentiate pulsations in the neck are enumerated as follows:

1) The jugular venous wave is sinuous

2) The jugular venous pressure varies with posture and respiration

3) The jugular venous wave is not palpable. (Remember that in pulmonary hypertension and tricuspid regurgitation the pressure may be so high that this may not apply)

4) The jugular venous pulse may be obliterated by compression at the root of the neck

5) The jugular venous pulse shows hepatojugular reflux

6) A venous hum may be heard

Carotid Pulse

Next, examine the carotid pulse. One may use the same format that was used for examination of the radial pulse. However, remember the carotid pulse may be visible and in addition it is important to listen for a bruit. Auscultation may be left till later and one may perform auscultation of the carotid artery at the same time as auscultation of the heart.

In summary examine the carotid pulse by:

♥ Inspection

♠ Palpation

♦ Auscultation

Trachea

The position of the trachea should be determined as this will show whether the mediastinum is displaced or not. Displacement of the apex beat will indicate cardiac enlargement only if the mediastinum is central. If not it reflects mediastinal shift.

Next, move on to examine the chest.

Chest

Examination of the chest should be performed in two stages. First, one should examine the chest wall and secondly one should examine the contents, in this case, the heart.

Chest Wall

Examine the chest wall. Note any deformity of the chest wall in general and the praecordium in particular. Note the state of the integument; note any scars, gynaecomastia or the presence of a pacemaker. Make a note of any obvious respiratory distress.

Heart

Next, one should examine the heart. The heart is examined with the patient assuming three positions.

Positions Assumed

The positions assumed by the patient during examination of the heart are the following:

♥ Semi-Recumbent

♠ Turning to the left side

♦ Seated up and leaning forward

Modalities Used

The following modalities are used in examination of the heart:

♥ Inspection

♠ Palpation

♦ Percussion

♣ Auscultation

Begin examination of the heart with the patient in the semi-recumbent position.

Inspection

On inspection one should look for:

♥ Position of the apex beat

♠ Pulsations over the praecordium and elsewhere in the chest

Palpation

Palpate and evaluate the following:

♥ Apex beat

♠ Left parasternal heave

♦ Pulsations over the praecordium or elsewhere in the chest

♣ Palpable heart sounds

♥ Thrills

Apex Beat

Definition

Remember the definition of the apex beat, which is as follows:

♠ The apex beat is the lowermost and outermost point at which the cardiac impulse is best seen, felt or heard.

Characteristics of the Apex Beat

Note the following characteristics of the apex beat:

♥ Position

♠ Rate and Rhythm

♦ Quantity

♣ Character

♥ Transmission

♠ Modifying factors

Position

Determine the position of the apex beat by inspection first and then palpation with the index and middle fingers of the right hand. This is the best way to localise it. Once the apex beat is localised, with the right hand maintaining position over the apex beat, localise the manubriosternal angle with the fingers of the left hand. The second costal cartilage articulates with the sternum at this level. Move the fingers of the left hand to the second intercostal space and count the intercostal spaces to the apex beat. Counting should proceed downwards and outwards to avoid the main muscle mass of pectoralis major. The intercostal space concerned is the first point of reference. The second point of reference is the relationship of the apex beat to the mid-clavicular line, which is the line drawn perpendicularly down from the mid-point of the clavicle. However, as the mid-point of the clavicle is difficult to determine one should use a line drawn perpendicularly down from a point mid-way between the middle of the suprasternal notch and the tip of the acromion. Thus, the position of the apex beat should be defined as the intercostal space in which it is best seen, felt or heard and by its relationship to the mid-clavicular line. In severe displacement of the apex, one may refer to its relationship to the anterior axillary line or even the mid-axillary line.

If it is difficult to palpate the apex beat because of obesity or chronic obstructive pulmonary disease, remember that one may use percussion or auscultation to define the position of the apex beat.

Rate and Rhythm

It is important to determine the apex rate and relate this to the pulse rate. However, this would be best done during auscultation of the heart sounds. The apex beat is not an important point at which rhythm is analysed.

Quantity

The quantification of the apex beat relates to cardiac size and this has already been determined by defining the position of the apex beat

Character

The character of the apex beat is best determined by palpation with the palm of the right hand. One's hand should be positioned so that the metacarpal heads overlie the apex beat.

The character of the apex beat is broadly divided into a:

- ♦ Normal impulse
- ♣ Left ventricular impulse
- ♥ Right ventricular impulse
- ♠ Tapping apex
- ♦ Double impulse

Left Ventricular Impulse

A left ventricular impulse is felt as a forceful impulse pushing on to the examining hand. It is a localised impulse. A left ventricular impulse is further divided into a:

- ♠ Thrust
- ♦ Heave

Thrust

A thrust is a quick in and out movement. A thrust is indicative of diastolic overload.

Heave

A heave is a sustained contraction. A heave indicates systolic overload.

Right Ventricular Impulse

A right ventricular impulse is felt as a more diffuse impulse than the left ventricular impulse, which is more localised. It is more difficult to appreciate and right ventricular hypertrophy is more readily appreciated by demonstrating left parasternal heave.

Tapping Apex

A tapping apex is really the palpable closure of the mitral valve. This occurs in mitral stenosis where the first heart sound is very loud. The tap is felt as an impulse distant from the examining hand.

Double Impulse

A double impulse is felt as two distinct impulses at the apex beat.

Transmission

Note any transmission at the apex beat. A loud murmur may be transmitted to the palpating hand as a thrill. Loud heart sounds may also be palpable.

Modifying Factors

Remember the use of modifying factors. Turning the patient onto the left lateral position brings the apex beat closer to the chest wall and thus makes evaluation of character easier. Thrills at the apex are felt more easily when the patient is in this position. However, one must remember that the position of the apex beat should not be defined in the left lateral position.

Parasternal Heave

Next, feel for a left parasternal heave. Place one's right hand over the praecordium with its radial border parallel to the left sternal border and the tips of the fingers pointing towards the patient's head. Exert gentle, sustained pressure. The hand would be felt to lift up if there is a left parasternal heave.

An alternative method is to place the tips of the fingers of one's right hand in the intercostal spaces to the left of the sternal border. The fingers would be felt to lift up if there is a left parasternal heave.

Pulsations

Palpate any pulsations that have been noted either over the praecordium or elsewhere.

Palpable Heart Sounds

When palpating the praecordium, note whether the heart sounds are of sufficient intensity to be palpable.

Thrills

Thrills that occur over the praecordium would have been felt whilst examining the apex beat and checking for left parasternal heave. On occasion one may have to palpate for thrills in other areas such as the infraclavicular and suprasternal areas.

Percussion

Percussion is not considered useful in examination of the praecordium but sometimes it may be necessary to use this method to define the position of the apex beat. In the presence of a pericardial effusion, a difference between the left cardiac border as defined by percussion and the apex as defined by inspection, palpation or auscultation will give a clue to the diagnosis.

When indicated percuss the left and right cardiac border.

Cardiac Auscultation

The key to successful auscultation of the heart is not keen hearing or a good stethoscope although keeping one's stethoscope free of wax and dirt is important. The key, as in any aspect of clinical medicine, is mindfulness. That is keeping the mind aware of the aspect of auscultation under consideration. Detailed explanation of this will be given.

Begin auscultation with the bell of the stethoscope over the apex of the heart. Simultaneously palpate the right carotid pulse with the fingers of the left hand in order to time the first heart sound. Go through all the defined auscultatory areas in turn using both the bell and the diaphragm of the stethoscope. The auscultatory areas are:

- ♣ Mitral Area
- ♥ Tricuspid Area
- ♠ Pulmonary Area
- ♦ Aortic Area

Mitral Area

The mitral area corresponds to the position of the apex beat.

Tricuspid Area

The tricuspid area is at the lower, left sternal edge.

Pulmonary Area

The pulmonary area is at the second, left intercostal space just lateral to the sternum.

Aortic Area

The aortic area is at the second, right intercostal space just lateral to the sternum.

When moving from one auscultatory area to the next, listen in the intervening areas as well because some murmurs, such as the murmur of mitral stenosis, are best heard in these intervening areas. Listen carefully to the heart sounds, any added sounds, murmurs and extra-cardiac sounds. If a murmur is heard note whether it radiates to the axilla in the case of apical murmurs and to the neck in the case of murmurs at the base of the heart.

Changes in Position

Next, ask the patient to turn on to the left hand side and repeat the examination, that is, palpation of the apex and auscultation. Following this ask the patient to sit up and lean forward. Ask the patient to breathe out and with the patient maintaining a phase of expiration, repeat palpation and feel for a thrill in the aortic area and then listen at the base of the heart for systolic murmurs and at the left sternal edge for early diastolic murmurs. Whilst doing this remember to ask the patient to breathe normally at intervals.

Analysis during Auscultation

When auscultating the heart one should analyse the following:

- ♣ Heart Sounds
- ♥ Added Sounds
- ♠ Murmurs
- ♦ Extra-Cardiac Sounds

Heart Sounds

When analysing heart sounds define the following:

- ♥ Position
- ♠ Rate
- ♦ Rhythm
- ♣ Quantity

♥ Character

Position

Define the position at which auscultation is performed

Rate

Count the rate. Compare this to the pulse rate.

Rhythm

When assessing rhythm one may define:

♣ Abnormalities of cardiac rhythm

♥ Abnormalities of the rhythm of the heart sounds

Abnormalities of Cardiac Rhythm

Either confirm an arrhythmia that has already been noted during examination of the pulse or detect an arrhythmia that was not noted earlier

Abnormalities of the Rhythm of the Heart Sounds

The normal rhythm of the heart sounds is a dual rhythm (I+II). The presence of added sounds may give a triple or rarely a quadruple rhythm.

Thus, the rhythm of the heart sounds may be:

♠ Dual rhythm

♦ Triple rhythm

♣ Quadruple rhythm

Quantity

Quantify the heart sounds. The intensity or loudness of each heart sound should be defined. Note whether the heart sounds are normal, soft or loud. Note any variation in intensity between beats.

Character

Make a note of the character of the heart sounds. The first heart sound is produced by closure of the mitral and tricuspid valve. The mitral valve closes just before the tricuspid. The second heart sound is produced by closure of the aortic and pulmonary valves. Normally the aortic valve closes first. If there is a variation in the timing of closure of the individual valves a split will result.

When analysing the character of the heart sounds make a note of whether the sound is single or split and if split whether the split varies with respiration. The character of the heart sounds may also vary if the patient has a prosthetic heart valve.

Thus, a change in the character of the heart sounds may be the presence of a:

♣ Split

♥ Prosthetic sound

Added Sounds

Added sounds may be:

♠ Diastolic

♦ Systolic

Diastolic Added Sounds

Diastolic added sounds may be:

♣ **Early Diastolic**

   Opening Snap

   Tumour Plop

   Diastolic Opening Click

♥ **Mid-Diastolic**

   Third Heart Sound

   Pericardial Knock

♠ **Late-Diastolic** (Pre-systolic)

Fourth Heart Sound

Opening Snap

An opening snap is caused by snapping open of a thickened mitral valve. It is heard in early diastole.

Tumour Plop

A tumour plop is caused by an atrial tumour plopping through the atrioventricular valve. It is heard in early diastole.

Diastolic Opening Click

A diastolic opening click is caused by the opening of a prosthetic mitral valve. It is heard in early diastole.

Third Heart Sound

A third heart sound is caused by vibrations produced by rapid ventricular filling in mid-diastole.

Pericardial Knock

A pericardial knock is caused by vibrations produced by the arrest of rapid ventricular filling in constrictive pericarditis. It is heard in mid-diastole.

Fourth Heart Sound

A fourth heart sound is produced by vibrations caused by forceful atrial contraction. It is pre-systolic.

Systolic Added Sounds

Systolic added sounds may be:

♠ **Early systolic**

Ejection Clicks

Systolic Opening Clicks

♦ **Mid-Systolic**

Mid-systolic clicks

Ejection Clicks

Ejection clicks are caused by snapping open of a sclerosed aortic or pulmonary valve or by blood flowing into a dilated aorta or pulmonary artery.

Systolic Opening Clicks

A systolic opening click is caused by opening of a prosthetic aortic valve

Mid-Systolic Clicks

Mid-systolic clicks are caused by prolapse of the mitral valve.

Murmurs

Next, one should concentrate on listening for murmurs. As the phase of the cardiac cycle in which the murmur occurs is of the utmost importance in identification of a lesion, one should very carefully define this. First, concentrate on systole; listen for a murmur and if one is present define it. Next, listen in diastole and repeat the process. If a murmur is heard define its:

♥ Position

♠ Timing

♦ Character

♣ Quantity

♥ Modifying Factors

♠ Transmission

Position

Define the position at which the murmur is best heard.

Timing

Ascertain the timing of the murmur. Murmurs should be timed accurately. First, are they systolic or diastolic? Next, the phase should be defined that is are they early, mid, late, holo (pan) systolic or diastolic.

Character

The character of the murmur should be described. Murmurs could be blowing, rumbling, rough or high-pitched

Quantity

Quantify the murmur. The intensity of the murmur should be noted. It could be graded from 1–6

1. Soft only heard with difficulty

2. Immediately audible

3. Easily audible

4. Associated with a thrill

5. So loud it can be heard by placing the edge of the diaphragm of the stethoscope over the chest

6. Can be heard when the stethoscope is not in contact with the chest wall

Most practising clinicians do not use this classification and simply use the words loud or soft to describe the intensity of a murmur.

Modifying Factors

Certain modifying factors influence the intensity of a murmur. Hence, one should note the effect of manoeuvres on the intensity of the murmur. These manoeuvres are the effect of respiration and the Valsalva manoeuvre, standing, squatting, change in position, exercise.

Transmission

Transmission or radiation of the murmur should be ascertained. The areas to which murmurs may transmit or radiate are the axilla, the neck and the back.

Extra-Cardiac Sounds

Next, note any extra-cardiac sounds. Extra-cardiac sounds may be:

- ♥ Pericardial rub
- ♠ Pericardial crunch
- ♦ Venous hum

Pericardial Rub

A pericardial rub has three components; a presystolic component during atrial contraction, a ventricular systolic component and a ventricular diastolic component. The systolic component is the loudest and most constant feature. The character is high-pitched and is similar to the sound made by lightly rubbing one's hands together.

Pericardial Crunch

A pericardial crunch is a crunching sound, synchronous with the heartbeat that may be heard in the presence of a left sided pneumothorax or pneumomediastinum.

Venous Hum

A venous hum may be heard in the neck or upper chest. It is a continuous sound that may be obliterated by pressure on the neck. It is caused by increased blood flow in the great veins.

Method of listening to Heart Sounds and Murmurs

♥ Count the rate of the heart sounds

♠ Note the rhythm of the heart sounds

♦ Listen to the first heart sound. Define whether it is normal in intensity, loud or soft. Ascertain whether the intensity of the sound varies between beats. Define its character. Define whether it is single or split and if split whether the split varies with respiration.

♣ Repeat for the second heart sound.

♥ Listen in early diastole for an opening snap, opening click or tumour plop

♠ Listen in mid diastole for the presence of a third heart sound or pericardial knock.

♦ Listen in late diastole for the presence of a fourth heart sound.

♣ Listen in early systole for an opening or ejection click.

♥ Listen in mid systole for the presence of a mid-systolic click

♠ Listen in systole for any murmurs. If a murmur is heard define it.

♦ Listen in diastole for any murmurs. If a murmur is heard define it.

♣ Listen for any extra-cardiac sounds.

Back

After the patient has gone through all the positional changes required for a thorough auscultation of the heart, he or she should be in a seated position. Next, ask the patient to lean forward and examine the patient from the back. One should note any abnormalities of the:

♥ Neck

♠ Spine

♦ Sacrum

♣ Scapula

♥ Lung bases

Examine the patient's neck. Palpate for enlarged lymph nodes if required.

Move the fingers of the examining hand down the patient's spine. This will help to remind one to look for any abnormalities of the spine that may be relevant. Palpate for sacral oedema. Examine the scapula. Percuss and auscultate the lung bases and take the opportunity to listen at the inferior angle of the left scapula for radiation of a mitral regurgitant murmur.

The remaining part of the examination is given for the sake of completeness. It is usually not required in a professional examination. However, if the patient has evidence of aortic regurgitation one should examine the femoral arteries and demonstrate the physical signs of relevance.

Abdomen

Examine the patient's abdomen in the usual manner.

Femoral Arteries

Examine the features of the pulse. Remember to auscultate over the femoral artery.

Lower Limbs

Examine the lower limbs in the usual manner. Remember to palpate the popliteal pulses.

Feet

Examine in a similar fashion to examination of the hands. Note the dimensions. Examine the dorsum of the feet. Look at the nails and the skin, examine the bones, joints, tendons, and muscles. Repeat the process for the plantar aspect. Palpate the peripheries and assess the state of the peripheral circulation. Check capillary refill. Palpate the dorsalis pedis and posterior tibial pulses. Examine the nervous system and locomotor system if required.

Buttocks, Perianal Region, Per Rectal Examination

In practice one should perform these examinations if required.

Spine

Examine the patient's spine if required.

Gait, Romberg's Sign, Standing from a Seated or Squatting Position

These tests would not be performed in a professional examination but they are sometimes required in practice.

Lesions of the Cardiovascular System

Before moving on to the findings that may be detected on clinical evaluation of the cardiovascular system, it would be prudent to consider the lesions that may occur. One should consider lesions of the:

♣ Heart

♥ Arteries

♠ Veins

Heart

The heart may be affected by disorders of the:

♦ Endocardium

♣ Valves

♥ Septum

♠ Myocardium

♦ Pericardium

♣ Great Vessels

Endocardium

Lesions that may affect the endocardium are:

- ♥ Thrombosis
- ♠ Endocarditis
- ♦ Tumours such as left atrial myxoma

Valves

Pathology of the valves could cause:

- ♣ Stenosis
- ♥ Regurgitation
- ♠ Combination of the two

Lesser degrees of involvement would result in:

- ♦ Sclerosis
- ♣ Floppy valves

Septum

The septum may be affected by defects such as:

- ♥ Atrial septal defect
- ♠ Ventricular septal defect

Myocardium

The heart muscle may be affected in:

- ♦ Ischaemic heart disease
- ♣ Myocarditis
- ♥ Cardiomyopathy

These conditions may result in heart failure.

Diseases of the Myocardium

Diseases of the myocardium may be classified according to the primary pathology affecting it. The pathology may be:

- ♥ Vascular Disorders
- ♠ Inflammation
- ♦ Degenerative Disorders

Vascular Disorders

By far the commonest disorder affecting the myocardium is ischaemic heart disease.

Inflammation

Myocarditis or inflammation of the myocardium has many causes. They are:

- ♠ **Biological Agents**

  Viruses: coxsackie, adenovirus, cytomegalovirus, echovirus, influenza, polio, hepatitis, HIV

  Bacteria: diphtheria, leptospira, borrelia

  Parasites: trypanosomes and toxoplasma

  Fungi and rickettsia

  Autoimmune disorders. This would include rheumatic fever.

- ♥ **Chemical Agents**

  Drugs: penicillin, sulphonamides

- ♠ **Physical Agents**

  Radiation

Degenerative Disorders

Under degenerative disorders one would consider the cardiomyopathies.

Cardiomyopathy may be:

- ♠ Dilated cardiomyopathy
- ♦ Hypertrophic cardiomyopathy
- ♣ Restrictive cardiomyopathy

Dilated Cardiomyopathy

Dilated cardiomyopathy may be due to:

- ♥ **Internal Factors**

  Genetic disorders: autosomal dominant dilated cardiomyopathy, X-linked cardiomyopathy

- ♠ **Systemic Factors**

  LMS systemic lupus erythematosus, systemic sclerosis

  E&M acromegaly, thyrotoxicosis, hypothyroidism, diabetes mellitus, haemochromatosis, thiamine deficiency, selenium deficiency

  CNS muscular dystrophy, Fiedreich's ataxia, mitochondrial myopathies

  HS sickle cell anaemia, thrombotic thrombocytopaenic purpura

  RAG puerperal (peri-partum) cardiomyopathy

  Toxins alcohol, cocaine

  Drugs doxorubicin, cyclophosphamide

Hypertrophic Obstructive Cardiomyopathy

Hypertrophic Obstructive Cardiomyopathy (HOCM) is usually due to autosomal dominant inheritance but sporadic cases may occur.

It may be associated with conditions affecting the:

- ♦ **CNS** Friedrich's ataxia, mitochondrial myopathy
- ♣ **E&M** glycogen storage disease
- ♥ **RAG** Noonan's syndrome

Restrictive Cardiomyopathy

Restrictive cardiomyopathy may be due to:

- ♠ **Internal Factors**

  Idiopathic

  Endomyocardial fibrosis

  Loeffler's endocarditis

- ♦ **Systemic Factors**

  HS amyloidosis

  RS sarcoidosis

  E&M haemochromatosis, glycogen storage disease

Pericardium

The pericardium may be affected by:

- ♦ Effusion
- ♣ Constriction

Great Vessels

Abnormalities of the great vessels may affect the

♥ **Great Arteries**

The great arteries may be:

Abnormal in position as in transposition of the great vessels

Affected by aneurysm formation.

♠ **Great Veins**

The great veins may be:

Abnormal in position as in anomalous pulmonary venous drainage

Obstructed (superior or inferior vena cava obstruction)

Aortic Aneurysm

An aortic aneurysm may be due to

♥ **Internal Factors**

Hypertension

♠ **Mural Factors**

Atheroma

Tertiary syphilis

♣ **Systemic Factors**

LMS Marfan's syndrome

Arteries

The causes of lesions in the arteries may be:

♣ **Internal Factors**

Changes in blood volume, changes in blood pressure, thromboembolism

♥ **Mural Factors**

The wall of the vessel may be:

Narrow due to atheroma, inflammation, Raynaud's phenomenon

Dilated due to an aneurysm

Veins

The causes of lesions in the veins may be:

♠ **Internal Factors**

Changes in blood volume, obstruction to outflow with resultant changes in pressure, thromboembolism

♦ **Mural Factors**

Thrombophlebitis

♣ **External Factors**

External compression from enlargement of neighbouring structures

Findings On History

The common findings that one may obtain on history taking are the following:

Chest Pain

The cardiac causes of chest pain are:

♥ **Internal Factors**

Factors within the blood vessels that may result in cardiac chest pain are:

Anaemia, hyperviscosity syndromes

♠ **Mural Factors**

Mural factors that may result in cardiac chest pain are:

Coronary artery disease, which may manifest as a result of spasm of the vessel, atheroma, thrombosis

Disease of the great vessels: dissecting aneurysm of the aorta

♦ **Extra Cardiac Factors**

Pericarditis

Dyspnoea

Dyspnoea or breathlessness of cardiac origin may be due to various factors. They are:

♣ **Internal Factors**

Internal factors refer to disorders of blood. These disorders may be:

Quality: anaemia or hyperviscosity

Quantity: hypervolaemia or hypovolaemia

Pressure: hypertension

♥ **Mural Factors**

Mural factors would include disorders of:

Valves: stenosis, regurgitation or a combination

Cardiac Muscle: ischaemic heart disease, cardiomyopathy, cardiac arrhythmias

♠ **Extra Cardiac Factors**

Pericardial tamponade, pericardial constriction

Swelling (dependent oedema or ascites)

Swelling may be due to:

♦ **Internal Factors**

Decreased colloid osmotic pressure (oncotic pressure), which may be due to cardiac cachexia or cardiac cirrhosis

Hypervolaemia, venous thromboembolism

♠ **Mural Factors**

Right heart failure

♥ **External Factors**

Pericardial tamponade, pericardial constriction

Palpitations

Palpitations or awareness of the heartbeat could be due to:

♠ **Internal Factors**

Anaemia

♦ **Mural Factors**

Tachyarrythmia

Mitral and aortic regurgitation can cause pounding of the heart. This may be described by the patient as "palpitation".

♣ **Systemic Factors**

Thyrotoxicosis

Claudication

Claudication refers to pain in the lower extremities on exertion. It may be due to:

♥ **Internal Factors**

Anaemia, hyperviscosity

♠ **Mural Factors**

Spasm of vessels, atheroma, inflammation (thrombangitis obliterans or vasculitis)

Cold Extremities

The causes of cold extremities are similar to those that result in claudication. Claudication and cold extremities may occur together.

Raynaud's Phenomenon

In Raynaud's phenomenon, the patient complains of white, cold peripheries, which become blue and then red. With time atrophy occurs. The causes are:

◆ **Internal Factors**

Cryoglobulinaemia

♣ **Mural Factors**

Idiopathic

♥ **Systemic Factors**

LMS connective tissue disease

Drugs ergotamine

Raynaud's phenomenon is discussed in more detail in the chapter on the locomotor system.

Syncope

Syncope refers to a transient loss of consciousness due to decreased cerebral perfusion. Syncope may be due to:

♠ **Internal Factors**

Ball valve thrombus, left atrial myxoma

Orthostatic hypotension, which may be secondary to autonomic neuropathy, drugs, hypovolaemia

◆ **Mural Factors**

Arrhythmia either tachy or brady arrhythmia or pacemaker malfunction

Hypertrophic obstructive cardiomyopathy

Pulmonary stenosis, aortic stenosis, aortic dissection, subclavian steal syndrome, carotid sinus syndrome

♣ **External Factors**

Cardiac tamponade

♥ **Systemic Factors**

CNS vasovagal attack, vertebrobasilar disease

RS cough syncope, pulmonary embolism, pulmonary hypertension

KUS micturition syncope

GIT deglutition syncope

Findings on Examination

The abnormalities that may be detected on clinical examination are as follows:

General Examination

On general examination of the patient one may note abnormalities of:

◆ Dimensions

♣ Integument

♥ Body temperature

Dimensions

On examination of the dimensions one may detect abnormalities of the following:

♠ Posture

◆ Height and proportions

♣ Weight and shape

Posture

One may note an abnormal posture of the patient. This could be:

- ♠ A marked kyphosis could indicate ankylosing spondylitis and suggest the presence of aortic incompetence.
- ♦ Orthopnoea would suggest left-heart failure.

Height

Variations in the height of the patient could be:

- ♠ Tall Stature
- ♥ Short Stature

Tall Stature

In a very tall patient it would be important to assess the proportions of the body. An increased height with eunuchoid proportions would suggest Marfan's syndrome or Klinefelter's syndrome.

Marfan's syndrome

Autosomal dominant inheritance. The striking feature is elongation of the tubular bones. The patient would be tall; the lower segment of the body from the soles of the feet to the pubis would be longer than the upper segment from the crown to the pubis. The arm span, measured between the tips of fingers with arms extended, would be greater than the height. The face would be elongated (dolicocephaly) and the digits of the hands would be long (arachnodactyly). Upward subluxation or dislocation of the lens may occur and the patient may have myopia and retinal detachment. A high arched palate would be observed. Due to elongation of the ribs there may be pectum excavatum or carinatum. Loose joints may cause recurrent joint dislocation. There would be kyphoscoliosis and pes planus. Pulmonary cysts may occur and this may result in spontaneous pneumothorax.

The cardiac complications are dissection of the aorta, aortic regurgitation and mitral regurgitation.

Homocystinuria

Homocystinuria is similar to Marfan's syndrome. The patient may have aortic regurgitation, mitral regurgitation. Vascular thromboses may occur. There is associated mental subnormality. Dislocation of the lens occurs and it would be a downward dislocation.

Klinefelter's syndrome

47 XXY commonly

The features of Klinefelter's syndrome are tall stature with the lower segment longer than the upper segment. Long extremities. There are learning difficulties, gynaecomastia and associated autoimmune endcorinopathies. Cardiac abnormalities may be atrial or ventricular septal defects, tetralogy of Fallot

Short Stature

Short stature could be due to:

♣ **Genetic Conditions**

Ellis van Creveld syndrome, Turner's syndrome, Noonan's syndrome, Down's syndrome

♥ **Chronic Disease of Childhood**

Congenital heart disease, rheumatic heart disease

Ellis van Creveld Syndrome

The features are skeletal deformities, abnormalities of the nails and mouth. The cardiac abnormalities may be atrial septal defect or single atrial chamber.

Turner's Syndrome

45 XO

The features of Turner's syndrome are short stature, increased carrying angle at the elbow, webbed neck, shield chest, amenorrhoea. The associated cardiac abnormalities could be coarctation of the aorta, bicuspid aortic valve, aortic stenosis

Noonan's Syndrome (Male Turner's)

Autosomal dominant inheritance

The features of Noonan's syndrome are short stature, mild mental retardation, hypertelorism, webbed neck, skeletal abnormalities. The associated cardiac abnormalities could be pulmonary stenosis, atrial septal defect, hypertrophic obstructive cardiomyopathy.

Weight

Weight could be:

♥ Increased

♠ Decreased

Increased Weight

Increased weight could be due to

♠ Oedema

♦ Obesity

♣ Endocrine disease

The shape of the patient would indicate what the increase in weight is due to.

Decreased Weight

Decreased weight would suggest cardiac cachexia.

♥ Cardiac cachexia is seen in end stage cardiac failure and results in nutritional failure with decompensation causing emaciation with ascites and oedema. The characteristic shape would be a thin upper body and upper limbs with protuberant belly and swollen ankles due to fluid retention. One should bear in mind that fluid retention may result in an increased weight and a normal body mass index (BMI).

Shape

Changes in the overall shape of the body may be:

♠ In coarctation of the aorta the upper body and limbs would be better developed than the lower body and limbs.

♦ In cardiac cachexia the patient would have a skeletal appearance with associated potbelly and dependent oedema.

Integument

When examining the integument one may note changes in the following:

♣ Colour

♥ Surface

♠ Consistency

Colour of the Skin

The colour of the patient may give a clue to underlying disease. The colour change may be:

♣ Pigmentation

♥ Pallor

♠ Cyanosis

Pigmentation

Pigmentation could suggest:

♦ Haemochromatosis, which may cause restrictive cardiomyopathy

♣ *Café au lait* spots are a feature of neurofibromatosis, which is associated with phaeochromo-cytoma and cardiac tumours

Pallor

Pallor could indicate:

♥ Anaemia

♠ Shock

♦ Dresden Doll Appearance

Anaemia

The associations are:

♣ Anaemia may exacerbate congestive cardiac failure or ischaemic heart disease.

♥ Anaemia would be a feature of subacute bacterial endocarditis.

♠ In aortic stenosis iron deficiency anaemia may occur due to associated angiodysplasia of the colon.

Shock

Shock may occur in:

♦ Myocardial infarction

♣ Pulmonary embolism.

179

Dresden Doll Appearance

A very pale appearance similar to a china doll may be associated with:

♥ Aortic stenosis.

Cyanosis

Cyanosis occurs in the presence of over 5 g/dl of deoxygenated haemoglobin in the blood. It may be either central or peripheral. The presence of methhaemoglobin or sulph-haemoglobin may give a similar appearance.

Types of Cyanosis

Cyanosis may be:

♣ Peripheral Cyanosis

♥ Central Cyanosis

Peripheral Cyanosis

Peripheral cyanosis is due to excessive uptake of oxygen from the blood and is due to poor peripheral perfusion and may occur in:

♠ Cardiovascular collapse with resultant intense vasoconstriction

♦ Peripheral vascular disease or Raynaud's phenomenon would cause localised areas of peripheral cyanosis

Central Cyanosis

Central cyanosis may be due to:

♣ Polycythaemia

♥ Pulmonary Oedema

♠ Cyanotic Heart Disease

Polycythaemia

Polycythaemia causes suffusion or reddening of the skin (plethora) with a cyanotic tinge to the nose lips, ears, hands and feet. Polycythaemia may be:

♦ Primary

♣ Consequent on cyanotic heart disease

♥ Indicate excessive smoking

Pulmonary Oedema

Pulmonary oedema occurs in:

♠ Left-heart failure

Cyanotic Heart Disease

Cyanotic heart disease could be due to:

♦ Right to left shunts

♣ Reversal of left to right shunts following development of pulmonary hypertension

Right to Left Shunts

Right to left shunts occur in:

♥ Fallot's tetralogy

♠ Transposition of the great vessels

Reversed Left to Right Shunts (Eisenmenger syndrome)

Reversal of left to right shunts occurs following development of pulmonary hypertension in:

♦ Atrial septal defect

♣ Ventricular septal defect

♥ Patent ductus arteriosus

Reversal of the shunt in patent ductus arteriosus results in differential cyanosis with cyanotic lower limbs and acyanotic upper limbs.

Surface of the Skin

Abnormalities that may be noted on the surface of the skin are:

♦ Excessive Sweating

♣ Dry Skin

♥ Oily Skin

Excessive Sweating

Excessive sweating would suggest:

♠ Thyrotoxic heart disease

♦ A cold sweat would suggest myocardial infraction. This would also occur in cardiogenic shock

Dry Skin

Dry skin would suggest:

♣ Hypothyroidism

Oily Skin

The skin would be oily in:

♥ Cushing's syndrome where the patient may be hypertensive.

Consistency of the Skin

The change that may be detected in the consistency of the skin is lax skin.

Lax Skin

Lax skin would suggest:

♠ Ehlers-Danlos syndrome

♦ Pseudoxanthoma elasticum.

The associated cardiac abnormalities could be dissection of the aorta, aneurysm of the sinus of Valsalva (aortic sinus), mitral valve prolapse. In pseudoxanthoma elasticum coronary artery disease and renovascular hypertension may occur.

Body Temperature

Fever

In relation to the cardiovascular system, fever would suggest:

♣ Bacterial endocarditis. This usually causes a low-grade fever but it may become a swinging fever if a paravalvar abscess develops

♥ Left atrial myxoma

♠ Dressler's syndrome or post-myocardial infarction syndrome. This occurs weeks or months after a myocardial infarction.

Regional Examination

The abnormalities that may be detected on regional examination are as follows:

Head

When examining the head in general one may note abnormalities of:

♦ Dimensions

♣ Integument

♥ Movement

Dimensions

On examination of the dimensions one may note abnormalities of the following:

♠ Size

♦ Length

♣ Shape

♥ Overall appearance

Size

Variations in the size of the head may be:

♦ A large head with prominent features would be seen in acromegaly where hypertension, cardiomyopathy and conduction defects may occur.

♣ The head would be bloated in superior vena cava obstruction

Length

The length of the head may be:

♥ Long (dolicocephaly) in Marfan's syndrome

♠ Short (brachycephaly) in Down's syndrome

Shape

The shape of the head would also give clues to associated disease.

♦ In acromegaly the facial features would be very prominent.

♣ In Cushing's syndrome and hypothyroidism the face would be rounded.

Cushing's syndrome is associated with hypertension

Hypothyroidism is associated with coronary artery disease, heart failure, pericardial effusion and bradycardia

♥ In Paget's disease of bone there may be enlargement of the vault of the skull. Paget's disease may cause high output cardiac failure.

♠ A gaunt or skeletal appearance would occur in cardiac cachexia

Overall Appearance of the Face

The overall appearance of the face may be characteristic of certain conditions.

♦ Hurler's syndrome (gargoylism). In this condition mitral or aortic valve disease may occur.

♣ A round, chubby face is associated with congenital pulmonary stenosis (valvular)

♥ An elfin face may be associated with congenital pulmonary artery stenosis and aortic stenosis (supra valvar), coarctation of the aorta, brachiocephalic artery stenosis. The elfin face is characterised by wide set eyes, cheeks that are baggy, thick lips, malformation of teeth and small chin. The patient may also have hypercalcaemia and may be mentally subnormal.

♠ Down's syndrome (Trisomy 21). The features would be a round face, prominent epicanthic fold, low nasal bridge, fissured tongue and hypoplastic ears. Associations are atrial septal defect, ventricular septal defect, tetralogy of Fallot, patent ductus arteriosus, coarctation of the aorta, transposition of the great vessels.

♦ Noonan's syndrome and Turner's syndrome have already been described.

Integument (Cover)

The skin over the face may be abnormal.

♣ The face would be discoloured in obstruction of the superior vena cava.

Movement

One may note abnormal movement of the head as a whole.

♥ Head nodding may occur in aortic incompetence. This is known as de Musset's sign

Nose

On examination of the nose one may note abnormalities of the following features:

Size

The size of the nose may be:

♠ Increased in acromegaly

Shape

The shape of the nose would change in certain conditions.

♦ A saddle nose may be seen in relapsing polychondritis. In this condition the associated feature would be aortic aneurysm.

♣ An upturned nose is a feature of elfin facies.

♥ A beak shaped nose occurs in scleroderma.

Eyes

On examination of the eyes one may note abnormalities of the following:

Orbits

One may note changes in:

Position

On examination of the orbits one may note variation in the position of the orbits.

♠ The orbits may be widely spaced. This is known as hypertelorism and is a feature of Turner's syndrome and Noonan's syndrome.

Eyeballs

When examining the eyeballs one may note change in:

Size

Abnormalities that may be noted in the size of the eyes are:

♦ An apparent increase in the size of the eyes would be seen in thyroid ophthalmopathy

♣ Enophthalmos may be noted in Horner's syndrome. Horner's syndrome may be caused by carotid or aortic aneurysms.

Eyelids

Abnormalities that may be noted in the eyelids are:

Position

The position of the eyelids may be abnormal:

♥ Ptosis would be observed in myotonia dystrophica

♠ Ptosis would occur in Horner's syndrome

Shape

The shape of the eyelids may be abnormal:

♠ A mongoloid slant occurs in Down's syndrome.

♦ An antimongoloid slant occurs in Noonan's syndrome.

♣ An epicanthic fold occurs in Down's syndrome

Surface

Lesions that may occur on the surface of the eyelids are:

♥ The surface may show plaques (xanthelasma) indicating hyper-lipidaemia and associated ischaemic heat disease

Consistency

The consistency of the eyelids may change with:

♠ Periorbital oedema in hypothy-roidism

Colour

Changes in the colour of the eyelids could be:

♦ Purple discoloration is seen in dermatomyositis where cardiomyopathy, conduction defects and pericarditis may occur

Lacrimal Glands

Abnormalities that may occur in the lacrimal glands are:

♣ The lacrimal glands may be enlarged in sarcoidosis where restrictive cardiomyopathy or conduction defects may occur.

Conjunctiva

The abnormalities that may occur in the conjunctiva are:

♦ A pale conjunctiva would be a feature of anaemia

♣ Conjunctival haemorrhage is a feature of infective endocarditis

Sclera

Changes that may be noted in the sclera are:

♥ The sclera would be blue in osteo-genesis imperfecta where mitral regurgitation may occur. It may also be blue in Ehlers-Danlos syndrome and Marfan's syndrome

♠ The sclera would be icteric in congestion of the liver consequent on congestive cardiac failure, tricuspid regurgitation, pericardial tamponade or constriction. Jaundice may also occur as a result of haemolysis caused by prosthetic heart valves.

Cornea

On examination of the cornea one may note:

♦ The presence of a white ring or arcus senilis would indicate hyperlipidaemia and consequent ischaemic heart disease.

Iris

Abnormalities of the iris could be:

♣ Coloboma of the iris refers to a defect in the iris and this may be associated with total anomalous pulmonary venous drainage.

♥ Brushfield spots are small, white areas that are seen in Down's syndrome.

Lens

Abnormalities that may be noted are:

- ♠ The lens may be dislocated from its normal site in Marfan's syndrome. The dislocation is upward.

- ♦ Homocystinuria also causes dislocation of the lens but here the dislocation is downward.

- ♣ In congenital rubella cataracts are seen. Other features that occur are deafness, patent ductus arteriosus, stenosis of the pulmonary artery

Fundus

Abnormalities that may be detected in the fundus are:

- ♥ Hypertensive retinopathy

- ♠ Roth spots are haemorrhages with central pale areas. They are seen in subacute bacterial endocarditis

- ♦ Angioid streaks occur in pseudoxanthoma elasticum.

Hypertensive Retinopathy

Hypertensive retinopathy may be graded as:

- ♣ **Grade 1**

  Where thickened vessels give a copper or silver wiring effect

- ♥ **Grade 2**

  Where features of grade 1 occur together with arteriovenous nipping

- ♠ **Grade 3**

Features of grade 2 together with flame shaped haemorrhages and soft or cotton wool exudates

- ♥ **Grade 4**

  Features of Grade 3 and papilloedema

3rd, 4th and 6th Cranial Nerves

On examination of cranial nerves 3, 4 and 6 one may detect:

- ♠ Argyll Robertson pupil in tertiary syphilis where aortic incompetence and aneurysm of the ascending aorta may occur

- ♦ Horner's syndrome may be caused by carotid or aortic aneurysm

Face

On examination of the face one may note abnormalities of the following:

Scalp

Abnormalities that may be noted on examination of the scalp are:

- ♦ Alopecia may occur in hypothyroidism, systemic lupus erythematosus, myotonia dystrophica. The pattern of balding may help to differentiate these conditions.

> Steinert disease is a condition in which myotonia dystrophica, conduction disorders and mitral valve prolapse occur.

- ♣ The sheen of the hair would be lost in hypothyroidism

185

Forehead

On examination of the forehead one may note:

- ♥ Thickened skin folds. They are a feature of acromegaly.

Eyebrows

Changes that may be seen are:

- ♠ Loss of the outer third of the eyebrows would suggest hypothyroidism

Malar Region

When examining the malar region one may note abnormalities of the following:

Surface

On the surface of the skin in the malar region one may note a rash.

Rash

Rashes that may occur over the malar region are:

- ♦ A butterfly rash may be observed in systemic lupus erythematosus where endocarditis, myocarditis and pericarditis may occur. Libmann-Sachs endocarditis or non-infective endocarditis of the mitral valve is rare. Treatment of this condition with steroids may ultimately lead to mitral stenosis.
- ♣ Adenoma sebaceum. In this condition intramural rhabdomyomata and pedunculated tumours of the heart may occur.

Circulation

Changes in the circulation over the malar region are:

- ♥ **Flush**

  A flush may occur in the malar region in mitral valve disease. Flushing would also be a feature of the carcinoid syndrome where tricuspid incompetence and pulmonary stenosis may occur.

- ♠ **Telangiectasia**

  Telangiectasia may be seen in:

  Cushing's syndrome, systemic sclerosis

Mouth

On examination of the mouth one may note abnormalities of the following:

Jaw

On examination of the jaw one may note changes in:

Size

One may observe variations in the size of the jaw.

- ♦ A large jaw or prognathos is seen in acromegaly
- ♣ A small jaw or agnatha is feature of the Pierre-Robin syndrome

Lips

When examining the lips one may note abnormalities of:

Size

The size of the lips may be:

- ♥ Small in systemic sclerosis where pulmonary hypertension, myocarditis and pericarditis could occur
- ♠ The lips may be thick and patulous in elfin facies.
- ♦ Thick lips would be a feature of acromegaly

Colour

The colour of the lips could differ from normal.

- ♣ Central cyanosis would be seen in the lips

Teeth

On examination of the teeth the abnormalities one may note are:

- ♥ The teeth would be widely separated in acromegaly.
- ♠ Dentogenesis imperfecta is the dental manifestation of osteogenesis imperfecta.

Tongue

Abnormalities that one may observe when examining the tongue are:

- ♦ Macroglossia. The tongue may be large in Down's syndrome, acromegaly, amyloidsosis. Restrictive cardiomyopathy may occur in amyloidsosis.
- ♣ Central cyanosis would be observed in the tongue

Palate

The palate would be high arched in:

- ♥ Marfan's syndrome
- ♠ Supravalvar aortic stenosis

Uvula

On examination of the uvula one may observe:

- ♦ Systolic pulsation of the uvula may occur in aortic regurgitation (Muller's sign)

Speech

Abnormalities that may be noted are:

- ♣ **Hoarse Voice**

  Hoarseness may be due to recurrent laryngeal nerve palsy caused by:

  Enlarged left atrium in mitral stenosis, aneurysm of the arch of the aorta

Ears

One may observe abnormalities of the:

Dimensions

Changes that may be detected in the dimensions of the ears are:

Size

Variations in size could be:

- ♥ Small ears would be seen in Down's syndrome.

Shape

Variations in shape could be:

- ♠ Deformity of the pinna may be observed in relapsing polychondritis

Surface

Abnormalities that may be detected on the surface of the ears are:

♦ An earlobe crease may be seen in patients with coronary artery disease

Upper Limbs

On general examination of the upper limbs one may note abnormalities of the:

Dimensions

Changes that one may observe are:

♣ Long upper limbs would be a feature of Marfan's syndrome

♥ Thin limbs in relation to the trunk would be a feature of Cushing's syndrome.

♠ Swollen upper limbs would occur in venous obstruction. In axillary vein thrombosis, the affected limb would be swollen, the superficial veins would be distended and the veins will not collapse when raised above the level of the heart. Bilateral changes would suggest superior vena cava (SVC) obstruction.

Hands

On examination of the hands one may note abnormalities of the:

Dorsum of the Hands

One may detect changes in the:

Dimensions

One may detect abnormalities of the size and shape of the hands.

Size

The size of the hands may be:

♠ Increased in acromegaly, obesity, hypothyroidism, primary amyloidosis and in those engaged in manual work.

♦ Unilateral enlargement occurs in oedema due to venous or lymphatic obstruction. Disuse after a hemiplegia may also cause oedema.

♣ An apparent contraction may be observed in scleroderma.

♥ Small hands and fingers are seen in Down's syndrome.

Shape

Variations in the shape of the hands that would be of significance are:

♠ Long spidery fingers or arachnodactyly are a feature of Marfan's syndrome.

♦ In scleroderma tapered fingers would be observed.

♣ In the Holt-Oram syndrome hypoplastic thumbs and accessory phalanges may be seen.

Nails

On examination of the nails one may note changes in the:

♥ Dimensions

♠ Colour

♦ Surface

♣ Connections

♥ Circulation

Dimensions

The main change in dimensions that would be of significance is a change in shape.

Shape

Significant changes in the shape of the nails are:

♥ Clubbing

♠ Koilonychia

Clubbing

Clubbing would suggest:

♦ Subacute infective endocarditis

♣ Cyanotic congenital heart disease

♥ Eisenmenger syndrome

♠ Unilateral clubbing occurs in arterio-venous malformations

Koilonychia

Koilonychia would indicate:

♦ Iron deficiency anaemia

Colour

Colour changes that one may observe in the nails are:

♦ Red lunulae would signify heart failure.

♣ Cyanosis may be observed in the nails

Surface

The surface of the nails may be abnormal.

♥ Beau's lines may be observed indicating growth arrest due to severe illness such as fever, cachexia, malnutrition.

Connections

Disturbance of the connections of the nails are:

♠ The attachment of the nail to the nail bed may be disrupted in onycholysis, which could indicate thyrotoxicosis.

Circulation

The blood vessels in the nail bed may show:

♦ Splinter haemorrhages, which could indicate infective endocarditis.

♣ Quincke's Sign

Quincke's sign is demonstrated by using the examining thumb to exert slight pressure on the distal extremity of the nail. This will cause blanching of the distal nail bed and thus create a line of demarcation between the blanched white region and the normal pink nail bed. In severe aortic regurgitation this line will pulsate with each heartbeat as blood flows in during systole and flows back with regurgitation in diastole.

Skin

The mobility of the skin over the dorsum of the hands may be abnormal.

♥ Contracted non-mobile skin occurs in scleroderma.

♠ Excess mobility may be due to pseudoxanthoma elasticum, Ehlers-Danlos syndrome.

Palms

The lesions that one may note on the palms of the hands are the following:

- ♦ A transverse palmar crease may be seen in Down's syndrome

- ♣ Erythematous macules or Janeway lesions may be seen on the palms in infective endocarditis.

- ♥ Palmar xanthomata are seen in hyperlipidaemia.

- ♠ Sweating and:

    Warm skin would indicate thyrotoxicosis or fever

    Cold skin would indicate cardiovascular collapse

    Normal temperature may be due to hyperhidrosis.

- ♦ Osler's nodes are tender, erythematous, nodules in the pulp of the fingers that may occur in infective endocarditis.

Joints

The lesions that may be observed in the joints of the hands are:

- ♣ Deformity and swelling of rheumatoid disease may indicate the presence of associated features such as coronary arteritis, pericarditis, myocarditis and valvular heart disease such as aortic and mitral regurgitation.

- ♥ Hyperextensible joints occur in Marfan's syndrome and in Ehlers-Danlos syndrome.

Tendons

One may note:

- ♠ Tendon xanthomata. These are nodules on the tendons and they are indicative of hyperlipidaemia.

Peripheral Circulation

When assessing the peripheral circulation one may note:

- ♦ Warm skin would indicate a hyperdynamic circulation as seen in thyrotoxicosis, fevers.

- ♣ Cold skin would indicate poor peripheral circulation due to:

    Localised insufficiency such as peripheral vascular disease or Raynaud's phenomenon

    Generalised changes due to a cardiovascular collapse or heart failure.

Poor peripheral circulation would be associated with an increase in capillary refill time.

Radial Pulse

On examination of the radial pulse one may note abnormalities of:

- ♥ Rate
- ♠ Rhythm
- ♦ Volume
- ♣ Character
- ♥ Transmission

Rate

Variations in the pulse rate could be:

- ♥ Bradycardia
- ♠ Tachycardia

Bradycardia

Bradycardia refers to a pulse rate of less than 60 beats per minute. Bradycardia may be:

♦ Sinus Bradycardia

♣ Atrioventricular block

Sinus Bradycardia

In sinus bradycardia the rhythm is regular. The causes of sinus bradycardia are conditions affecting the:

♥ **Sinoatrial Node**

Sinoatrial disease (sick sinus syndrome)

Myocardial infarction

♠ **Systemic Factors**

E&M hypothyroidism, hypothermia, hyperkalaemia

CNS raised intracranial pressure

GIT obstructive jaundice

Drugs beta-blockers, calcium antagonists

It could be physiological in athletes

Atrioventricular Block

Atrioventricular block or impairment of atrioventricular conduction may be:

♦ First-degree atrioventricular block

♣ Second-degree atrioventricular block

♥ Third-degree atrioventricular block (Complete heart block)

First-degree Atrioventricular Block

First-degree atrioventricular block refers to an increased PR interval. This cannot be detected on examination of the pulse. It may be physiological in young people and in well-trained athletes.

Second-degree Atrioventricular Block

Second-degree atrioventricular block causes intermittent loss of atrioventricular conduction. Second-degree atrioventricular block could be of two types:

♠ Type I varying PR interval (Wenckebach)

♦ Type II fixed PR interval

These conditions would result in dropped beats of the pulse.

Complete Heart Block

In complete heart block there is complete loss of atrioventricular conduction. In complete heart block the pulse rate is usually less than 40 beats per minute. The pulse volume would vary if atrial contraction were preserved as this would result in a variation in end-diastolic volume. The causes of heart block include conditions primarily affecting the:

♣ **CVS** endocarditis, calcific aortic stenosis, idiopathic fibrosis, ischaemic heart disease, cardiomyopathy

♥ **E&M** hypothyroidism, haemochromatosis

♠ **RS** sarcoidosis, diphtheria

♦ **LMS** rheumatic fever, ankylosing spondylitis, Reiter's syndrome

♣ **IS** systemic sclerosis

♥ **RAG** syphilis

♠ **Surgery** aortic valve replacement, repair of a congenital defect, AV ablation in patients with SVT, alcohol septal ablation in patients with HOCM

♦ **Drugs** digoxin, beta-blockers, calcium channel blockers

Tachycardia

Tachycardia refers to a pulse rate of more than 100 beats per minute. Tachycardia may be:

♠ Sinus Tachycardia

♦ Supra Ventricular Tachycardia

♣ Atrial Flutter

♥ Ventricular Tachycardia

Sinus Tachycardia

Sinus tachycardia is part of the cardiovascular response to stress and is a feature of any serious illness. It is regular in rhythm and is seen in conditions involving the:

♠ **E&M** fever, thyrotoxicosis

♦ **HS** anaemia

♣ **CVS** cardiac failure

♥ **Physiological** in anxiety

Supra Ventricular Tachycardia

In supra ventricular tachycardia the pulse rate is usually 120-200 beats per minute. The rhythm and volume may vary with varying degrees of atrio-ventricular block. The causes of supra-ventricular tachycardia are conditions involving the:

♠ **CVS** Wolfe-Parkinson-White syndrome, Lown-Ganong-Levine syndrome, ischaemic heart disease

♦ **E&M** thyrotoxicosis

♣ **Drugs** caffeine and tobacco

Atrial Flutter

In atrial flutter the atrial rate is between 250-350 beats per minute. However, due to associated atrioventricular block, which is usually 2:1 or 4:1 more rarely 3:1, 5:1, the ventricular rate is slower. In atrial flutter the pulse rate is usually about 150 due to this associated atrioventricular block. The causes are conditions involving the:

♥ **CVS** ischaemic heart disease,

♠ **E&M** thyrotoxicosis

♦ **Drugs** digoxin toxicity

Ventricular Tachycardia

In ventricular tachycardia the rate is usually 120-200 beats per minute. The pulse would be feeble and irregular.

Rhythm

Abnormalities that one may detect in cardiac rhythm are:

♣ Sinus Arrhythmia

♥ Dropped Beats

♠ Coupled Beats

♦ Atrial Fibrillation

Sinus Arrhythmia

In sinus arrhythmia the heart rate increases with inspiration and decreases with expiration. This is a normal variation in children and young adults.

Dropped Beats

Dropped beats may be due to:

♠ Atrial ectopics

♦ Ventricular ectopics

♣ Second-degree atrioventricular block

The causes of dropped beats are conditions involving the:

♥ **CVS** ischaemic heart disease, cardiomyopathy

♠ **E&M** thyrotoxicosis

Multiple ventricular ectopics can result in an irregularly irregular pulse. The rhythm becomes normal after exercise.

Coupled Beats

Coupled beats or pulsus bigeminus is usually due to:

♦ Digoxin toxicity.

Atrial Fibrillation

An irregularly irregular rhythm occurs in atrial fibrillation. A difference between the heart rate and the pulse rate, an apex-radial deficit, usually occurs. The rhythm does not become normal after exercise. The causes of atrial fibrillation are:

♣ **Internal Factors**

Hypertension

♥ **Mural Factors**

Valvular heart disease especially mitral, Ebstein's anomaly, ischaemic heart disease, cardiomyopathy, myocarditis, sinoatrial disease, Wolfe-Parkinson-White syndrome, atrial septal defect

♠ **External Factors**

Constrictive pericarditis

♦ **Systemic Factors**

E&M thyrotoxicosis, fevers due to any infection but especially pulmonary

Toxins alcohol

RS pulmonary embolism, carcinoma of the bronchus, pneumonia

Pulse Volume

On evaluation of the pulse volume one may note:

♣ Large Volume Pulse

♥ Small Volume Pulse

♠ Variation in Volume with Respiration

Large Volume Pulse

An increased volume occurs when there is a hyperdynamic circulation. This occurs in involvement of the:

♦ **CVS** aortic regurgitation, arteri-ovenous shunts

♣ **E&M** fever, thyrotoxicosis

♥ **HS** anaemia

Small Volume Pulse

A small volume would indicate problems due to:

♠ **Internal Factors**

Decreased venous return in hypovolaemia.

♦ **Mural Factors**

Aortic stenosis, mitral stenosis, pulmonary hypertension. It could also indicate decreased myocardial contractility in heart failure

Variation in Volume with Respiration

Normally the pulse volume decreases with inspiration due to decreased venous return to the left atrium. This is exaggerated in conditions affecting the:

- ♣ **CVS** pericardial tamponade, constrictive pericarditis
- ♥ **RS** severe obstructive airways disease

This is known as pulsus parodoxus. It is only seen if the systolic blood pressure falls by 10 mm of Hg. The paradox is that the patient has a heartbeat without a palpable pulse.

To check for pulsus paradox using measurement of blood pressure, ask the patient to breathe as normally as possible. Inflate a blood pressure cuff and occlude the pulse. Deflate the cuff whilst auscultating and note the pressure at which sounds are heard in expiration. Continue to deflate the cuff until sounds are heard in inspiration as well and note this pressure.

Character

Variations that may occur in the character of the pulse are:

- ♠ Anacrotic Pulse
- ♦ Collapsing Pulse
- ♣ Pulsus Alternans
- ♥ Bisferiens Pulse
- ♠ Jerky Upstroke

Anacrotic Pulse

An anacrotic pulse shows a slow rise or upstroke and has a small volume. This occurs in:

- ♦ Aortic stenosis.

Collapsing Pulse

In a collapsing pulse a quick rise and a quick fall are observed. The pulse pressure is widened to greater than normal, which is 50 mm of Hg. The causes of a collapsing pulse are conditions affecting the following:

- ♣ **CVS** aortic regurgitation, patent ductus arteriosus, arteriovenous fistula, complete heart block
- ♥ **E&M** fever, thyrotoxicosis, thiamine deficiency
- ♠ **HS** anaemia
- ♦ **RAG** pregnancy
- ♣ **LMS** Paget's disease of bone
- ♥ **GIT** cirrhosis of the liver
- ♠ **IS** exfoliative dermatitis

Pulsus Alternans

Pulsus alternans is an alternating high and low volume pulse. This occurs in:

- ♦ Left ventricular failure

Bisferiens Pulse

Bisferiens pulse has a double upstroke. This is seen in:

- ♣ Mixed aortic valve disease (stenosis and incompetence)

Jerky Upstroke

A jerky upstroke occurs in:

- ♥ Hypertrophic obstructive cardiomyopathy

Transmission

Abnormalities of transmission of the radial pulse are:

- ♠ Radio-Femoral Delay
- ♦ Radio-Radial Delay
- ♣ Absent Radial Pulse

Radio-Femoral Delay

Radio-femoral delay occurs in

- ♥ Coarctation of the aorta
- ♠ Delayed or absent femoral pulses may also occur in aortic dissection where the dissection involves the descending aorta

Radio-Radial Delay

Radio-radial delay or absence of the left radial pulse occurs in:

- ♦ Dissecting aneurysm of the aorta. The importance of checking all pulses in cardiovascular examination, especially in patients presenting with chest pain, can never be overemphasised.

Absent Radial Pulse

An absent radial pulse may be due to:

- ♣ Embolism
- ♥ Congenital abnormality
- ♠ Blalock shunt
- ♦ Takayasu's arteritis
- ♣ Subclavian artery stenosis

Involuntary Movements of the Hands

Involuntary movements that may be observed are:

- ♥ An exaggerated physiological tremor would be seen in thyrotoxicosis
- ♠ A flapping tremor occurs in heart failure.
- ♦ Choreiform movements may be observed in rheumatic fever

Forearm and Elbow

Abnormalities that may be noted in the forearm and elbow are:

- ♣ An increased carrying angle would indicate Turner's syndrome.
- ♥ Eruptive xanthoma may be seen in hyperlipidaemia

Upper Arm

In the upper arm one may note abnormalities of the:

- ♠ Integument
- ♦ Brachial artery

Integument

Skin elasticity would be decreased in:

- ♠ Ehlers-Danlos syndrome, pseudoxanthoma elasticum

Brachial Artery

On examination of the brachial artery one may detect abnormalities of the pulse and blood pressure.

Pulse

Abnormalities that may be detected are:

- ♦ A thickened tortuous brachial artery may be observed. This is called locomotor brachialis and indicates severe arteriosclerosis.

♣ Brachio-radial delay occurs in aortic stenosis.

Blood Pressure

Variations in blood pressure may be:

♥ Low blood pressure

♠ High blood pressure

Low Blood Pressure

The causes of low blood pressure are:

♦ **Shock**

Shock may be due to:

Internal factors

Hypovolaemic shock, septic shock

Systemic Factors:

CVS cardiogenic shock

CNS neurogenic shock

Or conditions affecting the:

♣ **CVS** arrhythmias, heart failure, cardiac tamponade

♥ **E&M** adrenal failure, hypothermia

♠ **CNS** autonomic neuropathy

♦ **RAG** pregnancy

♣ **Drugs** antihypertensives, diuretics, antidepressants

♥ **Toxins** alcohol

♠ **RS** pulmonary embolism

High Blood Pressure

High blood pressure may be:

♥ **Essential or Multifactorial**

The other causes of elevated blood pressure are conditions involving the:

♠ **KUS**

Renal: polycystic kidneys, glomerulonephritis, renin secreting tumour

Pre Renal: renal artery stenosis

Post Renal: hydronephrosis

♦ **E&M** acromegaly, hyperparathyroidism, hypothyroidism, Cushing's syndrome, Conn's syndrome, phaeochromocytoma

Porphyria

♣ **CVS** coarctation of the aorta

♥ **HS** polycythaemia rubra vera

♠ **RAG** pregnancy, oral contraceptive use

Neck

On examination of the neck one may detect abnormalities of the following:

♦ Dimensions

♣ Integument

♥ Jugular Venous Pressure

♠ Carotids

♦ Trachea

Dimensions

On examination of the dimensions of the neck one may note abnormalities of size and shape.

Size

The size of the neck could be:

♣ Increased

♥ Decreased

Increased

The size of the neck could be increased in:

♣ Obesity

♥ Superior vena cava obstruction

Decreased

The size of the neck would be decreased in:

♠ Cardiac cachexia

Shape

An abnormality of the shape of the neck that may be noted is:

♦ Webbed neck. This would be a feature of Noonan's syndrome and Turner's syndrome

Skin

The elasticity of the skin would be decreased in:

♣ Pseudoxanthoma elasticum (a chicken skin appearance may be observed)

Jugular Venous Pressure (JVP)

When evaluating the jugular venous pressure one may note abnormalities of:

♥ Height

♠ Character

♦ Transmission

♣ Modifying factors

Height

Elevated JVP

An elevated jugular venous pressure may be:

♥ Pulsatile elevation

♠ Non-pulsatile elevation

Pulsatile Elevation

Pulsatile elevation of the JVP may be due to:

♥ **Internal Factors**

Fluid overload

♠ **Mural Factors**

Tricuspid stenosis, tricuspid regurgitation, right heart failure, congestive cardiac failure

♦ **External Factors**

Pericardial tamponade or pericardial constriction

Severe elevation may cause pulsation of the ear.

Non-Pulsatile Elevation

Non-pulsatile elevation of the jugular venous pressure occurs in:

♣ Superior vena cava obstruction

Character of the JVP

When assessing the character of the JVP one may note abnormalities of the:

♥ **a** wave

♠ **V** wave

♦ **x** descent

♣ **y** descent

a wave

Abnormalities of the **a** wave are:

♥ 197

- ♦ Loss of the **a wave**
- ♣ Dominant **a wave**
- ♥ Canon **a waves**

Loss of the a wave

Loss of the **a wave** occurs in:

- ♠ Atrial fibrillation.

Dominant a wave

A dominant **a wave** indicates increased right atrial pressure. This occurs in:

- ♦ Tricuspid Stenosis
- ♣ Right Ventricular Hypertrophy. This causes a dominant **a wave** due to the resultant reduced compliance of the right ventricle. Right ventricular hypertrophy can occur in pulmonary hypertension and in pulmonary stenosis.
- ♥ Right Ventricular Strain. This may occur in pulmonary embolism

Canon a waves

A canon **a wave** occurs when the right atrium contracts against a closed atrioventricular valve in:

- ♠ Complete heart block. These canon waves are irregular in rhythm.
- ♦ Regular canon waves occur in nodal rhythm

V wave

A dominant systolic **V wave** occurs in:

- ♣ Tricuspid regurgitation

Differentiation

The differentiation of **a** waves from **V** waves is made on the basis of timing. The **a** wave is pre-systolic whilst the **V** wave is systolic. Another point to note is that the **a** wave is a pressure wave. The pressure in the right atrium rises but no change in volume occurs. Pressure may be represented by the height of a column of liquid. Thus, when the right atrial pressure rises the height of the jugular venous pulse increases. This would be seen as a vertical movement of the column of blood in the vein. This is best observed by looking directly at the vein from the right-hand side of the patient.

On the other hand the **V** wave of tricuspid regurgitation represents a change in pressure and volume in the right atrium. Thus, the height of the column of blood in the vein rises but at the same time due to the change in volume the vein distends as well. This would cause an outward movement of the vessel wall that would be best seen by looking across the vessel. This is done by leaning across the patient and looking at the vein in silhouette from the left-hand side of the patient.

x descent

The **x descent** may be:

- ♣ Prominent
- ♥ Blunted

Prominent

A prominent (exaggerated) **x descent** occurs in:

- ♠ Acute cardiac tamponade
- ♠ Constrictive pericarditis

Blunting

Blunting (absence) of the **x descent** occurs in:

♦ Atrial fibrillation

y descent

The **y descent** may be:

♣ Prominent

♥ Slow

Prominent

A prominent (sharp) **y descent** occurs in:

♠ Constrictive   pericarditis (Friedrich's sign)

♦ Tricuspid regurgitation

Slow

A slow **y descent** occurs in:

♠ Tricuspid stenosis

♥ Right atrial myxoma

Transmission

Loss of Hepatojugular Reflux

Hepatojugular reflux would be lost if there is an obstruction at any point between the hepatic veins and the superior vena cava. This would occur in:

♣ **Budd Chiari Syndrome** (hepatic venous thrombosis)

♥ **Superior Vena Cava Obstruction**

Superior vena cava obstruction may be caused by carcinoma of the bronchus, lymphoma, aortic aneurysm, mediastinal fibrosis, retrosternal goitre.

Modifying Factors

Kussmaul's Sign

The jugular venous pressure diminishes during inspiration due to negative intrathoracic pressure and rises during expiration as intrathoracic pressure increases. In constrictive pericarditis this is reversed and the jugular venous pressure is increased during inspiration. This paradoxical rise in the jugular venous pressure during inspiration is known as Kussmaul's sign.

Causes of Constrictive Pericarditis

The causes of constrictive pericarditis are as follows:

♣ **Internal Factors**

Post-purulent pericarditis, tuberculous pericarditis

♦ **Mural Factors**

Post haemorrhagic (following surgery), neoplastic infiltration (primary or secondary)

♣ **External Factors**

Radiation therapy

♥ **Systemic Factors**

LMS connective tissue disorders such as rheumatoid arthritis, systemic lupus erythematosus, systemic sclerosis, polyarteritis nodosa, giant cell arteritis, rheumatic fever

KUS uraemia

RS Churg-Strauss syndrome

Carotid Pulse

On examination of the carotid pulse one may note the following abnormalities:

- ♠ Exaggerated visible carotid pulsation is known as Corrigan's sign and indicates aortic regurgitation.
- ♦ Expansile pulsation may occur due to a kinked carotid, unfolding of the aorta or due to an aneurysm of the carotid artery.
- ♣ A bruit would indicate stenosis of the carotid arteries

Arterial Pulsations in the Neck

Arterial pulsations, other than carotid pulsations, that may be observed in the neck are:

- ♥ Visible arterial pulsation in the suprasternal notch in a young person would indicate coarctation of the aorta.

Trachea

The features to note are:

- ♠ Comment on the position of the apex beat only if the trachea is in the midline. Otherwise it may reflect mediastinal shift rather than enlargement of the heart.
- ♦ A tracheal tug, descent of the aorta with each heartbeat, may be observed in the presence of a large aortic aneurysm.

Chest Wall

On examination of the chest wall one may note abnormalities of the dimensions and skin.

Dimensions

When assessing the dimensions of the chest one may detect abnormalities in relation to the shape of the chest.

Shape

Variations in the shape of the chest that may be of significance are:

- ♠ Pectum excavatum, pectum carinatum, kyphoscoliosis are features of Marfan's syndrome.
- ♥ Cardiomegaly, which occurs as a consequence of congenital heart disease or heart disease occurring in childhood (rheumatic carditis), may cause a localised deformity.
- ♠ A shield chest, which is a broad chest with widely spaced nipples, may occur in Turner's syndrome.

Skin

Changes in the skin would be the same as those described earlier. However, this is a good place to assess skin elasticity especially in elderly patients who may have lax skin elsewhere.

In addition one should note the following:

- ♥ Scars
- ♠ Pacemaker
- ♦ Gynaecomastia

Scars

Scars on the chest could be:

- A median sternotomy scar could indicate valve surgery or coronary artery bypass grafting.

- A left lateral thoracotomy could indicate mitral valve surgery

- A left lateral thoracotomy may also indicate previous surgery for repair of coarctation of the aorta. The late complications of repair of coarctation of the aorta are:

  Aortic aneurysm, aortic valve disease (because of associated bicuspid aortic valve), ischaemic heart disease, hypertension, re-stenosis

Pacemaker

The presence of a pacemaker would suggest the patient has:

- An arrhythmia probably a bradyarrythmia but it could be a tachyarrythmia

Gynaecomastia

Gynaecomastia may be due to:

- Klinefelter's syndrome

- **Drugs** digoxin, spironolactone, methyldopa

Heart

On examination of the heart one may detect abnormalities in relation to the following:

- Praecordial pulsation

- Apex beat

- Left parasternal heave

- Pulsations in the second right intercostal space

- Palpable heart sounds

- Thrills

- Abnormalities on percussion

- Abnormalities on auscultation

Praecordial Pulsation

Praecordial pulsation may be seen in:

- Right ventricular hypertrophy

- Mitral regurgitation

- Ventricular aneurysm.

Apex Beat

On examination of the apex beat one may note abnormalities of the following:

- Position

- Rate

- Character

Position

When examining the site or position of the apex beat one may note:

- Displaced Apex Beat

- Absent Apex Beat

Displaced Apex Beat

Displacement of the apex beat may be:

- True Displacement

- Apparent Displacement

True Displacement

Displacement of the apex beat may be due to ventricular dilatation caused by:

♥ Diastolic overload, which is seen in aortic regurgitation, mitral regurgitation, ventricular septal defect. In systolic overload and hypertrophy of the ventricle the apex beat is not displaced much.

♠ Systolic heart failure

Apparent Displacement

The apex beat may be apparently displaced due to:

♦ Skeletal abnormalities such as pectum excavatum or scoliosis

♣ Mediastinal shift

Absent Apex Beat

Absence of the apex beat or an apex beat that is difficult to palpate may be due to problems in the:

♣ **Chest Wall**

Obesity

♥ **Lungs**

Emphysema

♠ **Pericardium**

Pericardial effusion or pericardial constriction

♦ **Heart**

Dextrocardia

Rate

On counting the apex rate one may note:

♣ Apex-radial deficit. A difference between the apex rate and the pulse rate would be noted in atrial fibrillation (usually done on auscultation of the heart)

Character

Variations in the character of the apex beat are the following:

♥ Thrusting apex

♠ Heaving apex

♦ Right ventricular impulse

♣ Tapping apex

♥ Double Impulse

Thrusting Apex

A thrusting apex beat is due to diastolic overload and is seen in:

♥ Mitral regurgitation

♠ Aortic regurgitation

♦ Ventricular septal defect

Heaving Apex

A heaving apex beat signifies systolic overload and occurs in:

♣ Aortic stenosis

♥ Coarctation of the aorta

♠ Hypertension

Right Ventricular Impulse

A diffuse apical impulse would be a feature of:

♦ Right ventricular hypertrophy

Tapping Apex

A tapping apex indicates:

♦ Mitral stenosis. A tapping apex beat is a palpable first heart sound.

Double Impulse

A double impulse could indicate:

♣ Ventricular aneurysm

♥ Hypertrophic obstructive cardiomyopathy

Left Parasternal Heave

Left parasternal heave could indicate:

♠ Right ventricular hypertrophy

♦ Mitral regurgitation

Pulsation in the Second Right Intercostal Space

Pulsation in the second right intercostal space could occur with:

♣ A large aneurysm of the aorta (tertiary syphilis)

Palpable Heart Sounds

Palpable heart sounds could be:

♥ Palpable S_1

♠ Palpable S_1 and S_2

♦ Palpable P_2

S_1

A palpable S_1 occurs in:

♣ Mitral stenosis. The tapping apex in mitral stenosis is the palpable closure of the mitral valve

S_1 and S_2

S_1 and S_2 may be palpable in:

♥ Tachycardia

Palpable P_2

Palpable pulmonary valve closure occurs in:

♠ Pulmonary hypertension

Thrills

Thrills are palpable vibrations caused by very loud murmurs. Thrills may occur in the following regions:

♣ Base

♥ Apex

♠ Left Parasternal Region

♦ Second Left Intercostal Space

♣ Second Right Intercostal Space

♥ Infraclavicular Region

♠ Suprasternal Region

Base

Thrills occur at the base of the heart in:

♠ Aortic stenosis

♦ Pulmonary stenosis

The surface marking of the heart on the anterior aspect of the chest may be likened to a triangle with the three corners of the triangle being the second right intercostal space (just lateral to the sternum), the second left intercostal space (just lateral to the sternum) and the apex beat. The base of this triangle is the line joining the second left and second right intercostal spaces; the apex of the triangle is the apex beat.

Apex

Thrills occur at the apex of the heart in:

♣ Mitral stenosis

♥ Mitral regurgitation

Left Parasternal Region

Thrills may be felt in the left parasternal region in:

♠ Ventricular septal defect

♦ Hypertrophic obstructive cardiomyopathy

Second Left Intercostal Space

Thrills occur in the second left inter-costal space in:

♣ Patent ductus arteriosus

♥ Pulmonary stenosis

Second Right Intercostal Space

Thrills occur in the second right intercostal space in:

♥ Aortic stenosis

Infraclavicular Region

Thrills occur in the infraclavicular region in:

♥ Subclavian artery stenosis

Suprasternal Region

Thrills occur in the suprasternal region in:

♠ Coarctation of the aorta

Percussion Note

Abnormalities that may be detected on percussion are:

♠ Right parasternal dullness may occur in pericardial effusion and in left atrial enlargement.

♦ A discrepancy between the left border of the heart on percussion and the apex beat on auscultation

could indicate a pericardial effusion.

♣ Absent praecordial dullness would occur in dextrocardia

Auscultation

On auscultation of the heart one may note abnormalities of the heart sounds and in addition one may detect added sounds, murmurs and extra-cardiac sounds. In summary, one may detect abnormalities of:

♥ Heart Sounds

♠ Added sounds

♦ Murmurs

♣ Extra-cardiac sounds

Heart Sounds

Abnormalities may be noted of:

♥ S_1

♠ S_2

♦ S_1 and S_2

S_1

On auscultation of the first heart sound one may note variations in:

♦ Quantity

♣ Character

Quantity

The intensity of the first heart sound depends on the position of the mitral valve prior to commencement of systole. Normally the valve leaflets float upwards during diastole. Stiffening of the valve prevents this. In addition forceful atrial contraction will drive the valve leaflets apart in end diastole. Hence, in any condition that results in either stiffening of the valve or forceful atrial contraction the valve will be closing from a greater distance and the intensity of the sound produced will be greater. An analogy is the noise made by shutting a door from a fully opened and a partially closed position. The noise will be greater when the door is shut from a fully opened position.

Abnormalities of the intensity of the first heart sound are the following:

♥ Loud First Sound

♠ Soft First Hear Sound

♦ Varying Intensity of the First Heart Sound

Loud First Sound

The causes of a loud first heart sound are:

♦ In mitral stenosis the first heart sound would be loud because stiff valves do not float up readily in diastole and the forceful atrial contraction that occurs would drive the leaflets apart prior to systole. Hence, a loud first heart sound would signify mitral stenosis.

♣ Ebstein's anomaly. In this condition the presence of a sail like anterior leaflet of the tricuspid valve produces a loud first heart sound.

Soft First Hear Sound

A soft first heart sound occurs in:

♥ Mitral regurgitation

Varying Intensity of the First Heart Sound

The first heart sound would vary in intensity in the following:

♠ In varying atrio-ventricular block the effect of atrial systole on the presystolic position of the atrioventricular valves would vary giving variable intensity of the first heart sound.

♦ In complete heart block with maintenance of sino-atrial function, as atrial contraction and ventricular contraction are not synchronised, the effect of atrial contraction on the pre-systolic position of the atrioventricular valves will vary. This would cause varying intensity of the first heart sound.

♣ In atrial fibrillation, the irregular heart rate and consequent variable filling of the ventricle in diastole would cause varying intensity of the first heart sound. Again this is due to the varying pre-systolic position of the atrioventricular valves.

Character

Variations in the character of the first heart sound are:

♥ Click

♠ Splitting

Click

A click (closing click) would be heard instead of a first heart sound in the presence of a:

♦ Prosthetic mitral valve

Splitting

Splitting of S_1 is a feature of:

♣ Ebstein's anomaly

S$_2$

On auscultation of the second heart sound one may note variations in:

- ♥ Quantity
- ♠ Character

Quantity

The intensity of the second heart sound is dependent on the systemic and pulmonary artery pressures. The greater the pressure the more forceful the closure of the valves and thus a louder second heart sound. Valve thickening will decrease the intensity of the sound.

The intensity of the second heart sound may be:

- ♦ Loud
- ♣ Soft

Loud

A loud second heart sound could signify:

- ♥ Systemic hypertension
- ♠ Pulmonary hypertension

Soft

A soft second sound would occur in:

- ♦ Aortic stenosis

Character

Variations in the character of the second heart sound could be:

- ♥ Splitting
- ♠ Single Second Sound
- ♦ Click

Splitting

The second heart sound is made up of closure of the aortic and pulmonary valves. The aortic valve closes first (A before P). Pulmonary valve closure may be delayed in right bundle branch block due to delayed depolarisation of the right ventricle and in atrial septal defect due to increased blood flow through the right ventricle. This would cause splitting of the second sound. The presence of a shunt in atrial septal defect would balance blood flow in inspiration and expiration and hence the split would not vary with respiration.

A split would also occur in pulmonary stenosis as the right ventricle empties slowly in this condition. Here the pulmonary component would be soft.

Types of Split Second Sound

The types of splitting of the second sound are:

- ♣ Varying Split
- ♥ Fixed Split
- ♠ Reversed Split

Varying Split

Varying splitting of the second heart sound occurs in:

- ♦ Right bundle branch block
- ♣ Pulmonary stenosis

Fixed Split

Fixed splitting of the second heart sound occurs in:

- ♥ Atrial septal defect

Reversed Split

Reversed splitting that is widening of the split in expiration and narrowing during inspiration occurs when the pulmonary valve closes before the aortic. This occurs in:

♠ Severe aortic stenosis

♦ Left bundle branch block

♣ Right ventricular pacing

♥ Left ventricular failure

♠ Patent ductus arteriosus

The cause of splitting is delayed or slower contraction of one ventricle in relation to the other. If the right ventricle is affected the split widens, if the left ventricle is affected the split reverses.

Single Second Sound

Splitting would be lost and the second sound would be loud and single in:

♦ Pulmonary hypertension. This is due to the high pulmonary artery pressure causing earlier and more forceful closure of the pulmonary valve.

A single second sound could also be heard in:

♣ Calcified aortic stenosis (soft A_2)

♥ Pulmonary stenosis (soft P_2)

♠ Common truncus arteriosus

Click

A click (closing click) would be heard instead of the second heart sound in the presence of a:

♦ Prosthetic aortic valve

S_1 and S_2

Abnormalities that affect both S_1 and S_2 are variations in the intensity of the heart sounds.

Soft S_1 and S_2

S_1 and S_2 would be soft in conditions affecting the:

♣ **Chest Wall**

Obesity

♥ **Lungs**

Emphysema

♠ **Pericardium**

Pericardial effusion or pericardial constriction

♦ **Heart**

Dextrocardia

Dextrocardia

The heart sounds would be best heard on the right side in:

♣ Dextrocardia

Kartagener's syndrome

Kartagener described patients with dextrocardia, bronchiectasis and sinusitis. Most clinicians would include situs inversus, dysplasia of the frontal sinuses, otitis media and infertility in their definition.

Added Sounds

When analysing added sounds one may detect abnormalities in relation to the following:

Diastole

♣ Diastolic Opening Sounds

♥ S_3

♠ S_4

♦ Pericardial Knock

Systole

♣ Systolic Clicks

Diastolic Opening Sounds

Diastolic opening sounds may be:

♥ Opening snap

♣ Opening click

♦ Tumour plop

Opening Snap

An opening snap is caused by a thickened mitral valve snapping open. Thickening of the mitral valve occurs in mitral stenosis. The opening snap occurs in early diastole. The gap between the opening snap and the second heart sound is related to the left atrial pressure, which is dependent on the degree of valve stenosis. Hence, the narrower the gap between the opening snap and the second heart sound, the greater the stenosis.

Diastolic Opening Click

A diastolic opening click would be heard if the patient has a prosthetic mitral valve.

Tumour Plop

A tumour plop is the sound caused by a left atrial myxoma plopping through the mitral valve in early diastole.

S_3

A third heart sound is caused by vibrations created by the rapid entry of blood into the ventricle in diastole. This can occur in the:

♥ Left ventricle

♠ Right ventricle

Left Ventricular S_3

A left ventricular S_3 is best heard at the apex and occurs in:

♦ Heart failure

♣ Diastolic overload in mitral regurgitation, aortic regurgitation, ventricular septal defect

♥ High output states such as anaemia, thyrotoxicosis, fever, pregnancy

♠ Normal in young people

Right Ventricular S_3

A right ventricular S_3 is best heard at the left sternal edge or in the epigastric region or over the xiphoid process in emphysematous patients. It occurs in:

♦ Right ventricular failure

♣ Tricuspid regurgitation

S_4

A fourth heart sound is caused by vibrations created by forceful atrial contraction in the pre-systolic phase. This forceful contraction is a consequence of reduced compliance of the ventricle due to hypertrophy or cardiomyopathy. Thus it can result from:

♥ **Internal Factors**

Hypertension; systemic or pulmonary

Right ventricular strain (pulmonary embolism)

♠ **Mural Factors**

Aortic or pulmonary stenosis, myocardial infarction, hypertrophic obstructive cardiomyopathy, restrictive cardiomyopathy

The fourth heart sound disappears when pressure is applied to the chest piece of the stethoscope.

Pericardial Knock

A pericardial knock is caused by the sudden arrest of ventricular filling as a consequence of pericardial constriction in constrictive pericarditis.

Systolic Clicks

Systolic clicks may be:

- Ejection clicks
- Opening clicks
- Mid Systolic clicks

Ejection Clicks

Systolic ejection clicks are heard in:

- Stenosis or sclerosis of the aortic or pulmonary valves
- Bicuspid aortic valve
- Dilatation of the root of the aorta or pulmonary arteries

Systolic Opening Click

An opening click is caused by opening of a:

- Prosthetic aortic valve

Mid Systolic Click

A mid-systolic click would be heard in:

- Mitral valve prolapse

Murmurs

When evaluating murmurs one may note abnormalities in relation to the following features:

- Position
- Timing
- Quantity
- Transmission
- Modifying Factors

Position

The site at which murmurs are best heard is not always a good guide to their site of origin.

Murmurs may be best heard at the following sites:

- Apex
- Left sternal edge
- Xiphisternum
- Pulmonary area
- Aortic area
- Left subclavian area

Apex

Murmurs at the apex usually originate from the:

- Mitral valve
- Aortic murmurs may be heard here as well. The murmur of aortic stenosis may be better heard at the apex rather than the base particularly in elderly patients. Rarely, the murmur of aortic regurgitation may be better heard at the apex or even in the left axilla (Cole-Cecil murmur).

Left Sternal Edge

Murmurs at the left sternal edge may be due to:

- Ventricular septal defect
- Hypertrophic obstructive cardiomyopathy
- Aortic Incompetence

♥ Tricuspid Incompetence

Xiphisternum

Murmurs heard over the xiphisternum are caused by:

♠ Tricuspid regurgitation

Pulmonary Area

Murmurs in the pulmonary area may be due to:

♦ Pulmonary valve lesions

♣ Flow murmurs

Aortic Area

Murmurs in the aortic area are due to:

♥ Aortic valve lesions

Left Subclavian Area

Murmurs in the left subclavian area are due to:

♠ Patent ductus arteriosus

Timing

In analysing murmurs the most important consideration is the timing of the murmur. Murmurs may be:

♦ Systolic Murmurs

♣ Diastolic Murmurs

♥ Combination Murmurs

♠ Continuous Murmurs

Systolic Murmurs

Systolic murmurs may be:

♥ Ejection systolic

♠ Late systolic

♦ Pan systolic

Ejection Systolic Murmurs

Ejection systolic murmurs may be heard due to abnormalities affecting the following:

♥ Blood (Flow Murmurs)

♣ Aorta

♦ Aortic Valve

♠ Pulmonary Valve

♥ Mitral Valve

♣ Myocardium

Blood (Flow Murmurs)

Flow murmurs are caused by turbulence due to increased flow of blood across a normal valve. It usually occurs in the left ventricular outflow tract but may sometimes occur in the right. Flow murmurs occur due to conditions involving the:

♥ **E&M** fever, thyrotoxicosis

♠ **HS** anaemia

♦ **CVS** atrial septal defect (pulmonary outflow tract), large arteriovenous fistulae.

Aorta

An ejection systolic murmur may occur due to lesions in the aorta:

♣ Coarctation of the aorta causes turbulence at the aortic valve and thus causes a murmur at the base of the heart. Coarctation may also result in aortic regurgitation due to hypertension or associated aortic valve disease.

Aortic Valve

An ejection systolic murmur may occur due to lesions such as:

♥ Aortic stenosis

♠ Aortic sclerosis

- Prosthetic aortic valve
- Aortic regurgitation. This causes an ejection systolic murmur due to increased flow across the valve in systole.

Pulmonary Valve

An ejection systolic murmur may be caused by lesions in the pulmonary valve such as:

- Pulmonary stenosis
- Pulmonary sclerosis
- Pulmonary regurgitation. This may also cause a flow murmur

Mitral Valve

Mitral valve lesions may cause ejection systolic murmurs especially:

- Papillary muscle dysfunction
- Rupture of the chordae tendinae

Myocardium

Disorders of the myocardium that cause ejection systolic murmurs are:

- Hypertrophic obstructive cardiomyopathy

Late Systolic Murmur

A late systolic murmur may be heard in:

- Mitral valve prolapse

Pan Systolic Murmurs

Pan systolic murmurs are heard in:

- Ventricular septal defect
- Mitral regurgitation
- Tricuspid regurgitation.

Diastolic Murmurs

Diastolic murmurs may be:

- Early diastolic

- Mid-diastolic
- Pre-systolic

Early Diastolic Murmurs

Early diastolic murmurs are heard in:

- Aortic regurgitation
- Pulmonary regurgitation

Mid-Diastolic Murmurs

Mid diastolic murmurs occur in:

- Mitral or tricuspid stenosis
- The Carey-Coombs murmur is caused by swelling of the mitral valve leaflets in acute rheumatic fever and causes a flow murmur in mid-diastole.
- A left atrial myxoma may also cause a mid-diastolic murmur by obstructing blood flow across the mitral valve.
- A prosthetic mitral valve may cause a flow murmur
- Severe mitral regurgitation may cause a flow murmur in mid-diastole
- Atrial Septal Defect. An increase in the flow of blood across the tricuspid valve in atrial septal defect may result in a mid-diastolic murmur
- Ventricular Septal Defect (VSD). In VSD an increase in the flow of blood across the mitral valve may result in a mid-diastolic murmur
- Patent Ductus Arteriosus. A mid diastolic murmur may be heard at the apex due to increased flow across the mitral valve

- Lutembacher's Syndrome. This is a combination of atrial septal defect and mitral stenosis

Mitral murmurs are best heard at the apex or medial to the apex whilst tricuspid murmurs are best heard at the left sternal edge or over the xiphisternum.

Silent Mitral Stenosis

In the presence of a very tight mitral stenosis and pulmonary hypertension, the flow across the mitral valve may be so small that the murmur may be inaudible.

Pre-Systolic Murmurs

In mitral stenosis in sinus rhythm, pre-systolic accentuation of the diastolic murmur occurs. This is caused by forceful left atrial contraction

Combination Murmurs

Combination murmurs refer to the presence of more than one murmur. These murmurs may be due to:

- ♥ Single lesions
- ♠ Multiple lesions

Single Lesions

Single lesions that may result in combination murmurs are the following:

- ♦ Aortic Regurgitation

  Ejection systolic and early diastolic murmurs

- ♣ Pulmonary Regurgitation

  Ejection systolic and early diastolic murmurs

- ♥ Mitral Regurgitation

Pan systolic and mid-diastolic murmurs

- ♣ Atrial Septal Defect

  Ejection systolic and mid-diastolic murmurs

- ♥ Ventricular Septal Defect

  Pan systolic and mid-diastolic murmurs

Multiple Lesions

Multiple lesions may cause a number of combinations of murmurs. One combination of particular interest is the combination of early-diastolic and mid-diastolic murmurs.

Combination Early Diastolic and Mid Diastolic Murmurs

Combination early diastolic and mid diastolic murmurs are the following:

- ♠ The Graham-Steele murmur occurs when pulmonary incompetence complicates pulmonary hypertension consequent on long standing mitral stenosis. Thus, it is a combination of an early and a mid diastolic murmur.

- ♦ The Austin-Flint murmur occurs in aortic regurgitation. The flow of blood back into the ventricle in diastole causes the anterior leaflet of the mitral valve to be pushed backwards causing functional mitral stenosis. Thus, this too is a combination of an early and a mid-diastolic murmur.

Aide Memoire

Austin FlInt -Aortic Incompetence (AI)

GrahaM Steele-Mitral Stenosis **(MS)**

Continuous Murmurs

Murmurs that are continuous throughout systole and diastole occur in:

♣ Patent Ductus Arteriosus

Patent ductus arteriosus causes a continuous murmur best heard in the left subclavian area. It increases in expiration.

♥ Arterio-Venous Shunts

♠ Ruptured Sinus of Valsalva.

An aneurysm of the sinus of Valsalva may rupture either into the right atrium or right ventricle. It causes a continuous murmur either at the left or right sternal edge.

♦ Sinus of Valsalva Fistula

Sinus of Valsalva fistula may occur in aortic root disease complicating bacterial endocarditis

♣ Coronary Artery Fistulae

Coronary artery fistulae occur as a result of congenital anomalies of the coronary arteries and result in a continuous murmur at the left sternal edge

♥ Coarctation of the Aorta

In coarctation of the aorta a continuous murmur may be heard over the back or in the interscapular region due to increased blood flow through collateral vessels.

Quantity

The intensity of a murmur is not a good guide to the degree of valvular narrowing.

♠ In fact in mitral stenosis severe narrowing with resultant atrial fibrillation and pulmonary hypertension may result in a paradoxical silent mitral stenosis due to very low flow across the valve.

♦ In ventricular septal defect a small defect may result in a very loud murmur. *Maladie de Roger* is a small haemodynamically insignificant hole that closes spontaneously

Transmission

Characteristic transmission of murmurs is as follows:

♣ Aortic stenosis radiates to the neck.

♥ Mitral regurgitation radiates to the axilla and to the inferior angle of the scapula.

♠ Rupture of the posterior leaflet of the mitral valve causes radiation of the murmur to the base of the heart as the regurgitant jet of blood strikes the atrial wall adjacent to the aortic root.

Modifying Factors

Factors that may modify the intensity of a murmur are:

♦ Position

♣ Posture

♥ Respiration

♠ Exercise

Position

Variations in position that may influence the intensity of a murmur are:

- The left lateral position increases the intensity of mitral valve murmurs such as mitral stenosis and mitral regurgitation.

- Asking the patient to lean forward and hold his or her breath in expiration accentuates the murmur of aortic incompetence.

- A change in position may alter the murmur in left atrial myxoma.

Posture

Changes in the intensity of a murmur may be caused by changes in posture such as:

- Standing

- Squatting

Standing

Standing reduces venous return and thus:

- Standing decreases the murmur in pulmonary stenosis and aortic stenosis.

- Standing increases the murmur of mitral valve prolapse and hypertrophic obstructive cardiomyopathy (decreased cardiac volume).

Squatting

Squatting increases afterload thus:

- Squatting increases the murmur of aortic regurgitation, pulmonary regurgitation and mitral regurgitation.

- Squatting decreases the intensity of the murmur in hypertrophic obstructive cardiomyopathy (it increases left ventricular cavity size and decreases obstruction- similar to a PEEP valve)

Fallot's Tetralogy

In Fallot's tetralogy, on squatting the resultant increase in systemic arterial pressure reduces the right to left shunt. Hence, the patient finds this posture the most comfortable to adopt.

Respiration

Variations in the intensity of a murmur may be caused by:

- Inspiration

- Expiration

Inspiration

Inspiration increases venous return to the right side of the heart and thereby increases right-sided murmurs.

Expiration

Expiration increases venous return to the left side of the heart and thereby increases left-sided murmurs.

Exercise

Variations in the intensity of a murmur following exercise occur in:

- Mitral stenosis where the intensity of the mid-diastolic murmur is increased

Aetiology of Lesions

The causes of cardiac lesions that may present with a murmur are as follows:

Mitral Regurgitation

Mitral regurgitation could be due to a lesion in a component of the mitral valve apparatus, it could be due to a lesion in one of the adjacent structures of the heart or it could be due to a systemic cause.

Hence, mitral regurgitation could be due to lesions in the:

♥ **Papillary Muscle**

Papillary muscle dysfunction

Rupture of the papillary muscle in myomalacia cordis following myocardial infarction

♠ **Chordae Tendinae**

Rupture of the chordae tendinae due to infective endocarditis, mitral valve prolapse, trauma, rheumatic mitral valve disease

♦ **Valve Leaflets**

Rheumatic carditis, infective endocarditis, valvotomy, floppy mitral valves, degenerative changes

Prosthetic valve dysfunction

♣ **Valve Ring**

Left ventricular dilatation in heart failure, fibrosis, degeneration

Paraprosthetic mitral regurgitation

♥ **Septum**

Atrial septal defect (ostium primum)

♠ **Muscle**

Hypertrophic obstructive cardiomyopathy, endomyocardial fibrosis

♦ **Systemic Causes**

LMS Marfan's syndrome, osteogenesis imperfecta, systemic lupus erythematosus, rheumatic fever

IS Ehlers-Danlos syndrome, pseudoxanthoma elasticum

Severity of Mitral Regurgitation

The severity of mitral regurgitation may be judged clinically by the presence of left ventricular dilatation and the presence of a third heart sound. These features indicate more severe disease.

Mitral Valve Prolapse

Mitral valve prolapse could be:

♣ **Primary**

Or

♥ **Secondary**

Mitral valve prolapse could be secondary to systemic conditions such as those affecting the:

LMS Marfan's syndrome, rheumatic fever, osteogenesis imperfecta, systemic lupus erythematosus

KUS polycystic kidneys

RAG Turner's syndrome

CVS coronary artery disease, hypertrophic obstructive cardiomyopathy, left atrial myxoma, mitral valve surgery, congestive cardiomyopathy, myocarditis

CNS muscular dystrophy

IS Ehlers-Danlos syndrome, pseudoxanthoma elasticum

Mitral Stenosis

The causes of mitral stenosis are:

- ♠ Rheumatic carditis
- ♦ Rarely mitral stenosis may be congenital.
- ♣ Systemic lupus erythematosus (following Libmann Sachs endocarditis)
- ♥ Calcification

Severity of Mitral Stenosis

The severity of mitral stenosis may be judged clinically by the gap between the second heart sound and the opening snap and the duration of the murmur. The shorter the gap between the second sound and the opening snap the tighter the stenosis (indicates greater left atrial pressure). Likewise the longer the murmur the tighter the stenosis.

Left Atrial Myxoma

In left atrial myxoma, the signs are similar to those in mitral stenosis but the signs may vary with changes in posture.

Aortic Regurgitation

Aortic regurgitation may be due to lesions at the level of the following:

- ♠ **Valve**

  Infective endocarditis, rheumatic fever

  Prosthetic valve dysfunction

- ♦ **Valve Ring**

  Dilatation in aneurysm of the aorta, dissecting aneurysm, hypertension, coarctation of the aorta

  Paraprosthetic aortic regurgitation

- ♣ **Septum**

  Ventricular septal defect where there is loss of support for the valve.

- ♥ **Systemic Causes**

  LMS ankylosing spondylitis other seronegative arthropathies, rheumatic fever, Reiter's syndrome, rheumatoid arthritis, Marfan's syndrome, Hurler's syndrome

  IS psoriasis

  GIT ulcerative colitis

  RAG tertiary syphilis

Severity of Aortic Regurgitation

The severity of aortic regurgitation may be judged clinically by the pulse pressure, the intensity of the second heart sound, the presence of a left ventricular third heart sound, duration of the diastolic murmur, the presence of an Austin-Flint murmur and signs of left ventricular failure. The signs of severe aortic regurgitation are; the pulse pressure would be wide, the second heart sound would be soft, the early diastolic murmur would be shorter (as aortic and ventricular pressure equalise earlier) a third heart sound may be heard, left ventricular failure may occur and an Austin-Flint murmur may be heard.

Aortic Stenosis

Aortic stenosis could be:

- ♠ Valvular

♦ Subvalvular

♣ Supravalvular

Valvular

Valvular aortic stenosis may be due to the following:

♥ Congenital

♠ Bicuspid aortic valve

♦ Rheumatic heart disease

♣ Degenerative calcification

Subvalvular

Subvalvular aortic stenosis is due to:

♥ Hypertrophic obstructive cardiomyopathy

Supravalvular

Supravalvular aortic stenosis is due to a ring of fibrous tissue.

♠ Supravalvular aortic stenosis is seen in William's syndrome. The features of William's syndrome are hypercalcaemia, mental retardation, elfin facies, supravalvular aortic stenosis

Severity of Aortic Stenosis

The severity of aortic stenosis may be judged clinically by the presence of a narrow pulse pressure, brachioradial delay, a systolic thrill, a soft second heart sound, a single second sound or reversed split of the second heart sound, a fourth heart sound, signs of cardiac failure

Tricuspid Regurgitation

Tricuspid regurgitation may be due to:

♥ Right Ventricular Dilatation

♠ Primary Tricuspid Regurgitation

Right Ventricular Dilatation

Right ventricular dilatation with resultant tricuspid regurgitation occurs in:

♦ Mitral valve disease

♣ Cor pulmonale

♥ Pulmonary embolism

♠ Primary pulmonary hypertension

♦ Right ventricular failure

♣ Right ventricular infarction

♥ Eisenmenger syndrome

♠ Atrial septal defect

♦ Thyrotoxicosis

Primary Tricuspid Regurgitation

Primary tricuspid regurgitation may be due to:

♠ Rheumatic heart disease

♦ Infective endocarditis

♣ Ebstein's anomaly

♥ Endomyocardial fibrosis

♠ Papillary muscle infarction

♦ Carcinoid syndrome

In Ebstein's anomaly the giant right atrium absorbs the regurgitant jet of blood and a V wave is not seen in the neck

Tricuspid Stenosis

Tricuspid stenosis is caused by:

♦ Rheumatic heart disease

Pulmonary Stenosis

Pulmonary stenosis may be:

217

♣ Valvular

♥ Supravalvular

♠ Subvalvular or Infundibular

The causes of pulmonary stenosis are:

♦ Congenital

♣ Rheumatic carditis

♥ Carcinoid syndrome

Associated Conditions

Pulmonary stenosis may be associated with:

♠ Noonan's syndrome

Pulmonary Regurgitation

Pulmonary regurgitation may be:

♦ Valvular

Or due to

♣ Dilatation of the valve ring

Valvular Pulmonary Regurgitation

Pulmonary regurgitation due to valvular lesions may be:

♥ Congenital

♠ Acquired

Acquired pulmonary regurgitation occurs following endocarditis, trauma, rheumatic carditis

Dilatation of the Valve Ring

Dilatation of the valve ring with resultant pulmonary regurgitation occurs in:

♦ Pulmonary hypertension

♣ Idiopathic dilatation of the pulmonary artery

♥ Patent ductus arteriosus

Prosthetic Valve Dysfunction

Prosthetic valve failure could be due to:

♠ Thrombosis

♦ Mechanical failure

♣ Tear or perforation of the valve

♥ Calcification

♠ Stiffening of the leaflets

♦ Suture line dehiscence

Thrombosis may occur acutely or may be due to organised clot (pannus) slowly occluding the valve. Thrombosis presents as acute or chronic heart failure. Disappearance of a closing click is an associated physical sign.

The other causes of valve failure present with features of stenosis or incompetence (regurgitation).

In addition to features of regurgitation mechanical failure can also result in embolisation of fragments.

Para-prosthetic leaks result in the clinical features of regurgitation (incompetence).

Atrial Septal Defect

The types of Atrial Septal Defect are:

♠ Ostium Secundum

♦ Ostium Primum

♣ Patent Foramen Ovale

Ostium Secundum

In ostium secundum atrial septal defect, the defect is usually in the middle of the septum (oval fossa defect). In some cases the defect may be close to the superior vena cava, the inferior vena cava or the coronary sinus.

Ostium Primum

In ostium primum atrial septal defect, the defect is in the lower part of the septum and there are associated defects in the mitral valve

Patent Foramen Ovale

Patent foramen ovale refers to retention of patency of the foramen ovale. It does not have the clinical features of atrial septal defect but it is associated with paradoxical embolism.

Associations of Atrial Septal Defect

Atrial Septal Defect may be:

♥ Isolated

♠ Associated with other cardiac defects

♦ Associated with somatic abnormalities

Isolated

Atrial septal defect may occur in isolation

Associated Cardiac abnormalities

Atrial septal defect may be associated with other cardiac abnormalities such as:

♣ Lutembacher's syndrome where there is associated mitral stenosis

Associated Somatic Abnormalities

Atrial septal defect may be associated with somatic abnormalities such as:

♥ **Holt-Oram syndrome** where the associated features could be hypoplastic thumbs, accessory phalanges and abnormalities of the forearm (autosomal dominant inheritance)

♠ It could also occur in Down's syndrome and Turner's syndrome.

Ventricular Septal Defect

Ventricular septal defect may be:

♦ Congenital

♣ Acquired

Acquired VSD occurs in myomalacia cordis following myocardial infarction

Congenital Ventricular Septal Defect

Congenital ventricular septal defect may be:

♥ Isolated

♠ Associated with other cardiac defects

♦ Associated with somatic abnormalities

Isolated

Ventricular septal defect may occur in isolation

Associated Cardiac Defects

Ventricular septal defect may be associated with other cardiac defects. They are:

♣ Syndromes in which the VSD is an integral part of the syndrome

♥ Syndromes in which the VSD is not an integral part of the syndrome

Syndromes in which the VSD is an integral part of the syndrome

The syndromes are:

- ♠ Fallot's tetralogy
- ♦ Truncus arteriosus
- ♣ Atrioventricular canal defects
- ♥ Double outlet right ventricle

Syndromes in which the VSD is not an integral part

The syndromes are:

- ♠ Patent ductus arteriosus
- ♦ Coarctation of the aorta
- ♣ Transposition of the great vessels
- ♥ Pulmonary Atresia
- ♠ Tricuspid Atresia

Somatic Abnormalities

Somatic abnormalities that are associated with VSD are:

- ♠ Down's syndrome, Turner's syndrome

Coarctation of the Aorta

Coarctation of the aorta may be:

- ♦ Isolated

Or associated with:

- ♣ Turner's syndrome

Patent Ductus Arteriosus

Patent ductus arteriosus may be:

- ♥ Isolated

Or associated with:

- ♠ Coarctation of the aorta
- ♦ Ventricular septal defect
- ♣ Pulmonary stenosis

Fallot's Tetralogy

Fallot's tetralogy consists of:

- ♥ Ventricular septal defect
- ♠ Overriding of the aorta
- ♦ Pulmonary stenosis
- ♠ Right ventricular hypertrophy

Differentiation of Mixed Valve Disease

In mixed valve disease where stenosis and regurgitation co-exist it may be necessary to determine the dominant lesion. For this one should analyse the features of valve disease as reflected in the pulse volume and character, the blood pressure, the position and character of the apex beat, the presence or absence of a thrill and the presence or absence of added heart sounds or opening snaps and clicks.

Mixed Mitral Valve Disease

The features that would help to determine the dominant lesion are as follows:

	Dominant Mitral Stenosis	Dominant Mitral Regurgitation
Pulse	Small volume	Sharp, quick
Apex beat	Not displaced, tapping	Displaced, thrusting
S_1	Loud	Soft
S_3	None	Present

Mixed Aortic Valve Disease

The features that would help to determine the dominant lesion are as follows:

	Dominant Aortic Stenosis	Dominant Aortic Regurgitation
Pulse	Small volume, slow rising	Collapsing
Pulse Pressure	Narrow	Wide
Apex beat	Not displaced, heaving	Displaced, thrusting
Thrill	Present	Absent
Murmurs	Loud	Soft

Aide Memoire

In summary when stenosis is dominant sizes are small, murmurs are loud (and there may be thrills). When incompetence (regurgitation) is dominant, sizes are large, murmurs are soft and there may be a 3rd heart sound.

This is true of life in general; small size is often associated with a lot of noise!

Combined Valve Disease

Lesions involving more than one valve are difficult to evaluate. There is difficulty in diagnosis and in determining the severity of individual lesions. Proceed as for mixed valve disease.

Extra-Cardiac Sounds

During auscultation one may hear the following extra-cardiac sounds:

- ♥ Pericardial Rub
- ♠ Pericardial Crunch
- ♦ Venous Hum

Pericardial Rub

A pericardial rub occurs in pericarditis.

Pericarditis

Pericarditis may be due to:

- ♠ **Internal Factors**

  Infection, which may be viral, purulent, tuberculous, fungal

- ♥ **Mural Factors**

  Trauma, idiopathic, rheumatic fever

- ♠ **External Factors**

  Acute transmural myocardial infarction, Dressler's syndrome, post-cardiotomy syndrome, dissecting aneurysm, local invasion by malignancy

- ♦ **Systemic Factors**

LMS rheumatoid arthritis, systemic lupus erythematosus, rheumatic fever, systemic sclerosis

KUS renal failure

RAG carcinoma of the breast

RS carcinoma of the bronchus

HS lymphoma, leukaemia

IS melanoma

Drugs doxorubicin, cyclophosphamide

Radiation therapy

Pericardial Effusion

The above conditions can also result in a pericardial effusion

Pericardial Crunch

A crunching sound may be heard in time with the heartbeat in:

- ♣ Pneumomediastinum
- ♥ Left sided pneumothorax

Venous Hum

A venous hum is a continuous sound, which may be heard at the base of the heart in the presence of a hyperkinetic jugular venous flow. It is abolished by pressure at the root of the neck.

Examination of the Back (Spine, Scapula, Sacrum, Lung Bases)

On examination of the back one may detect abnormalities of the following:

Spine

Abnormalities that may be noted in the spine are:

- ♠ Features of ankylosing spondylitis may be seen in association with aortic incompetence
- ♦ Kyphoscoliosis could be seen in Marfan's syndrome
- ♣ Kyphoscoliosis may be the cause of cor pulmonale
- ♥ Straight back syndrome. A systolic murmur may be heard in association with a straight spine. This is innocent.

Scapula

Abnormalities detectable in this region are:

- ♠ Prominent periscapular vessels may be seen in coarctation of the aorta.
- ♦ A continuous bruit best heard over the back may occur in coarctation of the aorta.
- ♣ A murmur conducted to the inferior angle of the scapula would suggest mitral incompetence.
- ♥ The murmur of coarctation of the aorta is often best heard over the back

Lower Back

In the lower back one may note:

- ♥ Sacral oedema in congestive cardiac failure.

Respiratory System

Abnormalities that one may note in the respiratory system are:

♥ Cheyne-Stokes respiration may occur in left ventricular failure

♠ Tachypnoea occurs in heart failure

♦ Bilateral basal crepitations occur in left ventricular failure.

♣ Bilateral pleural effusions may occur in congestive cardiac failure

♥ A left basal collapse may occur in pericardial effusion. This occurs as a result of compression by a large effusion.

If this occurs an area of dullness may be detected on percussion below the angle of the left scapula and this is known as Ewart's sign.

Abdomen

In the abdomen the abnormalities that occur are those that affect the following:

Liver

The liver may be enlarged in:

♣ Congestive cardiac failure, right ventricular failure, restrictive cardiomyopathy, tricuspid regurgitation, constrictive pericarditis, cardiac tamponade

♥ The liver may be pulsatile in tricuspid regurgitation.

Splenomegaly

Splenomegaly may occur in:

♠ Subacute bacterial endocarditis.

Palpable Kidneys

Palpable kidneys may represent the cause of hypertension as in the following:

♦ Polycystic kidneys

♣ Hypertrophied normal kidney in unilateral renal artery stenosis

♥ Hydronephrotic kidneys may also be palpable

Adrenal

Adrenal tumours are rarely palpable

Aortic Aneurysm

An abdominal aortic aneurysm may be present in patients with atherosclerosis. This presents as a pulsatile mass in the abdomen just to the left of the midline. The pulsation is expansile. A systolic bruit may be heard over it. Transmitted pulsation may be felt if thrombosis occurs in a saccular aneurysm.

Ascites

Ascites may occur in:

♠ Congestive cardiac failure

♦ Restrictive cardiomyopathy

♣ Constrictive pericarditis

Renal Artery Bruits

Renal artery bruits may be heard in patients with hypertension due to:

♥ Renal artery stenosis

Femoral Arteries

Abnormalities that one may note in the femoral arteries are:

223

♠ Radio-femoral delay would be a feature of coarctation of the aorta. It may also be a feature of dissecting aneurysm of the descending aorta.

♦ **Auscultation**

In severe aortic regurgitation, the flow of blood back into the ventricle in diastole causes the femoral artery to empty and the walls to collapse. In systole the jet of blood re-entering the artery causes the walls to be snapped apart giving rise to a sound either like a thud or a pistol shot.

Durosiez's murmur refers to systolic and diastolic bruits that may be heard when the femoral artery is lightly compressed with the bell of the stethoscope. The systolic bruit is due to the increased stroke volume. The diastolic bruit is due to reversal of blood flow due to the leak back into the ventricle.

Aortic Regurgitation

Auscultatory signs of aortic regurgitation that may be heard over the femoral artery are:

Femoral thud

Pistol shot

Durosiez's murmur

Thighs

Lesions that may occur in the thighs are:

♣ Erythema marginatum may occur in rheumatic fever

♥ Wasting of the muscles would be seen in cardiac cachexia.

Knees

Lesions that may occur in the knees are:

♠ Eruptive xanthoma may be seen in hyperlipidaemia

♦ Effusions may occur in rheumatic fever.

♣ Tendon xanthomata may occur in familial hypercholesterolaemia.

♥ An aneurysm may occur in the popliteal fossa.

Lower Legs

Lesions that may occur are:

♠ Erythema nodosum may occur in rheumatic fever and sarcoidosis.

♦ Varicose veins may cause a stasis ulcer over the medial malleolus

♣ Swelling, redness, dilated superficial veins, increased temperature would suggest the presence of deep venous thrombosis.

♥ Oedema would be observed in congestive cardiac failure.

♠ Dystrophic changes (wasting or hypertrophy) of muscles would be features of muscular dystrophy.

Ankles

Abnormalities that may occur are:

♦ Tendon xanthomata may be seen in hyperlipidaemia

Feet

The same features may be noted as in examination of the hand.   In addition:

♣ Peripheral vascular disease would cause pallor, the area would be cold and dystrophic skin changes and atrophy may be seen. Capillary refill time would be increased in peripheral vascular disease

♥ The dorsalis pedis and posterior tibial pulses may be absent in peripheral vascular disease.

Gait

If one were to observe gait one may note:

♠ Abnormalities of gait may be seen in tertiary syphilis where aortic aneurysm and aortic regurgitation may be features.

♦ In Freidrich's ataxia the associated cardiac features would be supra ventricular tachyarrythmia and cardiac failure.

Chapter 11

The Respiratory System

In the respiratory system one will study the air passages and their anatomical relationships, the lung parenchyma, the pleura, the chest wall and the diaphragm. Associated features of the causes and effects of respiratory disease reflected in other organs and organ systems will also be evaluated.

History Taking

The following symptoms would result from respiratory disease:

Upper Respiratory Tract

- ♥ Sneezing
- ♠ Blocked nose
- ♦ Nasal discharge
- ♣ Postnasal drip
- ♥ Epistaxis
- ♠ Facial pain
- ♦ Hoarseness
- ♣ Aphonia

Lower Respiratory Tract

- ♥ Dyspnoea
- ♠ Wheeze
- ♦ Cough
- ♣ Sputum
- ♥ Haemoptysis
- ♠ Chest pain

Next, one should perform a review of systems.

Personal History

Smoking

One pack year is the equivalent of smoking twenty cigarettes per day for a period of one year.

Physical Examination

Begin by performing a general examination

General Examination

Evaluate the position of the patient. This is very important in a patient with a respiratory condition as it would indicate if the patient is in any degree of respiratory distress. If the position of the patient is not suitable for examination, ask the patient if he or she would be comfortable with a change in position and then attempt to change the position of the patient so that his or her torso makes an angle of 45 degrees with the examination bed or couch. Next, assess growth and development and the metabolic state of the patient. Note any gross changes in the integument. Assess body temperature if required.

(Position, Height and Proportions, Weight and Shape, Integument, Body Temperature)

Regional Examination

Commence regional examination by examining the head. One may start by examining the hands if one wishes.

Head

Quickly evaluate cerebral cortical function if this has not being done already whilst taking the history. In a professional examination this would not be required. Assess the dimensions of the head and the integument. Following this examine the nose, the eyes, the face (scalp, forehead, eyebrows, malar region, chin), the mouth (jaw, lips, teeth, gums, buccal mucosa, tongue, palate, fauces, salivary glands) and the ears.

Remember the nose is used in the function of breathing and the mouth may also be used likewise. Hence, functional examination of the nose and mouth is important. When examining the nose observe if there is any evidence of respiratory distress (flaring of the alae nasi). Likewise when examining the lips observe if there is pursed lip breathing.

Do not forget that the mouth is also used in speech and this should be evaluated as well as lesions of the respiratory tract may rarely manifest as abnormalities of speech.

Upper Limbs

Perform a quick general examination of the upper limbs noting the dimensions and the state of the integument.

Hands

Note the dimensions. Next, examine the dorsum of the hands; the nails and skin, the bones, joints, tendons and muscles. Ask the patient to turn the hands over and examine the palms; the skin, the bones, the joints, the tendons and the muscles. Palpate the hands and note the state of the peripheral circulation and then examine the radial pulse. Ask the patient to stretch the arms out and look for a tremor. Next, ask the patient to extend the wrists with fingers spread wide apart. Look for a flapping tremor. Examine the nervous system and function of the locomotor system of the hands if required.

Quickly look at the forearms, the elbows, upper arms, shoulders and axillae. Examine these areas in detail only if required.

Neck

Assess the dimensions of the neck. Note the state of the integument. Note any enlargement of the thyroid gland. Note the state of contraction of the sternocleidomastoid muscle. Examine the jugular venous pulsation, examine the carotids if required and examine the trachea in detail. Lymph nodes should be examined later when one examines the back of the patient.

Trachea

On examination of the trachea one should note the following:

♦ Position

♣ Length

♥ Movement

♠ Stridor

Position

The position of the trachea should be determined. This should be performed by placing one's right index finger in the suprasternal notch with the pulp of the finger maintaining contact with the sternum. Note the direction of the trachea. Whilst maintaining the pulp of the finger in contact with the sternum, one should attempt to interpose the examining finger between the trachea and the sternocleidomastoid muscle on either side. Deviation of the trachea would be demonstrated by the gap being greater between the trachea and the muscle on one side and the gap diminishing on the other side.

An alternative method is to place one's middle finger in the suprasternal notch with the index finger and fourth finger lying flat on the sternum on either side. Palpate the direction the trachea takes and feel for a gap between the trachea and the sternocleidomastoid muscle on either side.

Length (the Suprasternal Length of the Trachea)

Place the fingers of one's right hand across the trachea with the long axes of the fingers lying at right angles to the long axis of the trachea. Normally three fingers may be interposed between the inferior margin of the cricoid cartilage and the sternum. A decrease in this length indicates hyperinflation of the lungs.

Movement (of the Trachea)

Note any movement of the trachea either with respiration or with the heartbeat.

Stridor

Note any stridor.

Chest

For convenience, examination of the chest may be divided into examination of the:

♦ Chest wall

♣ Examination of the lungs

Chest Wall

Inspection

Inspect the chest. Pay attention to the following:

♥ Structure

♠ Function

Structure

Assess the dimensions of the chest wall. Note size and shape and any discrepancy between the two sides of the chest wall. Note any changes in the skin and any gross changes in the breasts. Look for dilated blood vessels especially engorged veins.

Function

Observe movements of the chest wall and abdominal wall with respiration. Normally the chest wall and abdominal wall should expand with inspiration and contract with expiration. Movements should be equal on both sides. These observations should be repeated when one moves to the foot end of the bed to analyse respiration.

Palpation

Complete examination of the chest wall by paying attention to:

♦ Consistency

♣ Circulation

Consistency

Note the consistency of the chest wall. Crepitus may occur in subcutaneous emphysema

Circulation

Note any distension of the blood vessels. Dilated veins may be seen over the chest wall in obstruction of the superior vena cava. If dilated veins are observed, determine the direction of blood flow. Place the index fingers of both hands on a vein with the fingers in proximity to one another. Move one finger in either a cephalad or caudal direction and thus empty the vessel. Raise this finger and ascertain the direction of

blood flow by noting whether the vessel fills up with blood or remains empty. Repeat the procedure with the other finger now moving in the opposite direction. This will determine the direction of blood flow and should be from cephalad to caudal in obstruction of the superior vena cava.

This concludes examination of the chest wall.

Examination of the Lungs

Examination of the lungs is performed by undertaking the following:

♥ Analysis of respiration (inspection mainly)

♠ Palpation of the chest

♦ Percussion of the chest

♣ Auscultation of the chest

Respiration

When analysing respiration one should note the following:

♥ Position

♠ Rhythm

♦ Volume

♣ Character

♥ Transmission

♠ Rate

Move to the foot end of the bed and observe the following:

Position

Note the position of the patient. In a professional examination the patient should be positioned with the torso at an angle of 45 degrees to the bed or couch. In practice observing the position the patient adopts would give useful clues to the underlying condition. However, for ease of examination one should attempt to position the patient correctly.

Rhythm

The normal respiratory rhythm is inspiration followed by expiration and then a gap occurs before the next inspiration. Abnormalities of rhythm usually indicate serious disease.

Volume

Note the volume of chest expansion. A rough assessment may be made. Chest expansion may be measured with a tape at the level of the nipples, which are usually at the fourth inter-costal space. One should avoid breast tissue in females and either measure above or below the breasts. About 5 centimetres of expansion may be expected (the amount of expansion probably varies with the size of the patient). This is not an examination technique that is commonly adopted.

Character

Note the character of respiration. In normal respiration at rest, the respiratory movement is mainly diaphragmatic with gentle outward movement of the abdominal and chest walls in inspiration and the reverse in expiration.

Transmission

Look for evidence of respiratory distress such as the use of the accessory muscles of respiration and intercostal and subcostal indrawing with inspiration.

Now go back to the side of the patient and count the respiratory rate.

Rate

Count the respiratory rate. Place one's right hand on the patient's abdomen and allow it to rise and fall with the patient's respiration. Count the number of inspirations, ideally for a period of one minute, but in practice one may count for 15 seconds and multiply by four.

The respiratory rate may be counted either before moving to the foot end of the bed or after returning to the side of the patient. Most clinicians would do it after returning to the side of the patient as this would blend in better with the next step, which is palpation of the chest.

Palpation

Palpation of the chest should include:

♥ Position of the Apex Beat

♠ Respiratory Movements

♦ Tactile Vocal Fremitus

Apex Beat

Palpate the apex beat as described in the section on the cardiovascular system. Although strictly speaking this is not part of the examination of the respiratory system, it is important as it defines the position of the lower mediastinum.

Respiratory Movements

Clasp the patient's chest wall firmly with one's hands placed on either side of the chest. The thumbs should meet in the midline. Ask the patient to breathe actively and watch movement of the thumbs in relation to one another. Failure of movement or reduced movement on one side would indicate underlying disease. Ideally this should be performed over all three zones of the lungs; the upper, mid and lower. If analysis of respiratory movement is not performed over the upper zones important clues to underlying apical lesions may be missed.

To observe movements of the abdominal wall, place one's hands on the patient's upper abdomen with one's fingers pointing towards the patient's head. Normally the abdominal wall should move outwards with inspiration and inwards with expiration. In diaphragmatic palsy the reverse occurs.

Tactile Vocal Fremitus

Place the ulnar border of one's right hand over the chest wall and ask the patient to say ninety-nine. The palpating hand should feel the vibrations produced by the sound. Perform the procedure in the upper zones (left and right sides), the mid-zones (left and right sides) and the lower zones (left and right sides)

Next one should proceed to percuss the chest.

Percussion

In percussion one strikes the middle phalanx of one's left middle finger, the pleximeter, with the terminal phalanx of one's right middle finger, the plexor.

Good technique demands that the pleximeter is in close contact with the skin surface. The other fingers of the left hand should be close to the skin surface but ideally should not touch the surface. The plexor should strike the pleximeter at right angles to it. The movement of the right hand should be a free movement occurring at the wrist joint. The other fingers of the right hand should not be curled up

Begin with direct percussion over the clavicles and then proceed downwards and outwards and include the upper, mid and lower zones of the lungs. The initial direction of percussion is downwards and outwards to avoid the area of cardiac dullness. However, after this initial percussion one should always remember to analyse the extent of cardiac and liver dullness.

Following percussion one should move on to auscultation.

Auscultation

When auscultating breath sounds, ask the patient to keep the mouth partially open and breathe through the open mouth. This accentuates the breath sounds. Systematically examine all areas of both lung fields and compare corresponding areas of the two lungs. One should now:

♣ Analyse breath sounds

♥ Listen for any added sounds.

Breath Sounds

When analysing breath sounds one should define the following:

♥ Position

♠ Character

♦ Quantity

♣ Transmission

Position

Define the position at which the breath sounds are auscultated

Character

Define the character of the breath sounds. Two types of breath sounds are recognised.

Bronchial breath sounds are those sounds heard over large diameter bronchi. Vesicular breath sounds are those sounds heard over the distal air spaces or alveoli.

Definition of Breath Sounds

The following definitions of the types of breath sounds are important. Please memorise them.

♥ **Bronchial Breath Sounds**

Bronchial breath sounds are blowing in quality, the expiratory sound is as loud as or louder than, as long as or longer than, the inspiratory sound and there is a gap between the inspiratory sound and the expiratory sound.

♠ **Vesicular Breath Sounds**

Vesicular breath sounds are rustling in quality. The expiratory sound is shorter. There is no gap

between the inspiratory and expiratory phases.

Quantity

Quantify the breath sounds. This denotes the intensity of the breath sounds. They may be normal, increased, decreased or absent

Transmission

Note transmission. That is transmission of the spoken or whispered word to the examining ear via the stethoscope. The transmitted sounds that should be analysed are the following:

♦ Vocal Resonance

♣ Aegophony

♥ Whispering pectoriloquy

Vocal Resonance

To test for vocal resonance, ask the patient to say ninety-nine and listen with the stethoscope. Normally the sound is muffled. In increased vocal resonance the sound is clearly and loudly transmitted to the stethoscope.

Aegophony

Aegophony refers to a bleating sound that is heard when one elicits vocal resonance. (Like the bleating of a goat)

Whispering Pectoriloquy

To test for whispering pectoriloquy, ask the patient to whisper ninety-nine whilst listening with the stethoscope. Normally the whispered word cannot be heard clearly through the stethoscope. In whispering pectoriloquy the sound is heard clearly, as if the whisper is into the chest piece.

Added Sounds

The added sounds that may be heard are the following:

- ♠ Crepitations
- ♦ Rhonchi
- ♣ Squawks
- ♥ Stridor
- ♠ Pleural rubs

Crepitations or Crackles

Crepitations are discontinuous added sounds. Each individual sound is of short duration and is explosive in nature. When analysing crepitations one should define the following:

- ♠ Position
- ♦ Timing
- ♣ Quantity
- ♥ Character
- ♠ Modifying Factors

Position

Define the position at which the crepitations are heard

Timing

Define the timing that is whether they are early, mid or late inspiratory or whether they are heard in expiration.

- ♦ Early and mid inspiratory crepitations are caused by pathology in more proximal airways
- ♣ Late inspiratory crepitations are caused by pathology (either fibrosis or fluid) in the distal air

spaces. The fluid may be exudate, transudate or blood in the alveoli.

- ♥ Crepitations that occur during expiration are heard in patients with airflow obstruction

Quantity

Define whether the crepitations are loud or soft

Character

Define the character. Define whether the crepitations are fine or coarse.

- ♥ Fine crepitations signify alveolar origin
- ♠ Coarse crepitations suggest origin in the more proximal airways

Modifying Factors

Evaluate the effect of coughing on crepitations. Coughing may clear crepitations caused by secretions in more proximal airways.

Rhonchi or Wheeze

Rhonchi are continuous, longer, high-pitched musical, whistling sounds. They originate in the proximal tubular air passages. Remember, rhonchi from the bronchi. When analysing rhonchi one should define the following:

- ♦ Position
- ♣ Timing
- ♥ Quantity
- ♠ Character

Position

Define the position at which the rhonchi are heard

Timing

Define the timing. Rhonchi are expiratory usually but may occur in the inspiratory phase

Quantity

Define whether the rhonchi are loud or soft.

Character

Define the character of the rhonchi. Rhonchi may be:

♦ High pitched or sibilant

♣ Low pitched or sonorous

♥ Multiple pitches or tones are termed polyphonic rhonchi.

♠ A single tone or pitch is referred to as monophonic rhonchi

Very loud rhonchi may be heard without a stethoscope

Squawks

Squawks are high-pitched, squeaky sounds heard in inspiration. They are caused by opening up of airways that collapse during expiration. Squawks occur in pulmonary fibrosis.

Stridor

Stridor is caused by upper airway obstruction. When analysing stridor one should define:

♠ Timing

♦ Quantity

♣ Character

♥ Transmission

Timing

Stridor occurs during inspiration

Quantity

Define whether the stridor is loud or soft.

Character

Stridor is of lower pitch than rhonchi

Transmission

Stridor may be transmitted to the stethoscope. It should not be confused with rhonchi

Pleural Rub

A pleural rub is caused by rubbing together of inflamed pleural surfaces. When analysing a rub one should define:

♠ Position

♦ Timing

♣ Quantity

♥ Modifying Factors

♠ Character

♦ Transmission

Position

Define the position at which the rub is heard

Timing

Pleural rubs are inspiratory and expiratory

Quantity

If very severe the rub may be palpable.

Modifying Factors

Increasing pressure on the stethoscope may increase the loudness of the rub.

Character

A rub is a creaking or grating sound

Transmission

If severe, a rub may be transmitted to the palpating hand.

Differentiation of a Pleural Rub from Coarse Crepitations

Differentiation of a pleural rub from coarse crepitations can be quite difficult, the differentiating features are:

- ♣ A rub is usually localised

- ♥ A pleural rub is heard superficially whilst crepitations are deeper

- ♠ A pleural rub is usually louder

- ♦ A pleural rub is usually painful

- ♣ A rub is heard in both inspiration and expiration

- ♥ A pleural rub is accentuated by increasing pressure with the stethoscope

- ♠ A pleural rub does not change with coughing whilst crepitations may change

After completing examination of the patient from the anterior aspect, one should proceed to examine the patient from the posterior aspect. Ask the patient to sit up and lean forward. If the patient is able to, ask the patient to swing his or her legs over the side of the bed or couch and sit on the edge of the bed or couch as this makes access easier. Examine the following:

- ♥ Neck

- ♠ Spine

- ♦ Scapula

- ♣ Posterior aspect of the Chest Wall

- ♥ Posterior aspect of the Lungs

Neck

Palpate the lymph nodes of the neck

Spine

Examine the spine for abnormalities of shape. One should make a habit of running one's fingers down the patient's spine to remind oneself and emphasise this important aspect.

Scapula

Note the dimensions of the scapula. Position the patient so that the scapula moves forward and allows access to the back of the chest. Either ask the patient to reach forward or ask him or her to cross the arms in front of the chest.

Posterior Aspect of the Chest Wall and Lungs

The procedure that was used for the anterior aspect should be repeated. Examine the chest wall and then examine the lungs.

In a professional examination this would be all that is required. For the sake of completeness the remainder of the examination is described.

Lower Back

Examine the lower back (lumbar region) if required.

Abdomen

Examine the abdomen. Following this examine the inguinal region and genitals.

Lower Limbs

Perform a general examination of the lower limbs and then proceed to examine the hips, thighs, knees, lower legs, and feet. Examine the locomotor system and nervous system of the lower limbs if required.

Buttocks, Peri Anal Region and Per Rectal Examination

Examine the buttocks and perianal region and perform per rectal examination if required.

Spine

Ask the patient to stand and examine the spine.

Gait

Examine the patient's gait

Romberg's Sign, Standing from a Seated or Squatting Position

Look for Romberg's sign if required. If required observe the patient standing up from a seated or squatting position.

Lesions of the Respiratory System

In medical practice and in professional examinations the common lesions that may present are those that affect the following:

- ♠ Nose
- ♦ Paranasal Sinuses
- ♣ Pharynx
- ♥ Larynx
- ♠ Trachea
- ♦ Mediastinum
- ♣ Bronchi
- ♥ Alveoli
- ♠ Lung Parenchyma
- ♦ Pleura
- ♣ Chest Wall
- ♥ Diaphragm

Nose

The lesions that affect the nose are mainly vascular abnormalities presenting as epistaxis or the vasculitides such as Wegener's granulomatosis.

Rhinitis, which may be infective or allergic, may be part of the clinical picture.

Paranasal Sinuses

Lesions of the paranasal sinuses do not usually present to medical departments but inflammatory conditions of the para-nasal sinuses may be part of the general picture.

Pharynx

The pharynx may be affected by obstructive lesions such as the obstructive sleep apnoea syndrome.

Larynx

The larynx may be affected by obstructive lesions. Obstruction could be in the:

♠ **Lumen**

Epiglottitis, inhaled foreign body

♦ **Mural Factors**

Laryngitis, laryngeal carcinoma

♣ **External Factors**

Recurrent laryngeal nerve palsy

Trachea

The trachea may be affected by obstructive lesions. These may be in the:

♥ **Lumen**

Inhaled foreign body

♠ **Mural Factors**

Tracheal stenosis

♦ **External Factors**

Mediastinal lesions

Mediastinum

Lesions in the mediastinum usually present with features of obstruction of local structures such as the trachea and the superior vena cava. This may be due to:

♣ Lymph node enlargement

♥ Thymic tumours

♠ Retrosternal goitre

♦ Pericardial cysts

♣ Neurogenic tumours

♥ Idiopathic mediastinal fibrosis

Bronchi

Lesions of the bronchi either cause narrowing of the lumen or dilatation of the lumen. Hence, lesions of the bronchi could result in:

♠ Bronchial Narrowing

♦ Bronchial Dilatation (Bronchiectasis)

Bronchial Narrowing

Bronchial narrowing may be due to lesions in the:

♣ **Lumen**

Foreign body, resulting in a localised obstruction

♥ **Mural Factors**

Bronchial asthma, chronic bronchitis

♠ **External Factors**

Compression by a lymph node

♦ **Systemic Factors**

CVS cardiac asthma

HS asthmatic features occurring in association with eosinophilia in Churg-Strauss syndrome and in tropical pulmonary eosinophilia

Bronchiectasis

Bronchiectasis or fixed dilatation of the bronchi may be caused by conditions affecting the:

♣ **Lumen**

Obstruction by a mucous plug, tumour, inhaled foreign body.

♥ **Mural Factors**

Infections: especially childhood infections such as measles, whooping cough, other infections such as tuberculosis, pneumococcal pneumonia, adenovirus and AIDS

Mucociliary Clearance Defects

Cystic fibrosis, immotile cilia, Kartagener's syndrome

Miscellaneous

Marfan's syndrome, yellow nail syndrome

♠ **External Factors**

Fibrosis of the lungs, compression by a lymph node

♦ **Systemic Factors**

HS immune deficiency states like hypogammaglobulinaemia, complement deficiency, phagocyte defects, chronic granulomatous disease

RS hyperimmune states such as allergic bronchopulmonary aspergillosis or following lung transplantation

Alpha$_1$ antitrypsin deficiency, smoking related chronic obstructive pulmonary disease

GIT inflammatory bowel disease, gastric aspiration

LMS rheumatoid arthritis

Toxins heroin

Alveoli

Lesions of the alveoli result in either:

♣ Dilatation of the alveoli

♥ Collapse of the alveoli

Dilatation

Dilatation of the alveoli would be due to:

♣ Emphysema. Emphysema may be related to alpha-one antitrypsin deficiency or it may be multifactorial with smoking playing a major part in its pathogenesis.

Collapse

Collapse of the alveoli could be due to:

♠ Fibrosis

♦ Pulmonary oedema

Fibrosing Alveolitis

Fibrosing alveolitis may be:

♣ **Cryptogenic Fibrosing Alveolitis**

Where the cause is unknown.

♥ **Extrinsic Allergic Alveolitis**

Extrinsic allergic alveolitis is caused by external allergens such as:

Farmer's lung, bird fancier's lung and the many other named forms

♠ **Systemic Diseases**

Fibrosing alveolitis may be due to disease primarily affecting the:

LMS scleroderma, rheumatoid arthritis, Sjogren's syndrome, systemic lupus erythematosus, dermatomyositis, polymyositis

GIT autoimmune hepatitis, primary biliary cirrhosis, inflammatory bowel disease

KUS renal tubular acidosis

Pulmonary Oedema

When studying pulmonary oedema, consider the pulmonary capillary as the hollow structure. The causes of pulmonary oedema would then be conditions affecting:

Internal factors

Increased hydrostatic pressure within the pulmonary capillaries as a consequence of:

♦ Pulmonary venous hypertension

♣ Pulmonary arterial hypertension

♥ Decreased colloid oncotic pressure

♠ Fluid overload

Pulmonary venous hypertension

This may be:

♥ Cardiogenic

♠ Non-cardiogenic

Cardiogenic

Cardiogenic pulmonary venous hypertension may be caused by:

♦ Left ventricular failure, mitral valve disease, left atrial thrombosis, left atrial myxoma, cor triatrium, localised pericarditis

Non-cardiogenic

Non-cardiogenic pulmonary venous hypertension may be caused by:

♣ Congenital pulmonary venous stenosis, veno-occlusive disease, mediastinal masses, mediastinal granulomata, mediastinal fibrosis, neurogenic

Pulmonary arterial hypertension

Pulmonary arterial hypertension may be due to:

♥ Pulmonary emboli, hyperkinetic circulation (exercise, hypoxia, anaemia, thyrotoxicosis, left to right shunts), high altitude

Decreased colloid oncotic pressure

This is rare as a sole cause of pulmonary oedema but decreased colloid oncotic pressure due to hypoalbuminaemia may contribute to the pulmonary oedema occurring in:

♠ ARDS, hepatic failure, renal failure

Fluid overload

This may be iatrogenic or complicate failure of other organs

Mural factors

Factors that affect the wall are:

♦ Increased permeability

♣ Reduced alveolar septal interstitial pressure

Increased Permeability

Increased permeability of the alveolar septum could be due to:

- ♥ **Internal Factors** (consider the alveolus as the hollow structure)

  Aspiration of stomach contents, near drowning

  Inhalation of smoke, toxic gases

  Viral infection

- ♠ **External Factors**

  Radiation

- ♦ **Systemic Factors**

  GIT hepatic failure

  KUS renal failure, Goodpasture's syndrome

  RS ARDS

  IS Stevens-Johnson syndrome

  CNS neurogenic pulmonary oedema (thought to be the cause)

  Drugs aspirin, nitrofurantoin, bleomycin, heroin, morphine, methadone, dextropopxyphene

  Toxins paraquat

  Venoms coral snake venom

Reduced alveolar septal interstitial pressure

This is caused by upper airway obstruction, which could be:

- ♥ Acute
- ♠ Chronic

Acute upper airway obstruction

Acute upper airway obstruction could be due to:

- ♦ Epiglottitis, laryngospasm, strangulation, foreign body, tumour

Chronic upper airway obstruction:

Chronic upper airway obstruction could be due to:

- ♣ Obstructive sleep apnoea, goitre, acromegaly

External Factors

The external factor that causes pulmonary oedema is failure of lymphatic clearance.

Failure of lymphatic clearance

Failure of lymphatic clearance could be due to:

- ♥ Lymphangitis carcinomatosa, mediastinal obstruction, lung transplant

Lung Parenchyma

Lesions that occur in the lung parenchyma usually result in:

- ♦ Consolidation
- ♣ Collapse
- ♥ Cavitation
- ♠ Fibrosis

Consolidation

Consolidation of the lung may be due to:

- ♦ Pneumonia
- ♣ Carcinoma
- ♥ Pulmonary infarction

Carcinoma of the Bronchus

Carcinoma of the bronchus may be:

♥ **Small Cell Carcinoma**

♠ **Non-Small Cell Carcinoma**

Non-small cell carcinoma may be:

Squamous carcinoma

Large cell carcinoma

Adenocarcinoma

Alveolar cell carcinoma

Collapse

Collapse of the lung occurs due to obstruction of a bronchus by:

♣ **Internal Factors**

Carcinoma, mucous plug, inhaled foreign body

♥ **External Compression**

By lymph nodes, which may be enlarged due to cancer, lymphoma, tuberculosis

Cavitation

Cavitation of the lung may be due to:

♠ **Internal Factors**

Pyogenic infection, tuberculosis

♦ **Mural Factors**

Granulomatous disease like Wegener's granulomatosis, carcinoma of the bronchus

♣ **Systemic Factors**

Ankylosing spondylitis

Fibrosis

Fibrosis of the lung may be due to causes in the:

♥ **Lumen**

The pneumoconioses or inorganic dust diseases like asbestosis, silicosis, anthracosis (coal dust), berylliosis

♠ **Mural Factors**

Sarcoid, tuberculosis, adult respiratory distress syndrome (ARDS)

♦ **External Factors**

Radiation

♣ **Systemic Factors**

CVS mitral valve disease

KUS uraemia

Drugs amiodarone, busulphan, bleomycin, nitrofurantoin, methotrexate

Pleura

Lesions of the pleura usually result in:

♥ Effusion

♠ Pneumothorax

♦ Pleural thickening

Pleural Effusion

A pleural effusion may be a:

♣ Transudate

♥ Exudate

♠ Empyema

♦ Haemorrhagic effusion

♣ Chylous effusion

The causes of the different types of pleural lesions are as follows:

Pleural Effusion

Pleural effusion or fluid in the pleural space may be caused by:

♥ **Mural Factors**

  Secondary deposits, tuberculosis, lymphoma, mesothelioma

♠ **External Factors**

  Pneumonia, pulmonary embolism, bronchial carcinoma, subphrenic abscess, trauma

♦ **Systemic Factors**

  LMS rheumatoid arthritis, systemic lupus erythematosus

  CVS cardiac failure, Dressler's syndrome

  KUS nephrotic syndrome

  GIT cirrhosis, pancreatitis

  E&M hypothyroidism

  IS yellow nail syndrome

  RAG Meig's syndrome

  HS lymphoma

Empyema

Empyema refers to pus in the pleural space. The causes of empyema are:

♣ **Internal Factors**

  Primary infection of the pleural space may be caused by:

  Mycobacterium tuberculosis, Nocardia asteroides

♥ **External Factors**

  Bronchiectasis, bronchial obstruction, pneumonia, lung abscess, subphrenic abscess, penetrating injury or following thoracic surgery

♠ **Systemic Factors**

  GIT oesophageal perforation

E&M debilitating illness

Haemothorax

Haemothorax refers to blood in the pleural space. This may be caused by:

♦ **External Factors**

  Trauma

♣ **Systemic Factors**

  Drugs over-anticoagulation

  CVS rupture of a dissecting aneurysm of the aorta

  HS bleeding disorders

  RS pulmonary embolism

Chylothorax

Chylothorax refers to lymph in the pleural space. This may be caused by:

♥ **Mural Factors**

  Blockage of the lymphatics due to:

  Malignancy, lymphoma, filariasis, lymphangioleiomyomatosis

♠ **External Factors**

  Trauma

♦ **Systemic Factors**

  IS yellow nail syndrome

Pleural Thickening

Pleural thickening may be due to:

♣ Haemorrhage

♥ Infections such as tuberculosis, empyema

♠ Asbestosis

Pneumothorax

The causes of pneumothorax may be classified as:

♦ Traumatic

♣ Spontaneous

Spontaneous Pneumothorax

Spontaneous pneumothorax may be secondary to lesions in the lung such as the following:

♥ **Lumen**

Bacterial pneumonia, tuberculosis, *Pneumocystis carinii* pneumonia

♠ **Mural Factors**

Congenital cysts and bullae, sub-pleural blebs, bronchial asthma, chronic obstructive pulmonary disease, cystic fibrosis, whooping cough, sarcoidosis, bronchial carcinoma, lymphangioleiomyomatosis

♦ **External Factors**

Pleural malignancy

♣ **Systemic Factors**

LMS rheumatoid lung disease, Marfan's syndrome

CNS tuberose sclerosis

RAG endometriosis

GIT oesophageal rupture

Chest Wall

Lesions of the chest wall restrict respiration as a result of:

♥ **Deformity**

Kyphoscoliosis

♠ **Decreased Movement**

Decreased movement may be caused by ankylosis of joints in ankylosing spondylitis

♦ **Paradoxical Movement**

Paradoxical movement occurs in a flail segment

♣ **Muscle Weakness**

Muscle weakness occurs in ascending paralysis

Diaphragm

Lesions of the diaphragm that affect the respiratory system are those that cause diaphragmatic paralysis. Eventration and hernias are usually clinically silent and traumatic rupture presents to surgical units.

Weakness of the diaphragm may be:

♥ Unilateral

♠ Bilateral

Unilateral Weakness of the Diaphragm

Unilateral weakness of the diaphragm may be due to:

♥ Trauma including surgery

Other conditions that may cause unilateral weakness of the diaphragm are those affecting the:

♠ **RS** carcinoma of the bronchus, infections such as tuberculosis, pneumonia

♦ **CNS** poliomyelitis, herpes zoster, syphilis

Bilateral Weakness of the Diaphragm

Bilateral weakness of the diaphragm may be caused by conditions affecting the:

♣ **CNS** multiple sclerosis, poliomyelitis, Guillain-Barre

syndrome, quadriplegia, motor neurone disease

Findings on History

The findings that one may obtain on taking a history are as follows:

Epistaxis

Epistaxis may be due to:

♥ **Luminal Factors**

Foreign body

♠ **Mural Factors**

Vascular anomalies, vasculitides, infections, carcinoma

♦ **Systemic Factors**

HS blood dyscrasias

CVS hypertension

Dyspnoea

Dyspnoea may be due to conditions involving the:

♣ **Pharynx**

Obstructive sleep apnoea syndrome

♥ **Epiglottis**

Epiglottitis

♠ **Trachea**

Foreign body, tracheal stenosis

♦ **Mediastinum**

Enlarged lymph nodes, retrosternal goitre, thymoma

♣ **Bronchi**

Narrowing due to bronchial asthma, chronic bronchitis, bronchial carcinoma

Dilatation due to bronchiectasis

♥ **Alveoli**

Collapse due to fibrosing alveolitis or pulmonary oedema

Dilatation due to emphysema

♠ **Lung Parenchyma**

Consolidation, collapse, cavitation, infarction, fibrosis

♦ **Pleura**

Pneumothorax, effusion, thickening

♣ **Chest Wall**

Lesions that result in:

Deformity: kyphoscoliosis

Ankylosis of joints: ankylosing spondylitis

Muscle weakness: ascending paralysis in the Guillain-Barre syndrome

♥ **Diaphragm**

Unilateral or bilateral weakness of the diaphragm

♠ **Systemic Conditions**

HS anaemia

E&M fever, thyrotoxicosis, acidosis

CVS heart failure

KUS uraemia resulting in acidosis

Wheeze

Wheezing is caused by lesions that result in narrowing of the bronchi. Wheezing could be due to:

♦ **Luminal Factors**

Inhaled foreign body

♣ **Mural Factors**

Bronchial asthma, chronic bronchitis, bronchial carcinoma

♥ **External Factors**

Compression by an enlarged lymph node

♠ **Systemic Factors**

CVS left ventricular failure (cardiac asthma)

LMS vasculitides such as polyarteritis nodosa, Churg-Strauss syndrome

HS tropical pulmonary eosinophilia

Cough

Cough may be due to lesions in the:

♦ **Para Nasal Sinuses**

Chronic sinusitis

♣ **Pharynx and Larynx**

Upper respiratory tract infections

♥ **Trachea**

Tracheitis

♠ **Bronchi**

Bronchial asthma, bronchitis (acute and chronic), bronchial carcinoma, bronchiectasis

♦ **Lung Parenchyma**

Consolidation, collapse, fibrosis, cavitation,

♣ **Systemic Factors**

Systemic factors that result in cough are conditions affecting the:

GIT gastro-oesophageal reflux

CVS cardiac failure

Character of the Cough

The types of cough that may occur are:

♥ **Short Cough**

A short cough is usually due to upper respiratory tract infections or pain due to pleurisy. Pain inhibits coughing

♠ **Paroxysmal Coughing**

Paroxysmal coughing is due to conditions where there is narrowing of the air passages such as chronic bronchitis, whooping cough, inhaled foreign body

♦ **Brassy or Metallic Quality**

A brassy or metallic quality would be caused by tracheal compression

♣ **Bovine**

A bovine cough would be caused by recurrent laryngeal palsy

Modifying Factors

Factors that may affect coughing are:

♥ **Nocturnal Cough**

A nocturnal cough may be due to bronchial asthma, heart failure, sinusitis, gastro-oesophageal reflux

♠ **Early Morning Cough or Cough Related to a Change in Posture**

A cough on waking up in the morning or a cough with a change in posture occurs in bronchiectasis or chronic bronchitis. It is probably due to movement of secretions.

Sputum Production

Sputum production may be from the:

- ◆ **Bronchi**

  Chronic bronchitis, bronchiectasis

- ♣ **Alveoli**

  Pulmonary oedema

- ♥ **Lung Parenchyma**

  Consolidation, cavitation

- ♠ **External Factors**

  Hepatobronchial fistula

Character of the Sputum

Variations in the character of sputum could be:

- ♠ **Viscid Sputum with Bronchial Casts**

  Viscid sputum with bronchial casts occurs in bronchial asthma

- ◆ **Frothy Sputum with Pink Staining**

  Frothy sputum with pink staining occurs in pulmonary oedema

- ♣ **Rusty Sputum**

  Rusty sputum occurs in pneumonia

- ♥ **Green Sputum**

  Green sputum would indicate infection

- ♠ **Yellow Sputum**

  Yellow sputum may be due to pus or a high eosinophil content in asthma

- ◆ **Anchovy Sauce Sputum**

  Anchovy sauce sputum refers to the expectoration of brown, necrotic material in hepato-bronchial fistula complicating amoebic liver abscess.

Haemoptysis

Haemoptysis may be from the:

- ♣ **Bronchi**

  Carcinoma of the bronchus, chronic bronchitis, bronchiectasis

- ♥ **Alveoli**

  Alveolar haemorrhage occurs in:

  RS idiopathic pulmonary haemosiderosis

  CVS mitral stenosis, left ventricular failure

  LMS SLE, systemic vasculitides

  KUS Goodpasture's syndrome, rapidly progressive glomerulonephritis

- ♠ **Lung Parenchyma**

  Consolidation, collapse, cavitation, infarction

- ◆ **External factors**

  Thoracic trauma

- ♣ **Systemic factors**

  RAG endometriosis

  HS coagulation disorders

Chest Pain

In relation to the respiratory system, chest pain may be due to lesions in the:

- ◆ **Pleura**

  Pleurisy or inflammation of the pleura may be caused by underlying pneumonia, pulmonary embolism

♣ **Chest Wall**

Chest wall lesions that result in pain are myalgia, fractures, secondary deposits

Findings on Examination

The abnormalities that one may detect on clinical examination of the patient are as follows:

General Examination

On general examination one may detect abnormalities of the:

♥ Dimensions

♠ Integument

Dimensions

On examination of the dimensions one may note changes in the following:

♦ Posture

♣ Height

♥ Weight

♠ Shape

Posture

The abnormalities that one may note in the posture of the patient are:

♥ Severe kyphoscoliosis may be associated with respiratory disease.

♠ Ankylosing spondylitis may be associated with apical fibrosis.

Height

The variations that one may note in the height of the patient are:

♦ **Tall Stature**

Marfan's syndrome is associated with spontaneous pneumothorax.

♣ **Short Stature**

Short stature may reflect:

Chronic lung disease affecting growth in childhood

Pancreatic insufficiency in cystic fibrosis

Weight

On assessment of the patient's weight one may note:

♥ **Decreased Weight**

Emaciation could be a reflection of underlying lung disease especially tuberculosis, emphysema, cystic fibrosis, advanced malignancy.

♠ **Increased Weight**

Increased weight may be due to:

Obesity

Obesity is associated with the obstructive sleep apnoea syndrome

Salt and Water Retention

Salt and water retention occurs in cor pulmonale. It could also occur in ventilatory failure and carbon dioxide retention

Endocrine Causes

Endocrine causes of increased weight may have the following associations:

Hypothyroidism may occur in association with pleural effusions

Cushing's syndrome may represent a non-metastatic manifestation of bronchial carcinoma or it could be iatrogenic

Shape

Noting the overall shape of the patient would be useful as:

♦ The shape of the patient would enable one to differentiate the cause of increased weight.

♣ In cachexia a skeletal appearance would be seen. Associated ascites and dependent oedema would be a feature of nutritional decompensation.

Integument

On examination of the integument one may note changes in:

Colour

Changes in colour that would be of significance are:

♥ **Cyanosis**

Cyanosis would occur in respiratory insufficiency

♠ **Flushing**

Flushing would be a feature of emphysema or it may be due to the carcinoid syndrome.

Pink Puffer

The pink puffer refers to an emphysematous patient who is breathless and has pursed lip breathing and a flushed appearance.

Blue Bloater

The blue bloater refers to a patient, who is cyanosed and oedematous due to cor pulmonale as a consequence of chronic bronchitis.

♦ **Suffusion (Plethora)**

Diffuse reddening of the skin may occur in polycythaemia. This would be associated with cyanosis.

♣ **Pigmentation**

Pigmentation may be due to:

Addison's disease, which may occur in tuberculosis

Non-metastatic manifestations of bronchial carcinoma may also result in pigmentation.

Head

On examination of the head one may note changes in the:

♣ Mental state

♥ Dimensions

♠ Integument

Mental State

Changes in the mental state that would be of significance are:

♣ A confusional state may occur due to carbon dioxide narcosis or hypoxia.

♥ Encephalopathy may occur as a non-metastatic manifestation of bronchial carcinoma.

Dimensions

The changes that may occur in the dimensions are changes in:

♣ Size

♥ Shape

Size

Changes that one may observe in the size of the head are:

♠ Swelling would be seen in patients with obstruction of the superior vena cava.

Shape

Changes in the shape of the head that could be of significance are:

♦ A thin skeletal appearance would be observed in cachectic states like tuberculosis, advanced malignancies.

♣ A moon face may occur in Cushing's syndrome occurring as a result of steroid use or as a non-metastatic manifestation of carcinoma of the bronchus.

Integument

The colour of the skin may be:

♠ Darker and suffused in obstruction of the superior vena cava

Nose

On examination of the nose one may note changes in the:

♠ Dimensions

♦ Integument

♣ Function

Dimensions

Shape

Abnormalities that may be observed in the shape of the nose are:

♥ A saddle nose may occur as a result of destruction of cartilage in Wegener's granulomatosis

♠ In systemic sclerosis a beaked appearance would be observed.

Skin (Cover)

On examination of the skin over the nose one may note a:

Rash

The types of rash that would be of significance are:

♦ Lupus pernio (violaceous plaques) may occur in sarcoidosis

♣ Lupus vulgaris may occur in tuberculosis

Function

Abnormalities of function of the nose that may be noted are:

♥ Flaring of the alae nasi would be observed in respiratory distress

Eyes

On examination of the eyes one may note abnormalities of the following:

Size

The size of the eyes may show an:

♠ Apparent increase in size due to proptosis caused by hypercapnoea.

♦ Enophthalmos may be observed in Horner's syndrome

Eyelids

When examining the eyelids one may note changes in:

Size

The eyelids may be:

♣ Swollen due to oedema in hypercapnoea

Colour

The colour of the eyelids may change due to:

♥ Dermatomyositis, which may occur in carcinoma of the bronchus

Lacrimal Glands

Abnormalities that may occur in the lacrimal glands are:

♠ Dacryoadenitis occurs in sarcoidosis and tuberculosis

♦ Lacrimal gland swelling may occur as part of the Mikulicz syndrome.

Conjunctiva

Abnormalities that could occur in the conjunctiva are:

♣ The conjunctiva may be oedematous. This is known as chemosis and occurs in carbon dioxide retention.

♥ Phlyctenular conjunctivitis may be observed in primary tuberculosis. This presents as a waxy nodule on the conjunctiva with a sheaf of blood vessels radiating from it.

♠ Conjunctivitis may occur in sarcoidosis.

♦ Sjogren's syndrome may be associated with fibrosing alveolitis.

Iris

Lesions that may occur in the iris are:

♣ Uveitis may occur in sarcoidosis and tuberculosis

Fundus

Lesions that may occur in the fundus are the following:

♥ Papilloedema may occur in hypercapnoea

♠ Papilloedema could be due to secondary deposits from a bronchial cancer increasing intracranial pressure

♦ A choroid tubercle may be seen in primary tuberculosis

3rd, 4th and 6th Nerves

The abnormalities that may occur are:

♦ Ptosis would occur in Horner's syndrome

♣ A small pupil would be seen in Horner's syndrome, which could occur due to cervical sympathetic involvement in apical bronchial cancer (Pancoast's syndrome). Horner's syndrome may also occur in malignant cervical lymphadenopathy, which may complicate carcinoma of the bronchus.

Face

When examining the face one may note abnormalities of the following:

Forehead

Abnormalities in this region are not common. Very rarely one may see:

♥ Hypertrichosis lanuginosa. This refers to hair growth on the forehead that may occur in bronchial carcinoma.

Malar Region

On examination of the malar region one may note changes in the following:

- ♦ Surface
- ♣ Circulation

Surface

Rash

A rash may be seen in the malar region in:

- ♦ Systemic lupus erythematosus, which is associated with fibrosing alveolitis, pleural effusion

Circulation

Abnormalities that one may note in the circulation in the malar region are:

- ♣ **Flush**

  A flush could occur in the carcinoid syndrome caused by a bronchial carcinoid.

- ♥ **Telangiectasia**

  Telangiectasia may occur in scleroderma.

Mouth

On examination of the mouth one may note abnormalities of the following:

Jaw

On examination of the jaw one may observe:

- ♣ A small jaw. This may be associated with obstructive sleep apnoea.

Lips

When examining the lips one may note changes in:

- ♦ Size
- ♣ Colour
- ♥ Circulation

Size

The lips may be:

- ♦ Small in scleroderma

Colour

The colour of the lips may be abnormal and one may observe:

- ♣ Central cyanosis

Circulation

Lesions that may affect the blood vessels of the lips are:

- ♥ **Telangiectasia**

  Telangiectasia may occur in the Osler-Rendu-Weber syndrome, which may be associated with pulmonary arterio-venous fistulae. Pulmonary arterio-venous fistulae may cause clubbing, cyanosis and bruits over the lung fields.

Tongue

On examination of the tongue one may note abnormalities of:

Colour

The colour of the tongue may change and:

- ♣ Central cyanosis may be observed in the tongue

Palate

The palate may be:

♥ High arched in Marfan's syndrome

Buccal Mucosa

The buccal mucosa may be:

♠ Dry in Sjogren's syndrome, which is associated with fibrosing alveolitis

♦ Pigmented in adrenal insufficiency

Salivary Glands

Lesions that one may note in the salivary glands are:

♠ Parotid enlargement may occur in sarcoidosis, tuberculosis, Sjogren's syndrome

♦ Mikulicz syndrome refers to bilateral salivary and lachrymal gland swelling. This may be due to sarcoidosis, lymphoma, leukaemia.

Functions

Functional abnormalities that one may detect on examination of the mouth may be in relation to:

♠ **Breathing**

Fish mouth or pursed lip breathing would be observed in emphysema.

♦ **Speech**

The voice may be hoarse due to laryngitis or recurrent laryngeal palsy

Hoarseness may be due to granulomata on the vocal cords in Wegener's granulomatosis.

Aphonia may be caused by laryngitis

If the patient has a hoarse voice ask the patient to cough and listen for the bovine cough of recurrent laryngeal nerve palsy

Upper Limbs

On general examination of the upper limbs one may note changes in the:

Dimensions

The changes that may occur are:

♣ An increased arm span would be observed in Marfan's syndrome.

♥ In Cushing's syndrome thin (matchstick) arms would be seen in association with truncal obesity.

Hands

On examination of the hands one may note abnormalities of the following:

Dimensions

On examination of the dimensions one may note changes in:

♣ Size

♥ Shape

Size

Abnormalities that one may observe in the size of the hands are:

♠ In scleroderma the hands would appear small and have a distinctive shape.

Shape

Abnormalities that may be observed in the shape of the hands are:

- ◆ Arachnodactyly would be seen in Marfan's syndrome.
- ♣ Rheumatoid deformity of the hands. Rheumatoid arthritis may be associated with pulmonary fibrosis, pleural effusion.
- ♥ Dactylitis may occur in sarcoidosis and tuberculosis. This results in sausage shaped fingers.

Nails

When examining the nails one may note changes in:

- ♠ Shape
- ◆ Colour
- ♣ Circulation

Shape

Significant changes in the shape of the nails would be:

Clubbing

Clubbing would be seen in lesions of the:

- ♠ **Bronchi**

  Bronchiectasis, bronchial carcinoma

- ◆ **Alveoli**

  Fibrosing alveolitis

- ♣ **Lung Parenchyma**

  Lung abscess, asbestosis

- ♥ **Pulmonary Vasculature**

  Arteriovenous fistulae in hereditary haemorrhagic telangiectasia (Osler-Rendu-Weber syndrome)

- ♠ **Pleura**

  Mesothelioma, empyema

Colour

Changes that one may observe in the colour of the nails are:

Tar Staining

Tar staining indicates cigarette smoking, which may result in:

- ◆ Cancer of the bronchus, chronic obstructive pulmonary disease

Circulation

Nail Fold and Nail Edge Infarcts

Nail fold and nail edge infarcts may be seen in:

- ♣ Vasculitis, which may occur in association with fibrosing alveolitis

Skin

Abnormalities that one may observe in the skin over the hands are:

- ♥ Cyanosis would occur in any condition that causes ventilatory failure.
- ♠ Dermatomyositis may occur in association with carcinoma of the bronchus

Peripheral Circulation

When assessing the peripheral circulation one may note:

- ◆ Warm skin in carbon dioxide narcosis

Radial Pulse

On examination of the radial pulse one may note changes in:

- ♣ Rate
- ♥ Rhythm
- ♠ Volume

Rate

Variations in the pulse rate could be:

- ♣ Tachycardia may occur in any acute respiratory condition or decompensation of any chronic respiratory condition
- ♥ Tachycardia may be a reflection of treatment with beta agonists

Rhythm

Variations in the rhythm of the radial pulse could be:

- ♠ Atrial fibrillation. This complicates chest infections especially in the elderly.
- ♦ Atrial fibrillation may occur in malignancies of the lung infiltrating the heart.

Volume

Variations in the pulse volume could be:

- ♣ A high-volume, bounding pulse would occur when there is carbon dioxide retention.
- ♥ Pulsus paradoxus occurs in severe asthma

CNS

On examination of the nervous system of the hands, the abnormalities that one may note are:

Muscle Wasting

Wasting of the small muscles of the hand would be seen in:

- ♠ T_1 lesions caused by an apical bronchial carcinoma (Pancoast's syndrome)

Involuntary Movements

The involuntary movements that may occur are:

- ♦ A flapping tremor which would signify hypercapnoea
- ♣ Physiological tremor may reflect treatment with beta agonists

Forearm

Lesions that may occur in the forearm are:

- ♥ Hypertrophic pulmonary osteoarthropathy would present as tenderness and swelling of the wrist. It is the most severe form of clubbing.

Upper Arms

In the upper arms one may note changes in:

Blood Pressure

The changes that may occur are:

- ♠ Elevated blood pressure occurs with ectopic ACTH production in bronchial carcinoma
- ♦ Hypotension occurs in severe pneumonia

Shoulders

In the shoulders the abnormalities that may occur are:

- ♣ A buffalo-hump shaped deposition of fat would be observed in Cushing's syndrome.
- ♥ Tenderness and weakness of the shoulder girdle would occur in dermatomyositis, which may be associated with bronchial carcinoma.
- ♠ Proximal myopathy may occur in the ectopic ACTH syndrome complicating bronchial cancer.

Axillae

In the axillae one may observe:

- ♦ Acanthosis nigricans, which may occur in carcinoma of the bronchus

Neck

On examination of the neck one may note changes in the following:

Size

The size of the neck may be:

- ♣ **Increased**

  In superior vena cava obstruction and in subcutaneous emphysema

- ♥ **Decreased**

  In emaciation as a result of pulmonary tuberculosis, cystic fibrosis, malignancy

Integument

On examination of the integument one may note:

- ♠ A scar across the trachea. This could indicate a previous tracheostomy
- ♦ A scar across the suprasternal notch. This may indicate that the patient has undergone a mediastinoscopy.

Consistency

The consistency of the tissues of the neck may be abnormal.

- ♠ The consistency would change due to air in subcutaneous emphysema and this would result in crepitus.

Sternocleidomastoid Muscle

On examination of the sternocleido-mastoid muscle one may note:

- ♦ The sternocleidomastoid muscle would be in a state of contraction in respiratory distress.

Jugular Venous Pressure

When examining the jugular venous pressure one may note abnormalities of the following:

- ♣ Height
- ♥ Character
- ♠ Transmission

Height

Abnormalities of the height of the jugular venous pressure are:

♣ The jugular venous pressure would be raised in pulmonary hypertension and in cor pulmonale.

♥ Non-pulsatile elevation occurs in obstruction of the superior vena cava.

The causes of obstruction of the superior vena cava are bronchial carcinoma, enlargement of mediastinal lymph nodes, retrosternal goitre, thymic tumour, neurogenic tumour, mediastinal fibrosis.

Character

Variations in the character of the jugular venous pressure are:

♠ A dominant **a** wave would be seen in pulmonary hypertension.

♦ A dominant **V** wave would be seen in cor pulmonale and tricuspid regurgitation

Transmission

Lack of transmission or absent hepato-jugular reflux would occur in:

♣ Obstruction of the superior vena cava

Trachea

On examination of the trachea one may note abnormalities of the following:

♥ Site

♠ Length

♦ Movement

♣ Stridor

♥ Rattling

♠ Stertorous breathing

♦ Sighing

Site

The trachea may be:

♥ **Pushed**

Pushed to the opposite side by a pneumothorax or pleural effusion

♠ **Pulled**

Pulled to the same side by fibrosis, collapse of the lung, pneumonectcomy.

The only exception to this is in carcinoma of the bronchus where malignant infiltration may cause the trachea to be deviated to the same side as a pleural effusion.

Length

Normally three fingers may be interposed between the cricoid cartilage and the sternum. This gap would be decreased:

♦ In hyperinflation of the chest in emphysema

♣ During an attack of asthma

Movement

The abnormalities that may be detected are:

♥ Inspiratory descent of the trachea occurs in severe obstructive airways disease and in other forms of respiratory distress.

Stridor

Stridor occurs in:

♣ Epiglottitis

♥ Laryngeal carcinoma

- ♠ Tracheal compression
- ♦ Tracheal stenosis which may be:

  Congenital, following tracheostomy, post intubation

- ♣ Tracheal stenosis may occur due to vasculitis in Wegener's granulomatosis
- ♥ Recurrent laryngeal palsy

Rattling

Rattling occurs due to accumulation of secretions in the upper airways of patients who are unable to cough due to:

- ♠ Suppression of the cough reflex
- ♦ General debilitation

Stertorous Breathing

Stertorous breathing occurs due to vibration of the soft tissues of the pharynx, larynx and cheeks.

Sighing

Sighing occurs when a patient takes deep breaths as a compensation for acidosis in:

- ♣ Diabetic ketoacidosis
- ♥ Uraemia
- ♠ Salicylate poisoning

Chest Wall

On examination of the chest wall one may note abnormalities of the:

- ♥ Dimensions
- ♠ Integument
- ♦ Breasts
- ♣ Blood vessels

Dimensions

On examination of the dimensions one may note changes in:

- ♥ Size
- ♠ Shape

Size

The size of the chest would be:

- ♦ Increased and the chest would be barrel shaped due to hyperinflation in obstructive airways disease.
- ♣ An apparent increase in size may occur in subcutaneous emphysema

Shape

Abnormalities in the shape of the chest could be:

- ♥ **Barrel Shaped Chest**

  In a barrel shaped chest the antero-posterior diameter and the transverse diameter would be about equal. It signifies chronic obstruction of the airways.

- ♠ **Pectum Excavatum**

  Pectum excavatum is a funnel shaped deformity of the chest. It is usually congenital.

- ♦ **Pectum Carinatum**

  Pectum carinatum or pigeon chest is a prominent upper sternum. It can be caused by rickets and chronic chest infections.

- ♣ **Rickety Rosary**

  A rickety rosary refers to prominent costochondral

junctions. This occurs in childhood rickets.

♥ **Harrison's Sulcus**

Harrison's sulcus refers to indrawing of the ribs below the nipples. It indicates childhood asthma or rickets

♠ **Localised Retraction**

Localised retraction of the chest wall may occur due to underlying fibrosis. Apical retraction would suggest tuberculosis.

♦ **Chest Wall Retraction**

Retraction of the chest wall would be seen if the patient has had a pneumonectomy

♣ **Bulging**

Bulging of one side may be caused by a pneumothorax.

♥ **Prominence of the Intercostal Spaces**

Prominence of the intercostal spaces may be seen in pleural effusion.

Integument

Abnormalities that one may note in the skin over the chest wall are the following:

♥ A thoracotomy scar could indicate a pneumonectcomy.

♠ A midline sternotomy scar could indicate a double lung transplant.

♦ A thoracotomy scar could indicate a single lung transplant

♣ Radiotherapy marks could indicate underlying malignancy or pulmonary fibrosis

Breasts

On examination of the breasts one may note:

♠ In a male gynaecomastia may be a non-metastatic manifestation of carcinoma of the bronchus

♦ Mastectomy could suggest the cause of a metastatic lesion or pleural effusion

Blood Vessels

Dilated veins would be seen in obstruction of the superior vena cava. The flow of blood would be from cephalic to caudal.

Respiration

When examining respiration one may note abnormalities of the following:

♣ Position

♥ Rate

♠ Rhythm

♦ Volume

♣ Character

♥ Transmission

Position

In a professional examination the patient would be positioned with the torso at an angle of 45 degrees to the bed or couch. In practice observing the position the patient adopts would give useful clues to the underlying condition. The following abnormalities may be noted:

♣ **Orthopnoea**

In orthopnoea the patient must remain in the upright position to maintain respiration. This occurs in most forms of respiratory disease. In severe respiratory distress, the patient may hold on to items of furniture to facilitate contraction of the accessory muscles of respiration.

♥ **Platypnoea**

In platypnoea the patient finds breathing more comfortable when supine. This is seen in patients with the hepato-pulmonary syndrome.

♠ **Trepopnoea**

In trepopnoea the patient is more comfortable lying on a side. This occurs in congestive heart failure. These patients prefer the right lateral decubitus position.

Rate

The normal respiratory rate is between 10-19 respirations per minute.

Tachypnoea

An increased respiratory rate or tachypnoea indicates conditions involving the:

♦ **RS** pneumonia, asthma, exacerbation of chronic obstructive pulmonary disease, pulmonary embolism

♣ **E&M** fever, thyrotoxicosis, diabetic ketoacidosis

♥ **KUS** uraemia causing acidosis

♠ **CVS** heart failure

♦ **HS** anaemia

♣ **CNS** anxiety states

Decreased Respiratory Rate (Bradypnoea)

A decreased respiratory rate or bradypnoea is not common. The causes are:

♥ **Drugs**

Narcotic analgesics

Sedatives

Incorrect oxygen therapy in patients with chronic respiratory disease and carbon dioxide retention. This would take away the hypoxic respiratory drive required to maintain ventilation.

♠ **E&M** hypothermia, metabolic alkalosis

♦ **Physiological** in well-trained athletes

Rhythm

The normal rhythm of respiration is inspiration followed by expiration, which is followed by a gap. Inspiration is normally longer than expiration. Abnormalities of rhythm usually indicate serious disease.

♥ Expiration is longer than inspiration in obstructive airways disease

♠ In Cheyne-Stokes breathing a cyclical variation in the respiratory rate occurs. The nadir of the cycle is a period of apnoea and the zenith is a period of tachypnoea. The causes are cerebrovascular disease, uraemia, cardiac failure.

♦ Central hyperventilation occurs in lesions of the pons and midbrain

♣ Ataxic irregular breathing occurs in medullary depression

♥ Ondine's curse refers to failure of the automatic control of respiration by the brainstem. Whilst awake the patient is able to breathe but when the patient falls asleep hypoventilation or even apnoea occur. The cause may be congenital or occur following stroke, multiple sclerosis, tumour compression, surgery, infection.

Volume

Changes in respiratory volume are as follows:

♣ In most respiratory illness chest expansion diminishes.

♦ An increase in volume would be seen in Kussmaul's respiration or deep sighing respiration. This occurs when there is respiratory compensation for metabolic acidosis

Character

In normal respiration at rest, the respiratory movement is mainly diaphragmatic with gentle outward movement of the abdominal and chest walls in inspiration and the reverse in expiration.

♣ Paradoxical movement of the abdominal wall, moving in during inspiration and out during expiration occurs in phrenic nerve palsy.

♥ Flail segment of the chest, following trauma, results in a segment of the chest wall moving in a direction opposite to that of the rest of the chest wall.

Transmission

Other features that would be associated with abnormal respiration are the following

♠ Intercostal indrawing denotes increased negative intrathoracic pressure (decreased intrathoracic pressure) and occurs in obstructive airways disease.

♦ The use of the accessory muscles of respiration would be observed when the patient is in a state of respiratory distress.

Respiratory Movements (by palpation)

The abnormalities that may be detected are:

♣ Reduced Movement

♥ Paradoxical Movement

Reduced Movement

Reduced movement on one side would indicate disease underlying that area. This could be a lesion in the:

♣ **Lung Parenchyma**

Consolidation, collapse, fibrosis, pneumonectomy

♥ **Pleura**

Pleurisy, pleural effusion, pneumothorax

Paradoxical Movement

Paradoxical movement occurs in:

♣ Diaphragmatic paralysis

♦ Flail segment

Vocal Fremitus

Variations that may be noted are:

* ♣ Increased Vocal Fremitus
* ♥ Decreased Vocal Fremitus

Increased Vocal Fremitus

Increased vocal fremitus would indicate that the transmission of sound from the bronchi to the chest wall has increased. This could be due to:

* ♣ The underlying lung becoming solid (consolidation) and conducting sound better
* ♥ The bronchi coming closer to the chest wall due to collapse (peripheral) or localised fibrosis of the lung

Decreased Vocal Fremitus

Decreased vocal fremitus implies separation of the bronchi from the chest wall due to lesions in the:

* ♠ **Lung parenchyma**

  Collapse (central), pneumonectomy

* ♦ **Pleura**

  Pneumothorax, pleural effusion

Percussion Note

Abnormalities that may be detected on percussion are the following:

* ♣ Hyper-Resonant Percussion Note
* ♥ Decreased Cardiac Dullness
* ♠ Decreased Liver Dullness
* ♦ Dull Percussion Note
* ♠ Stony Dull Percussion Note

Hyper-Resonant Percussion Note

A hyper-resonant percussion note indicates:

* ♥ Pneumothorax
* ♠ Emphysema.

Decreased Cardiac Dullness

Decreased cardiac dullness (resonance over the praecordium) occurs in:

* ♦ Emphysema
* ♣ Pneumothorax
* ♥ Dextrocardia

Decreased Liver Dullness

Decreased liver dullness (resonance below the fifth right intercostal space in the mid-clavicular line) occurs in:

* ♠ Emphysema
* ♦ Pneumothorax

Dull Percussion Note

The percussion note would be dull in conditions involving the:

* ♣ **Lung parenchyma**

  Pneumonia, collapse, fibrosis, pneumonectcomy

Stony Dull Percussion Note

A stony dull percussion note occurs in conditions involving the:

* ♥ **Pleura**

  Pleural effusion

Breath Sounds

Abnormalities that occur may affect the following:

- ♥ Quantity
- ♠ Character
- ♦ Transmission

Quantity

The abnormality that could occur is:

Diminished Breath Sounds

Diminished breath sounds would occur when there is an increased distance between the distal air spaces and the chest wall or where conduction of sound is decreased. This occurs in conditions involving the:

- ♥ **Alveoli**

  Emphysema

- ♠ **Lung Parenchyma**

  Central collapse, diffuse pulmonary fibrosis, pneumonectcomy

- ♦ **Pleura**

  Pleural effusion, pneumothorax

Character

Abnormalities in the character of the breath sounds are as follows:

Bronchial Breath Sounds

Bronchial breath sounds are heard when there is increased transmission of sound from the bronchial tubes to the chest wall. This occurs in conditions involving the:

- ♣ **Lung Parenchyma**

Peripheral collapse, localised pulmonary fibrosis (the bronchi come close to the chest wall)

Consolidation (solid lung between the bronchi and the chest wall)

Following pneumonectomy bronchial breath sounds may be heard over the displaced trachea.

Amphoric Breath Sounds

Amphoric breath sounds are a variety of bronchial breath sounds. In amphoric breath sounds, the sound is hollow, similar to the sound made if one were to blow over the top of a narrow mouthed flask.

- ♥ Amphoric breath sounds are heard when a bronchus is in communication with a large cavity or with a pneumothorax.

Transmission

Variations in sound transmission could be noted when examining:

- ♠ Vocal resonance
- ♦ Whispering pectoriloquy

Vocal Resonance

The variations that may occur in vocal resonance are the following:

- ♣ **Increased Vocal Resonance**

  Increased vocal resonance occurs in conditions where conduction of sound from the bronchi to the chest wall is increased or where the bronchi come closer to the chest wall as in:

  Consolidation, collapse (peripheral), localised pulmonary fibrosis

♥ **Decreased Vocal Resonance**

Decreased vocal resonance occurs in conditions where conduction of sound from the bronchi to the chest wall is decreased or where the bronchi move away from the chest wall as in:

Central collapse, pneumonectomy, emphysema, pleural effusion, pleural thickening, pneumothorax

♠ **Aegophony**

Aegophony is heard at the upper level of a pleural effusion. It is due to differential conduction of sound through air and fluid and reflected sound at the fluid level.

Whispering Pectoriloquy

Whispering pectoriloquy is a confirmatory sign of bronchial breathing. No comment should be made regarding the presence of bronchial breathing without eliciting this sign to confirm it.

Added Sounds

When listening for added sounds one may detect the following:

♦ Crepitations

♣ Rhonchi

♥ Squawks

♠ Pleural rub

Crepitations

If crepitations are heard one would note the following:

♦ Character

♣ Timing

♥ Position

♠ Modifying factors

Character

The character of crepitations may be:

♦ **Coarse Crepitations**

Coarse crepitations are caused by conditions affecting the bronchi such as bronchiectasis and chronic bronchitis

♠ **Fine Crepitations**

Fine crepitations are caused by conditions affecting the alveoli such as left ventricular failure, fibrosing alveolitis, pneumonia, pulmonary fibrosis

Timing

One would note the timing of the crepitations. The timing may be:

♥ **Early and Mid-Inspiratory**

Early and mid-inspiratory crepitations are caused by pathology in more proximal airways

♠ **Late Inspiratory Crepitations**

Late inspiratory crepitations are caused by pathology in the distal air spaces either fibrosis or fluid (exudate, transudate or blood) in the alveoli

♦ **Expiratory Crepitations**

Expiratory crepitations occur in airflow obstruction

Position

The position at which the crepitations are heard would be a guide to the underlying pathology.

Fine Crepitations

Fine crepitations may be heard at the:

♦ **Base**

Fine basal crepitations are caused by left ventricular failure, fibrosing alveolitis

♣ **Apex**

Fine apical crepitations may be caused by tuberculosis, ankylosing spondylitis, radiation fibrosis

♥ **Localised**

Localised fine crepitations are caused by pneumonia

Coarse Crepitations

Coarse crepitations may be heard at the:

♠ **Base**

Coarse basal crepitations may be caused by bronchiectasis, hypostasis

♦ **Scattered**

Scattered coarse crepitations may be caused by chronic bronchitis, bronchiectasis

Modifying Factors

Crepitations may be modified by:

♣ **Coughing**

Coughing clears coarse crepitations

Rhonchi (Wheezing)

When analysing rhonchi one should note the following:

♥ Position

♠ Character

Position

The position at which rhonchi are heard may give a clue to the cause.

♥ **Scattered Rhonchi**

Scattered rhonchi are heard in:

Bronchial asthma and chronic bronchitis

♠ **Localised Rhonchi**

Localised rhonchi occur in:

Airway obstruction due to a tumour, foreign body, mucous plug

Character

Variations in character could occur. Rhonchi may be:

♦ **Sibilant Rhonchi**

High pitched (sibilant) rhonchi occur in narrowing of smaller airways

♣ **Sonorous Rhonchi**

Low pitched (sonorous rhonchi) occur in narrowing of larger airways

♥ **Polyphonic Rhonchi**

Polyphonic rhonchi or rhonchi with multiple pitches occur in asthma and chronic obstructive pulmonary disease

♠ **Monophonic Rhonchi**

Monophonic rhonchi or rhonchi with a single pitch occur in localised narrowing of a single air passage due to a tumour or foreign body

Squawk

A squawk is a high-pitched inspiratory sound that occurs due to opening up of airways that close in expiration.

* Squawks occur in pulmonary fibrosis and they are often preceded by crepitations.

Pleural Rub

A pleural rub may be caused by underlying:

* Pneumonia
* Pulmonary infarction

Heart

Lesions that occur in the heart in relation to respiratory disease are conditions that affect the:

* Apex beat
* Left parasternal heave
* Heart sounds
* Murmurs
* Extra-cardiac sounds
* Bruits

Apex Beat

The abnormalities that may be detected on examination of the apex beat are:

* The apex beat may be displaced with severe mediastinal shift.
* Dextrocardia may be associated with bronchiectasis in Kartagener's syndrome.
* The apex beat may be difficult to palpate in:

Chronic obstructive pulmonary disease with hyperinflated lungs, left-sided pleural effusion, pericardial effusion complicating bronchial cancer

Left Parasternal Heave

Left parasternal heave occurs in:

* Right ventricular hypertrophy consequent on pulmonary hypertension

Heart Sounds

Abnormalities in relation to the heart sounds are those that may be detected on:

* Palpation
* Auscultation

Palpation

On palpation of the heart sounds one may detect:

* A palpable P_2 in pulmonary hypertension

Auscultation

On auscultation of the heart sounds one may detect the following:

* The heart sounds would be better heard on the right side of the thorax in dextrocardia, severe mediastinal shift.
* A loud single P_2 would be heard in pulmonary hypertension.
* A split second sound would occur in right bundle branch block.
* An ejection click would be heard if there is dilatation of the pulmonary artery.

♥ A fourth heart sound would occur in pulmonary hypertension, right ventricular hypertrophy, right ventricular strain.

Murmurs

Murmurs that would be of significance in pulmonary disease are:

♠ An early diastolic murmur would occur in pulmonary regurgitation consequent on pulmonary hypertension

♦ A pan systolic murmur would be heard in tricuspid regurgitation due to right ventricular failure consequent on long-standing respiratory disease.

Extra-Cardiac Sounds

Extra-cardiac sounds that may be heard in relation to respiratory disease are:

♠ **Pericardial Crunch**

A crunching sound may be heard in time with the heartbeat in:

Left sided pneumothorax, pneumomediastinum

♦ **Pericardial Rub**

A pericardial rub may be heard in pericarditis complicating bronchial cancer

Bruits

Bruits may be heard over the lung fields in:

♠ Hereditary haemorrhagic telangiectasia (Osler-Rendu-Weber syndrome)

Posterior Aspect of the Neck

On examination of the posterior aspect of the neck one may note:

♥ Lymphadenopathy, which could be due to tuberculosis, carcinoma of the bronchus, sarcoidosis, AIDS

♠ Subcutaneous emphysema occurs in rib fractures, rupture of the oesophagus, as a complication of medical or surgical interventions, gas gangrene. It gives a characteristic crackling sensation.

Spine

On examination of the spine one may note:

♦ Kyphoscoliosis, which may be associated with ventilatory insufficiency and bronchiectasis.

♣ Kyphoscoliosis may be a feature of Marfan's syndrome.

♥ Ankylosing spondylitis may be associated with apical fibrosis or cavitation.

Abdomen

Abnormalities that one may note on examination of the abdomen are those in relation to the following:

Liver

Abnormalities of the liver that may occur in relation to respiratory disease are:

♠ Hepatomegaly may occur due to cor pulmonale or metastases in the liver.

♦ Autoimmune hepatitis is associated with fibrosing alveolitis

♣ A pulsatile liver may occur due to tricuspid regurgitation in cor pulmonale

Spleen

Abnormalities of the spleen that may occur in relation to respiratory disease are:

♥ Hepatosplenomegaly may occur in sarcoidosis

Kidneys

Abnormalities of the kidneys that may occur in relation to respiratory disease are:

♠ A kidney tumour may explain pulmonary secondaries.

Ascites

The presence of ascites may explain the cause of:

♦ A right-sided pleural effusion. This could be the result of fluid passing through tracts in the diaphragm

Lower Limbs

Abnormalities of the lower limbs could be those affecting the following:

Hips

Lesions that may occur in the hips are:

♣ Proximal myopathy could be a non-metastatic manifestation of bronchial cancer.

Lower Leg

Lesions that may occur in the lower legs are the following:

♥ Erythema nodosum may occur due to sarcoidosis or tuberculosis.

♠ Oedema may be due to:

Cor pulmonale, ventilatory failure and carbon dioxide retention

♦ Thrombophlebitis migrans may occur in carcinoma of the bronchus

Gait

Abnormalities of gait that occur in relation to the respiratory system are:

♣ Cerebellar ataxia may be caused by a secondary deposit or it may be a non-metastatic manifestation of bronchial cancer

♥ Eaton-Lambert syndrome, caused by small cell lung cancer, may present with gait abnormalities due to limb girdle weakness

♠ A waddling gait may occur if the patient has a proximal myopathy

Standing from a Seated or Squatting Position

Standing from a seated or squatting position would be difficult for patients with:

♦ Proximal myopathy complicating bronchial cancer

Chapter 12

The Digestive System

In this system one will study the digestive tract, the associated glands of the digestive tract and the hepato-biliary system. The causes and effects of diseases that involve the digestive system but are reflected by clinical features in other systems will also be studied.

History Taking

One should enquire about symptoms related to the:

- ♥ Digestive Tract
- ♠ Hepato-Biliary System

Digestive Tract

One would analyse the digestive tract by starting at the cephalic end and moving systematically down to the caudal end.

One should enquire about:

- ♥ Appetite
- ♠ Mastication
- ♦ Pain or soreness of the mouth
- ♣ Swallowing:

  Enquire about difficulty in swallowing or pain.
- ♥ Heartburn
- ♠ Reflux
- ♦ Belching
- ♣ Abdominal Pain
- ♥ Early Satiety
- ♠ Bloating or Distension
- ♦ Swelling

- ♣ Bowel Movements:

  Number of motions

  Consistency

  Blood

  Mucous
- ♥ Evacuation of Faeces:

  Enquire about rectal sensation, continence and adequacy of evacuation (complete or incomplete evacuation). Ask about ease of commencement of evacuation and whether there is a need to strain.
- ♠ Prolapse of rectum
- ♦ Perianal Problems:

  Discharge, pain, lump

Hepato-Biliary System

One should enquire about:

- ♣ Pain
- ♥ Jaundice
- ♠ Itch
- ♦ Discoloration of Urine
- ♣ Colour of Stool
- ♥ Lack of Energy

♠ Swelling (of the abdomen and the limbs)

One should then proceed to perform a review of systems.

Physical Examination

One should begin with a general examination and then proceed to perform regional examination.

General Examination

Evaluate the position of the patient. Next, assess the state of growth and development and the metabolic state of the patient. Note any gross changes in the integument. Assess the body temperature if required. (Position, Height and Proportions, Weight and Shape, Integument, Body Temperature)

Regional Examination

Commence regional examination by starting with the head. One may commence by examining the hands if one prefers.

Head

Note the mental state. Assess the dimensions of the head. Examine the regions of the head; the nose, the eyes, the face (scalp, forehead, eyebrows, malar region, chin), the mouth (jaw, lips, teeth, gums, buccal mucosa, tongue, palate, fauces, salivary glands) and the ears.

Upper Limbs

Perform a quick general examination of the upper limbs noting the dimensions and the state of the integument.

Hands

Assess the dimensions. Next, examine the dorsum of the hands; the nails and skin, the bones, joints, tendons and muscles. Ask the patient to turn the hands over and examine the skin, the bones, joints, tendons and muscles. Palpate the hands and assess the state of the peripheral circulation and examine the radial pulse. Ask the patient to stretch the arms out and look for tremors. Next, ask the patient to extend the wrists and spread the fingers apart. Look for a flapping tremor. If the patient is unable to maintain this position, hold the patient's forearm, just above the wrist, with one hand. With one's other hand hold the patient's hand, wind it around a few times and push the patient's wrist into the dorsi-flexed position and maintain this position. If present, the flapping tremor will be felt against the examining hand.

Examine the nervous system and function of the locomotor system of the hands if required.

Perform a quick examination of the forearms, the elbows, the shoulders and the axillae. In practice, if required, one should examine the locomotor system and the nervous system of the upper limbs. This would not be expected in professional examinations.

Neck

Quickly examine the neck. Note the dimensions, look for any changes in the integument. Look for elevation of the jugular venous pressure. In a professional examination, mention to the examiners that one would perform a thorough examination of the lymph nodes when the patient is asked to sit up to examine the back of the patient. If they ask you to examine the lymph nodes then ask the patient to sit up and examine the lymph nodes using the method described in the chapter on the haematological system.

In practice one should examine the dimensions, the integument, the thyroid, the sternocleidomastoid, the jugular venous pressure, the carotids, the trachea and the lymph nodes. The lymph nodes should be examined when the patient sits up for one to examine the back of the patient.

Chest

Examine the chest wall. Quickly note the dimensions of the chest wall and the state of the integument. In a male one should note the presence of gynaecomastia. In a professional examination one should avoid exposing a female patient's breasts but in practice one should examine the breasts if indicated.

In practice one should examine the contents of the chest, and then examine the back of the patient before moving on to the abdomen.

Abdomen

Examination of the abdomen should follow the usual routine of inspection, palpation, percussion and auscultation. Examine the abdominal wall and then examine the contents of the abdomen. Begin by positioning the patient correctly. The patient should be asked to lie as flat as possible. However, remember the patient's comfort is paramount. One thin pillow should be provided although, ideally, dispensing with this is better. Some clinicians ask the patient to bend the knees and facilitate this by placing a pillow under the knees. One may do this if one wishes. The patient's legs should not be crossed.

The abdomen should be exposed correctly. Ideally exposure should be from the upper chest to the inguinal region. But, care should be taken to avoid unnecessary exposure especially where female patients are concerned. The breasts and genitals should not be exposed. The patient should be asked to keep the mouth partially open and breathe gently. The patient's arms should rest by his or her side.

One should be satisfied that the patient is comfortable prior to commencing examination. An enquiry should be made whether there are any painful areas in the abdomen before commencing examination.

Abdominal Wall

Note the dimensions of the abdominal wall in particular the size and the shape. The general shape of the abdomen and any localised deformity should be noted. Study the integument in detail making a special note of any scars of previous abdominal surgery or stoma. Note the position, size and shape of the umbilicus. Note any distended veins. If distended veins are observed, ascertain the direction of blood flow in these vessels. If surgical scars are observed, ask the patient to lift the head off the pillow or cough and look for herniae. Ideally, herniae are examined with the patient standing.

Observe movements of the abdominal wall with respiration. The abdominal wall should rise gently with inspiration and fall with expiration. Note any visible peristaltic movement. Visible peristalsis is best observed by lowering one's head to the level of the abdomen by bending one's knees, kneeling or sitting. Make a note of any visible pulsation.

Further examination of the abdominal wall would be palpation of the abdominal wall and making a note of any areas of rigidity, guarding, and tenderness or rebound tenderness. This will be discussed further when describing the method of examination of the contents of the abdomen.

If required one may perform neurological examination and test movements of the abdominal wall, reflexes and sensation.

Contents of the Abdomen

The following techniques would be used in examination of the contents of the abdomen:

- ♥ Palpation
- ♠ Percussion
- ♦ Auscultation

Palpation of the Abdomen

Palpation of the abdomen is an important clinical skill. It allows one to derive a lot of useful information pertaining to diagnosis. In addition it clearly demonstrates the level of one's clinical skill. Skilful palpation is immediately obvious and is a pleasure to watch. Poor skill in palpation in addition to being obvious is also painful to watch and indeed painful for the unfortunate patient. Poor skill also leads to pain of mind for the candidate at professional examinations, as he or she will surely fail!

Technique

The crucial point in technique is that the forearm of the examining upper limb, the right, should be horizontal. The examining forearm should be brought into the horizontal position by bending one's knees, kneeling or sitting. The forearms, wrists, hands and fingers should be in a straight line. The palm of the hand and the palmar aspect of the fingers must be in firm, yet gentle, contact with the abdominal wall. The palpating movement must be at the metacarpophalangeal joints. Movement must be gentle and concur with the respiratory movements of the abdominal wall. The examining fingers should rise with the abdominal wall in inspiration and move in with the abdominal wall in expiration. Palpation should be performed with the pulp of the fingers. When defining the edges of enlarged organs or masses either the radial border of the index finger or the tips of the fingers may be used. For deeper palpation place the left hand over the right. This allows more force to be applied and thus one may reach deeper and achieve the objective of deep palpation.

Left-handed individuals may modify the technique to suit themselves but in a professional examination it would be important to point out to the examiners that one is left-handed.

Dipping

Dipping is employed in the presence of ascites where ordinary palpation is inadequate. The palpating hand is placed over the area of concern and a quick in-and-out movement is made at the metacarpophalangeal joints. This sudden movement displaces the underlying fluid and allows the enlarged organ or mass to be felt as the palpating fingers give it a tap.

A variation of the dipping technique is to use the tips of the examining fingers, moving them in a direction perpendicular to the abdominal wall to achieve the dipping movement. (A stabbing movement with the tips of the fingers)

Routine

Ask the patient whether there is any pain in the abdomen and identify the area or areas concerned if any.

Warm one's hands by rubbing them together, assume the position required to make the examining forearm horizontal (bending one's knees, kneeling, sitting) and place the hand on the abdominal wall. Rest the hand on the abdominal wall and observe the movement of the abdominal wall with respiration. Allow the fingers to be pushed out as the patient breathes in and the abdominal wall moves outwards. As the patient breathes out follow the movement of the abdominal wall inwards. Gently explore all the areas of the abdomen, note any abnormality of the abdominal wall as discussed earlier and feel for any obvious masses or tender areas. If a mass is felt, define the characteristics of the mass. Next, palpate the liver and spleen. When doing this one examines the right and left hypochondrium. Next, examine the lumbar region using bimanual palpation. Following this examine the epigastrium, the central abdomen, the left iliac fossa, the suprapubic region and the right iliac fossa.

Remember one should actively examine for enlargement of the liver, the spleen, the kidneys, pancreas, the aorta, para-aortic nodes, the bladder and in the female, masses arising out of the pelvis (uterine or ovarian) and for any other lump. One should not expect physical signs to demonstrate themselves.

In summary, look for enlargement of the intra-abdominal organs and feel for masses in the defined regions of the abdomen.

Regions of the Abdomen

The abdomen may be divided into nine regions. This is achieved by thinking of two vertical planes that pass upwards from the femoral artery to cross the costal margin close to the tip of the ninth costal cartilage. Two horizontal planes pass across the abdomen. They are the subcostal plane, which connects the lowest points of the costal cartilages and the interiliac plane, which connects the tubercles of the iliac crests.

The resulting nine regions are:

♠ Right and left hypochondrium

♦ Epigastric region

♣ Right and left lumbar regions

♥ Umbilical region

♠ Right and left iliac fossae

♦ Suprapubic region

Note On Palpation

It is important to have a routine of examination to ensure that all areas are palpated and no region is missed. Do it with an awareness of what is being examined and this will make it more likely that no physical sign is missed.

Many routines are described .Use whichever one finds most suitable to oneself. A routine is described below.

Routine of Palpation

Begin at the left hypochondrium then palpate the epigastrium, the right hypochondrium, the right lumbar region, the central abdomen (umbilical region), the left lumbar region, the left iliac fossa, the hypogastric region (suprapubic) and finally the right iliac fossa. This gives a rough S shape.

From the right iliac fossa proceed to palpate the liver, then the spleen. Feel for the kidneys (perform bimanual palpation), then palpate the epigastrium for any masses. Examine the central abdomen and the aorta and para-aortic nodes. Next examine the left iliac fossa, the suprapubic region for enlargement of the bladder and for masses arising from the pelvis and then the right iliac fossa.

A detailed description of examination of the liver and spleen will be given in this chapter. Examination of the kidneys will be described in detail in the chapter on the kidneys and urinary system and examination of the aorta and para-aortic nodes will be described in the chapter on the haematological system.

Liver

Begin palpation in the right iliac fossa. Allow the hand to move with respiration. As the patient breathes out move the palpating fingers in following the natural movement of the anterior abdominal wall. As the patient breathes in, allow the palpating fingers to be pushed outwards by the abdominal wall. When the patient breathes in movement of the diaphragm will carry the liver in a caudal direction and if it is enlarged, the palpating fingers should feel the liver as they ride over the liver edge. If the liver is not felt this low gradually move the palpating hand in a cephalic direction until it meets the costal margin. Allow at least one cycle of inspiration and expiration to be completed before moving the palpating hand to the next position. If the edge of the liver is felt follow it and define it clearly. Next, move the hand on to the surface of the liver and continue palpation. Note the characteristics of the surface, note the consistency and whether the liver is tender. Note whether the liver is pulsatile (some clinicians employ bimanual palpation to demonstrate a pulsatile liver). Move the hand along to the costal margin, confirm that the palpating fingers cannot be interposed between the costal margin and the liver.

Spleen

The spleen enlarges downwards and towards the right iliac fossa. Hence, one should commence palpation in the right iliac fossa. One's left hand should be placed over the lower left ribs. The left hand performs two functions. The first is to restrict movement of the lower ribs during respiration. It is hoped that this would encourage movement of the diaphragm and thereby increase the excursion made by the spleen during respiration. Secondly, the left hand exerts traction on the abdominal wall in a medial direction. This relaxes the abdominal wall and makes palpation easier. The right hand should make firm, yet gentle, contact with the abdominal wall and as the patient breathes out the fingers should follow the inward movement of the abdominal wall. As the patient breathes in the examining fingers should rise up to meet the edge of the spleen, as it is pushed down with inspiration, and if it is enlarged the fingers will be felt to ride over its edge. If the spleen is not felt on initial palpation one should gently work one's way upwards and towards the left costal margin. Remember, palpate for at least one cycle of respiration before moving the hand to the next position. If the spleen is not palpable upon reaching the costal margin, the patient should be asked to turn onto his or her right side. The patient's right lower limb should be extended and the left knee should be flexed. The left knee should rest on the bed. The patient should be asked to place the left arm near his or her head so that it will not obstruct palpation. Continue palpation as before.

If the spleen is palpable, the edge should be palpated and an attempt should be made to define the splenic notch. Next, palpate the surface and note the consistency of the spleen. One should confirm inability to interpose the palpating fingers between the spleen and the costal margin, in other words one should not be able to get above the spleen.

Following palpation of the spleen one should complete palpation of the contents of the abdomen as described earlier. When performing bimanual palpation of the loins, one should take the opportunity to note that if the liver and spleen were palpable they are not ballotable. Perform deep palpation if indicated.

Employ dipping if required.

(The technique of ballotment is described in the chapter on the kidneys and urinary system)

Percussion of the Abdomen

The technique is the same as that employed in percussion of the chest. The crucial points are close contact of the pleximeter with the surface of the abdominal wall with no contact by the other fingers. The other fingers should be slightly raised. The plexor should strike the middle phalanx of the pleximeter firmly and perpendicularly.

Percussion should be performed with the long axis of the pleximeter lying parallel to the edge of the organ or fluid level being percussed. Percussion should always begin in a resonant area and move towards the area where dullness would be expected.

Percussion of the Liver

First, percuss and define the upper border of the liver. Palpate the manubriosternal angle, which articulates with the second costal cartilage, and thereby define the second-right intercostal space. Place the pleximeter in this space with the middle phalanx in the mid-clavicular line. Begin percussion and move down from the second intercostal space until dullness is reached. Normally the upper border of the liver is at the fifth intercostal space in the mid-clavicular line. Percuss the lower border of the liver by beginning in a resonant area below the lower border and proceeding in a cephalic direction. Normally the lower border of liver dullness is at or just below the costal margin. If the liver is enlarged demonstrate that the dullness over it is continuous with the normal liver dullness.

Percussion of the Spleen

Begin percussion below the edge of the spleen and percuss towards it. Demonstrate dullness over an enlarged spleen and demonstrate that this dullness is continuous with the splenic dullness over the lower costal cartilages. If the spleen is not enlarged one may demonstrate resonance over the left eighth and ninth ribs in the anterior axillary line with the patient in the supine position.

Percussion of an Abdominal Mass

When using percussion to define a mass in the abdomen, always begin percussion in a resonant area away from the mass and move towards it. Do so from all directions.

Percussion of Ascites

To diagnose ascites clinically one should demonstrate:

- Flank dullness or horseshoe dullness
- Shifting dullness

If a large quantity of ascites is present one may also demonstrate a:

- Fluid thrill

Flank Dullness and Horseshoe Dullness

Percuss in the centre of the abdomen and demonstrate an area of resonance, then continue percussion into the flanks. If ascites is present one may demonstrate flank dullness. From the centre of the abdomen percuss inferiorly towards the symphysis pubis. If a significant quantity of ascites is present one may demonstrate an area of dullness in the suprapubic region. Thus, one may demonstrate a horseshoe shaped area of dullness.

Shifting Dullness

If flank dullness has been detected one may test for shifting dullness. Percuss the left flank. Whilst maintaining position with the pleximeter, ask the patient to turn on to the right-hand side, percuss and demonstrate that the dullness in the left flank is no longer present. Percuss towards the right flank and demonstrate that the area of dullness in the right flank has shifted towards the mid line. Maintain the pleximeter in this position and ask

the patient to lie flat once more. Demonstrate that this area is resonant once again. Demonstrate dullness in the left flank once more. Repeat the process on the other side this time asking the patient to turn to the left hand side.

Fluid Thrill

An assistant or the patient should place the ulnar border of his or her hand over the centre of the abdomen with the long axis of the hand lying in a cephalo-caudal direction. The clinician's left hand should be placed over the left flank of the patient with the palm making close contact with the abdominal wall. With the middle finger of one's right hand tap the right flank with a flick of the finger. In the presence of a large quantity of ascites a ripple will be felt striking the left palm.

Routine for Percussion

- Define any lump that has been detected
- Percuss the liver
- Percuss the spleen
- Percuss the centre of the abdomen
- Percuss the flanks
- Percuss the suprapubic region
- Demonstrate shifting dullness if flank dullness is detected
- Demonstrate fluid thrill if possible

Auscultation

On auscultation of the abdomen one should listen for the following:

♥ Succussion Splash

♠ Bowel Sounds

♦ Bruits

♣ Venous hum

Succussion Splash

Firmly grasp the patient's pelvis with one's right hand over the left iliac bone and one's left hand over the right iliac bone. Next, lower one's head so that one's left ear is close to, but does not touch, the epigastric region of the patient. Give the pelvis a firm shake. A splashing sound would be heard in the epigastric region in the presence of gastric outlet obstruction. The stethoscope may be used if desired. This test is not performed routinely and should be performed only if symptoms suggest gastric outlet obstruction

Bowel Sounds

Listen with the bell of the stethoscope over the anatomical listening post of the abdomen. The anatomical listening post is a few centimetres away from the umbilicus along a line joining the umbilicus to the anterior superior iliac spine. It is approximately one third of the distance from the umbilicus to the anterior superior iliac spine.

Bruits

Listen with the bell. Auscultate over the liver, the spleen and over any lumps that have been detected. Listen over the aorta and follow the line of the aorta inferiorly. At about the level of the umbilicus follow the expected line of the iliac vessels.

Venous Hum

Venous hums are heard over the upper abdomen. Exert gentle pressure with the chest piece of the stethoscope. A continuous humming sound will be heard.

This concludes examination of the abdomen.

Liver

Features that should be demonstrated to confirm that a mass in the right hypochondrium is an enlarged liver:

♥ The liver is palpable in the right hypochondrium; the rare exception is situs inversus

♠ It is superficial

♦ The edge is usually well defined, although in some instances it may be rounded

♣ The upper border is not palpable or in other words it is not possible to get above the liver

♥ It moves with respiration

♠ It is not ballotable

♦ The percussion note over it is dull and this dullness is continuous with the normal liver dullness

♣ A bruit may be heard over it

Spleen

Features that should be demonstrated to confirm that a mass in the left hypochondrium is an enlarged spleen:

- ♥ The spleen is palpable below the left costal margin
- ♠ It is felt superficially
- ♦ It has a well-defined edge
- ♣ A notch may be palpable
- ♥ The upper border cannot be defined or in other words it is not possible to get above the spleen
- ♠ It moves with respiration
- ♦ It is usually not ballotable although a massive spleen may be ballotable
- ♣ The percussion note over it is dull and this dullness is continuous with the normal splenic dullness
- ♥ A rub may be heard over it

Inguinal Region and Genitals

Next, one should examine the inguinal region. In particular take note of enlarged lymph nodes and examine the hernial orifices (inguinal and femoral). This may be performed at the same time as the rest of the abdominal examination if one wishes.

Ideally one should examine the genitalia as well. Remember that examination of the hernial orifices and the male external genitalia is best done with the patient standing.

However, it would be unwise to ask to examine the male genitalia in the erect position!

The inguinal region and genitals are not examined in professional examinations but it would be wise to mention to the examiners that it is one's usual practice to do so.

Buttocks, Perianal Region and Per Rectal Examination

Examination of the abdomen should include examination of the buttocks, the perianal region and per rectal examination. This would not be expected in a professional examination but it is standard practice to mention to the examiners that one would perform these examinations.

Similarly, one should mention that it is one's practice to examine the patient's neck, spine, back of chest and lower back.

Per Rectal Examination

Although not required in professional examinations the method is described below for the sake of completeness.

Ask the patient to assume the left lateral position with the lower limbs flexed as much as possible. Separate the patent's buttocks and examine the perianal region.

Put on a pair of gloves and lubricate one's right index finger generously. Raise the patient's right buttock with one's left hand and place one's gloved, lubricated, right index finger on the patient's anus with the pulp of the finger lying flat on it. Gently exert pressure with this finger and the anal sphincter will relax and allow entry.

Feel the wall of the anal canal by rotating one's finger through 360 degrees and then assess the tone of the anal sphincter. Ask the patient to contract the sphincter and assess squeeze pressure.

Pass the finger into the rectum and examine the wall of the rectum by performing 360-degree rotations with the finger at incremental levels.

Next, examine the exterior relationships of the rectum; posteriorly the sacrum and coccyx, laterally the side walls of the pelvis. Anteriorly in the male the prostate, seminal vesicles and the rectovesical pouch, in the female the cervix and uterus, the ovaries and the pouch of Douglas.

Lower Limbs

For the sake of completeness one should consider examination of the lower limbs. If required perform a general examination and then examine the hips, thighs, knees, lower legs and feet. Examine the nervous system and locomotor system if required.

Spine

Ideally one should also ask the patient to stand and examine the spine.

Gait, Romberg's Sign, Trendelenburg Test, Standing from a Seated or Squatting Position

Finally when indicated one should examine the patient's gait, look for Romberg's sign, perform the Trendelenburg test and assess the patient's ability to stand from a seated or squatting position.

Lesions of the Gastrointestinal Tract

When studying lesions of the gastrointestinal tract it would be easy if one were to consider the gastrointestinal tract as a hollow tube, connecting the mouth to the anus, with three solid appendages, the salivary glands, the pancreas and the liver attached to this tube. In addition one should also consider lesions affecting the peritoneal cavity.

Hence one should consider lesions of the:

♦ Hollow Organs

♣ Solid Organs

♥ Hepato-biliary system

♠ Peritoneal cavity

Hollow Organs

Lesions of the hollow organs usually cause local effects, effects due to obstruction, increased movement of intestinal contents or reversed movement of intestinal contents, haemorrhage.

Mouth

The common lesions that affect the mouth are:

♦ **Ulcers**

Ulcers may be malignant, consequent on bad dentition or due to coeliac disease or inflammatory bowel disease.

Other causes of mouth ulcers include infections such as syphilis and chronic inflammatory disorders such as Behcet's disease

Pharynx

Lesions of the pharynx could be in the:

♣ **Lumen**

Foreign body impaction

♥ **Mural**

Pharyngeal pouch

♠ **Systemic Factors**

CNS bulbar or suprabulbar palsy

Oesophagus

Lesions of the oesophagus could be in the:

♦ **Lumen**

Foreign body impaction

♣ **Mural**

Oesophagitis may be due to gastro-oesophageal reflux, ingestion of corrosives or infections such as candida, cytomegalovirus

Strictures could be benign or malignant

Fistulae may be:

Congenital (paediatric practice)

Malignant (bronchial or oesophageal malignancies. It could also occur following treatment of malignancies)

Motility Disorders that affect the oesophagus are corkscrew oesophagus, achalasia of the cardia, nutcracker oesophagus and non-specific oesophageal dysmotility. These conditions usually result in dysphagia and may be remembered by using the acronym CANNOD which stands for Corkscrew, Achalasia, Nutcracker, Non-specific Oesophageal Dysmotility. (These patients CANNOD swallow)

♥ **External Factors**

External factors cause dysphagia and could be an:

Enlarged left atrium, aortic aneurysm, enlarged lymph node, bronchial carcinoma

♠ **Systemic Factors**

LMS systemic sclerosis, which may cause dysphagia

Stomach

Lesions that occur in the stomach could be lesions in the:

♦ **Lumen**

Gastric bezoars

♣ **Mural Lesions**

Gastritis, ulcers benign or malignant, diffuse lesions such as infiltration by cancer, lymphoma,

281

Menetriere's disease, vascular anomalies, surgical reconstruction of the stomach (trauma)

♥ **Systemic Conditions**

E&M diabetic autonomic neuropathy

Duodenum

Lesions that occur in the duodenum could be:

♠ Ulcers

♦ Tumours (rarely)

Small Intestine

Conditions that affect the small intestine are lesions in the:

♦ **Lumen**

Gallstones, worms

♣ **Mural Lesions**

Coeliac disease, Crohn's disease, Whipple's disease, intestinal lymphangiectasia, tumours such as adenoma, lymphoma, carcinoid, hollow visceral myopathy

♥ **External Factors**

Adhesions, peritoneal bands

♠ **Systemic Factors**

E&M diabetic autonomic neuropathy

HS amyloidosis

Large Intestine

Conditions that affect the large intestine are those involving the:

♦ **Lumen**

Impacted faeces, worm infestations

♣ **Mural Factors**

Inflammatory conditions like ulcerative colitis, Crohn's disease, tumours, which may be carcinoma, polyps, diverticular disease, motility disorders such as Hirschprung's disease, acquired megacolon, hollow visceral myopathy

♥ **External Factors**

Volvulus

♠ **Systemic Factors**

HS amyloidosis

Perianal Lesions

In medical practice involvement in this region is usually due to:

♦ Inflammatory bowel disease

Solid Organs

One should consider lesions affecting the:

♦ Salivary Glands

♣ Pancreas

Salivary Glands

The main concern in the context of medical conditions would be conditions that cause enlargement of the salivary glands.

Enlargement may be:

♦ Unilateral

♣ Bilateral

Unilateral Enlargement

Unilateral enlargement of the salivary glands could be due to problems in the:

♦ **Lumen**

Obstruction due to calculi

♣ **Mural**

Mixed parotid tumour

Bilateral Enlargement

Bilateral enlargement of the salivary glands could be due to conditions affecting the:

♥ **GIT** alcohol abuse

♠ **RS** sarcoidosis

♦ **LMS** Sjogren's syndrome

♣ **Infections**: mumps parotitis. Parotitis can also occur in the elderly and in debilitated patients on account of poor oral hygiene as a consequence of inadequate mouth care.

Pancreas

Lesions that commonly occur in the pancreas are:

♥ **Mural Lesions**

Pancreatitis (acute and chronic), exocrine tumours, endocrine tumours

♠ **External Lesions**

Pancreatic pseudocyst

Hepato-Biliary Lesions

Problems in the hepato-biliary system may be due to lesions affecting the:

♦ Bile ducts

♣ Liver cells (hepatocellular)

♥ Vasculature

Bile Ducts

Problems in the bile ducts may be due to lesions in the:

♦ **Lumen**

Gallstones

♣ **Mural Lesions**

Strictures, which may be benign or malignant

Cholangitis, which may be infective, primary sclerosing cholangitis, secondary sclerosing cholangitis, primary biliary cirrhosis

♥ **External Lesions**

Enlarged lymph node, carcinoma head of pancreas

Hepatocellular

Damage to the liver cells may be due to:

♠ Biological Agents

♦ Chemical Agents

Biological Agents

Biological agents that result in hepatocellular damage are:

♠ **Viruses**: hepatitis A, B, C, E

♦ **Immune reactions**: Auto Immune Hepatitis

Chemical Agents

Chemical agents that result in hepatocellular damage are:

♣ **Metabolic problems**: Wilson's disease, haemochromatosis, alpha$_1$ antitrypsin deficiency

- ♥ **Toxins**: alcohol
- ♠ **Drugs**: paracetamol, antibiotics, immunosuppressive agents, anaesthetic agents

Vascular Lesions

Vascular lesions of the liver may be caused by problems in the:

- ♦ Hepatic Veins
- ♣ Portal Veins
- ♥ Hepatic Artery

Hepatic Veins

The lesions that may occur are:

- ♠ Thrombosis in the Budd-Chiari syndrome
- ♦ Congestion in tricuspid regurgitation, congestive cardiac failure, right ventricular failure, restrictive cardiomyopathy, constrictive pericarditis, cardiac tamponade

Portal Veins

Lesions that occur are:

- ♣ Portal vein thrombosis

Hepatic Artery

The condition that may be caused by involvement of the hepatic artery is:

- ♥ Shocked liver

Peritoneal Cavity

Ascites is the main problem encountered in clinical practice. This could be due to:

- ♠ **Internal Factors**

Tuberculous peritonitis, fungal peritonitis (cryptococcus, candida), parasitic infestation (*Endamoeba histolytica, Stongyloides stercoralis*)

- ♦ **Mural Factors**

Secondary deposits, lymphoma, leukaemia, mesothelioma, pseudomyxoma peritonei

- ♣ **External Factors**

Lymphatic obstruction resulting in chylous ascites

- ♥ **Systemic Factors**

Conditions involving the:

GIT

Portal hypertension: Budd-Chiari syndrome, veno-occlusive disease, cirrhosis of the liver, portal vein thrombosis

Biliary tract: bile ascites

Pancreas: pancreatic ascites

Intestine: eosinophilic gastroenteritis, Whipple's disease, protein losing enteropathy, nutritional failure

CVS congestive cardiac failure, right ventricular failure, constrictive pericarditis, cardiac tamponade

KUS nephrotic syndrome, urinary ascites

E&M hypothyroidism

RAG ovarian cancer, Meig's syndrome

RS sarcoidosis

LMS systemic lupus erythematosus

Findings on History

The common findings that may be obtained on taking a history are problems related to the following:

Appetite

Loss of appetite or anorexia is not a specific feature.

- ♠ Appetite may be decreased in any lesion of the digestive system.
- ♦ Severe anorexia is a feature of carcinoma of the stomach

Thirst

Excessive thirst would reflect:

- ♣ Salt and water loss consequent on severe diarrhoea or vomiting.

Dry Mouth

A dry mouth would reflect:

- ♥ Destruction of salivary glandular tissue

Excess Salivation

Excess salivation may be due to:

- ♠ An irritant lesion in the mouth.
- ♦ Difficulty in swallowing (failure to swallow saliva)

Water Brash

Water brash is a sudden increase in salivation.

- ♣ It is associated with reflux and nausea

Sore Mouth

Soreness in the mouth may be due to:

- ♥ Mouth ulcers
- ♠ Stomatitis

Mastication

Problems with mastication may be due to:

- ♦ **Mural Factors**

  Dental caries and ill-fitting dental prostheses

- ♣ **External Factors**

  Arthritis of the temperomandibular joint

- ♥ **Systemic Factors**

  LMS jaw claudication in giant cell arteritis

Swallowing

Symptoms related to swallowing may be:

- ♠ Dysphagia
- ♦ Odynophagia

Dysphagia

Difficulty in swallowing (food sticking) may be due to:

- ♠ **Luminal Factors**

  Impacted foreign body

- ♦ **Mural Factors**

  Diverticulum, pharyngeal pouch, oesophageal web, Schatzki ring, stricture either benign or malignant, oesophageal dysmotility

♣ **External Factors**

Compression by a:

Lymph node, aortic aneurysm, enlarged left atrium, bronchial cancer

♥ **Systemic Factors**

Conditions affecting the:

CNS bulbar palsies

LMS systemic sclerosis

Odynophagia

Pain on swallowing may be due to:

- ♠ Oesophagitis
- ♦ Oesophageal dysmotility

Heartburn, Reflux, Belching

Heartburn, reflux, belching are features of:

- ♣ Gastro-oesophageal reflux

Vomiting

Vomiting may be due to:

♣ **Luminal Factors**

Toxins, poisons, impacted foreign body, gallstone ileus

♥ **Mural Factors**

Gastric surgery, pyloric obstruction due to peptic stricture or malignancy, intestinal obstruction due to inflammatory bowel disease, tumours, infarction of the small bowel

♠ **External Factors**

Intestinal obstruction due to:

Adhesions, peritoneal bands, volvulus

♦ **Systemic Factors**

Conditions affecting the:

CNS increased intra cranial pressure, vestibular lesions

E&M diabetic ketoacidosis

Drugs almost any drug may cause vomiting

Liver pathology in the liver may cause vomiting

RAG pregnancy

Toxins alcohol

Abdominal Pain

Abdominal pain could be due to lesions affecting the gastrointestinal tract such as the following:

♣ **Luminal Factors**

Stones, parasites like roundworms

♥ **Mural Factors**

Ulcers, inflammation, strictures either inflammatory or malignant, ischaemia, infarction, dysmotility

♠ **External Factors**

Adhesions, peritoneal bands, inflammatory masses, peritonitis, herniae

Pancreatitis

Hepatobiliary disease (see later section)

♦ **Systemic Factors**

Conditions affecting the:

E&M hyperparathyroidism (stones, bones and abdominal groans), porphyria

Toxins lead poisoning

Haematemesis

Haematemesis could be due to:

♣ **Arterial Bleeding**

Mallory-Weiss tears, ulcers, vascular malformations like Dieulafoy lesions

♥ **Venous Bleeding**

Oesophageal or gastric varices

♠ **Telangiectasia**

Hereditary haemorrhagic telangiectasia

Early Satiety

Any lesion in the upper gastrointestinal tract may cause early satiety.

Bloating or Distension

Bloating or distension are common features of:

♣ Functional disorders.

♥ Their presence may suggest intestinal obstruction.

Swelling

Swelling of the abdomen may be due to:

♠ Intestinal obstruction

♦ Ascites

♣ Tumours

Bowel Movements

The changes that may occur in relation to bowel habit are:

♥ Constipation

♠ Diarrhoea

Constipation

Constipation could be due to:

♥ **Luminal Factors**

Impacted faeces

♠ **Mural Factors**

Strictures (which may be inflammatory, ischaemic, malignant) or dysmotility

♦ **External Factors**

Adhesions, volvulus

♣ **Systemic Factors**

Conditions affecting the:

E&M diabetic autonomic neuropathy, hypothyroidism, hypercalcaemia

CNS lesions of the pudendal nerve, sacral plexus, cauda equina and spinal cord

Parkinsonism

Drugs opioid analgesics, anticholinergics, iron

LMS systemic sclerosis

Diarrhoea

Diarrhoea could be due to:

♥ **Luminal Factors**

Toxins, bacterial infections, viral infections, parasitic infestations, bile acid malabsorption, bacterial overgrowth

♠ **Mural Factors**

287

Inflammatory bowel disease, coeliac disease, Whipple's disease, intestinal lymphangiectasia, lymphoma, infectious diarrhoea, pseudomembranous colitis

♦ **External Factors**

Pancreatic insufficiency

♣ **Systemic Factors**

Conditions affecting the

E&M thyrotoxicosis, gastrinoma, vipoma, carcinoid syndrome

Drugs antihypertensives, diuretics, antibiotics, proton pump inhibitors

Toxins beer

Spurious Diarrhoea

Constipation caused by impacted faeces or stricture may result in spurious diarrhoea due to liquefaction of the retained stools.

Bleeding Per Rectum

Bleeding per rectum may be due to:

♠ **Luminal Factors**

Foreign body

♦ **Mural Factors**

Inflammatory bowel disease, tumours benign or malignant, vascular malformations

Tenesmus

Tenesmus refers to the sensation of a desire to defaecate without the production of a significant amount of faeces. It may be a continuous sensation or recur frequently. It may be caused by:

♣ Proctitis

♥ Rectal prolapse

♠ Rectal tumour

Evacuation of Faeces

Problems with evacuation of faeces could be due to:

♥ **Luminal Factors**

Impacted faeces

♠ **Mural Factors**

Stricture, fissure

♦ **Systemic Factors**

CNS lesions of the sacral plexus, cauda equina and spinal cord

Pneumaturia or Faecal Discharge Per Vaginum

Pneumaturia or faecal discharge per vaginum would suggest fistulae either due to:

♣ Inflammatory bowel disease

♥ Diverticular disease

♠ Malignancy

Perianal Problems

Perianal problems such as a lump, pain or discharge are usually due to:

♦ Inflammatory bowel disease

Hepato-Biliary Symptoms

Symptoms that may arise in relation to the hepato-biliary system are as follows:

Pain

The types of pain that arise in relation to the hepato-biliary system are:

- ◆ Biliary Pain
- ♣ Capsular Pain
- ♥ Pericapsular Pain

Biliary Pain

Biliary pain may be due to

- ♠ **Luminal Factors**

  Stones

- ◆ **Mural Factors**

  Cholangitis, cholecystitis or rarely sphincter of Oddi dysfunction

Capsular Pain

Capsular pain refers to pain caused by the liver capsule being stretched. This could be due to

- ♣ Congestion
- ♥ Inflammation
- ♠ Tumour

Congestion

Congestion could be due to:

- ♠ Heart failure, cardiac tamponade, constrictive pericarditis
- ◆ Budd-Chiari syndrome

Inflammation

Inflammation of the liver resulting in pain occurs in:

- ♣ Acute hepatitis

Tumour

Tumours within the liver that result in pain are:

- ♥ Hepatoma
- ♠ Cholangiocarcinoma (peripheral intrahepatic type)
- ◆ Secondary deposits

Pericapsular Pain

Pericapsular inflammation may also cause pain in the right hypochondrium. Pericapsular pain occurs in:

- ♠ Perihepatitis (Fitz-Hugh-Curtis syndrome)

Jaundice

Jaundice could be:

- ◆ Obstructive
- ♣ Hepatocellular
- ♥ Haemolytic

Obstructive Jaundice

Obstructive jaundice may be due to lesions affecting the bile ducts such as the following:

- ♠ **Luminal Factors**

  Stones

- ◆ **Mural Factors**

  Strictures (benign and malignant), cholangitis, primary sclerosing cholangitis, secondary sclerosing cholangitis, primary biliary cirrhosis

- ♣ **External Factors**

  Compression of the bile duct by lymph nodes or carcinoma of the head of the pancreas

289

Intrahepatic cholestasis

Hepatocellular Jaundice

Hepatocellular jaundice is caused by damage to the liver cells.

♥ The causes of liver cell damage have already been discussed

Haemolytic Jaundice

This refers to jaundice caused by excessive destruction of red cells.

♠ The causes of haemolysis will be discussed later in the chapter on the haematological system

Itch

Itch could be caused by:

♦ Intra or extra-hepatic biliary obstruction

Discolouration of Urine

Discolouration of urine could occur in:

♣ Obstructive, hepato-cellular or haemolytic jaundice

Pale Stools

Pale stools would be a feature of:

♥ Obstructive jaundice

Lack of Energy

Lack of energy is a feature of:

♠ Any chronic liver disease

Findings on Examination

The abnormalities that may be detected on clinical examination are as follows:

General Examination

When performing a general examination one may note abnormalities of the following:

♣ Dimensions

♥ Integument

♠ Body Temperature

Dimensions

On examination of the dimensions one may note abnormalities of:

♣ Height

♥ Weight

♠ Shape

Height

Variations in height may be:

♦ **Short Stature**

   Short stature could indicate nutritional failure occurring in childhood

Weight

Variations in weight could be:

♣ **Decreased Weight**

   Decreased weight would occur in nutritional failure

♥ **Obesity**

   Obesity could be associated with non-alcoholic steato hepatitis,

gallstones, gastro-oesophageal reflux

Shape

Variations in the shape of the patient that would be of significance are:

♠ Skeletal Appearance

A skeletal appearance would suggest chronic nutritional failure. However, one should remember that with decompensation fluid retention would occur with resultant change in shape with a potbelly and ankle oedema and a spurious increase in body weight.

♦ Pseudocushings

A Cushingoid appearance may occur in those who abuse alcohol.

Nutritional Failure

Nutritional failure may be caused by:

♣ Luminal Factors

Lack of food, which could be due to socio-economic causes, psychiatric disorders such as anorexia nervosa, dysphagia

Parasites in the lumen and bacterial overgrowth could also result in nutritional failure.

♥ Mural Factors

The short bowel syndrome where the effective area for digestion and absorption is reduced

Mucosal diseases of the small intestine such as coeliac disease, Crohn's disease, Whipple's disease, intestinal lymphangiectasia, lymphoma, amyloidosis, tuberculosis

Motility disorders such as hollow visceral myopathy

♠ External Factors

Pancreatic insufficiency

♦ Systemic Factors

Conditions affecting the:

E&M thyrotoxicosis, diabetes mellitus

HS hypogammaglobulinaemia

LMS scleroderma

Any chronic disease, which results in over-expression of cytokines, would result in cachexia.

Integument

On examination of the integument one may note changes in the following:

- ♣ Colour
- ♥ Surface
- ♠ Circulation

Colour

Variations in the colour of the skin that may be of significance are:

♣ Increased Pigmentation

Increased pigmentation occurs in:

Haemochromatosis, primary biliary cirrhosis, chronic liver disease, porphyria, nutritional failure, Whipple's disease

♥ Jaundice

Jaundice would be seen in hepato-biliary disease, hepatocellular failure

♠ Vitiligo

Vitiligo occurs in autoimmune hepatitis, pernicious anaemia.

- ♦ **Cyanosis**

  Cyanosis may occur due to pulmonary arterio-venous shunts in cirrhosis.

- ♣ **Tattoos**

  Tattoos may indicate viral infection of the liver caused by contaminated needles

Surface

On examination of the surface of the skin one may observe:

- ♥ Scratch marks. They occur in obstructive jaundice either intra or extra-hepatic.

- ♠ In porphyria cutanea tarda fragile skin, which blisters easily, may be seen

Rash

Rashes that may occur in relation to the digestive system are:

- ♦ Dermatitis herpetiformis may occur in coeliac disease.

- ♣ Rose spots may be seen in typhoid fever

- ♥ Deficiency of zinc could result in dermatitis especially at the extremities.

- ♠ Petechiae and bruising may be seen in liver disease and in alcohol abuse

Circulation

Circulatory changes that may be observed in the skin are:

- ♦ Telangiectasia may be seen in chronic liver disease

Body Temperature

Fever may be due to an:

- ♣ Infective aetiology of gastrointestinal disease

- ♥ A septic complication of gastrointestinal disease

- ♠ Bacterial translocation across a diseased gut

Regional Examination

On regional examination one may detect abnormalities of the following:

Head

On examination of the head one may detect abnormalities of the:

- ♥ Mental state

- ♠ Dimensions

Mental State

The changes that may occur are:

- ♦ Portosystemic encephalopathy. This refers to a neuropsychiatric syndrome due to chronic liver disease. A similar condition may also occur in fulminant liver failure. The features are changes in personality, intellect, mood, reversal of sleep rhythm. This may progress to confusion, drowsiness and coma.

  Associated features of portosystemic encephalopathy are:

- ♣ Foetor hepaticus

- ♥ Inability to draw a five-pointed star

- ♠ Asterixis (flapping tremor)

Dimensions of the Head

Shape

Variations in the overall shape of the head that would be significant are:

♣ **Skeletal Appearance**

A skeletal appearance would be observed in cachexia.

♥ **Cushingoid Facies**

Cushingoid facies would occur in alcoholic pseudocushings, iatrogenic Cushing's

Nose

On examination of the nose one may observe abnormalities of:

Structure

Abnormalities that may occur are:

♠ Rhinophyma, a complication of acne rosacea, is commoner in alcoholics.

Function

Examination of the functions of the nose is an instance where the sense of smell plays a part in examination of a patient.

♦ Foetor hepaticus may occur in liver failure.

♣ The smell of alcohol may be noted in patients who abuse alcohol.

Eyes

When examining the eyes one may note abnormalities of the following:

Dimensions

The eyes would be:

♥ Sunken in malnutrition

Eyelids

Surface

Abnormalities that may occur on the surface of the eyelids are:

♠ Xanthelasma would occur on the surface of the eyelids in primary biliary cirrhosis.

Conjunctiva

On examination of the conjunctiva one may note changes on the:

Surface

The surface of the conjunctiva may show abnormalities such as:

♦ **Conjunctivitis**

Conjunctivitis occurs in inflammatory bowel disease

♣ **Dry Eyes**

Dry eyes occur in Sjogren's syndrome, Xerophthalmia occurs in vitamin A deficiency

♥ **Bitot's Spots**

Bitot's spots occur in vitamin A deficiency.

♠ **Episcleritis**

Episcleritis may occur in inflammatory bowel disease

Sclera

When examining the sclera one may note changes in the:

Colour

Variations that may be noted are:

Jaundice

A yellow discolouration or jaundice becomes clinically detectable if the serum bilirubin is more than 50 micromoles per litre.

Cornea

On examination of the cornea one may note changes in the:

Colour

Variations that one may note are:

♦ Kayser-Fleischer rings may be seen in Wilson's disease. They appear as a ring of greenish-brown pigment deposition at the junction of the cornea and sclera, just within the cornea.

♣ The cornea may become opacified in keratomalacia

Surface

The surface may be:

♥ Dry in keratomalacia

Anterior Chamber

The anterior chamber of the eye may be:

♠ Cloudy or display a hypopyon in anterior uveitis, which can complicate inflammatory bowel disease.

Iris

Abnormalities that may occur are:

♦ Anterior uveitis may complicate inflammatory bowel disease.

Lens

Abnormalities that may occur are:

♣ Sunflower cataract may occur in Wilson's disease

Optic Fundus

Lesions that may occur are:

♥ Congenital hypertrophy of retinal pigment epithelium may be seen in familial adenomatous polyposis coli.

Face

On examination of the face one may note abnormalities of the following:

Scalp

Abnormalities that may occur are:

♠ Loss of scalp hair would be observed in malnutrition.

♦ Decreased pigmentation of hair would occur in malnutrition.

♣ White hair is a feature of pernicious anaemia.

♥ Hair would be brittle and easy pluckability may be demonstrated in malnutrition.

Malar Region

In the malar region one may note the following:

♠ In malnutrition a skeletal appearance would be best seen here

♦ A malar flush occurs in the carcinoid syndrome.

♣ Telangiectasia may occur in the carcinoid syndrome

Chin

Over the chin one may note the following:

♥ Decreased beard growth may occur in males with hepatocellular failure.

Mouth

On examination of the mouth one may note abnormalities of the following:

Lips

On examination of the lips one may note changes in:

♠ Size

♦ Colour

♣ Surface

♥ Circulation

Size

The lips may be:

♠ Small in systemic sclerosis

♦ Thickened lips may occur in Crohn's disease

Colour

Variations in the colour of the lips that may be significant are:

♣ Pallor would signify anaemia.

♥ Pigmented macules would be seen in the Peutz-Jeghers syndrome

Surface

Abnormalities that one may note on the surface of the lips are:

♠ Chelosis or inflammation of the lips would be seen in malnutrition.

♦ Angular stomatitis occurs in vitamin deficiency

Circulation

When assessing the blood vessels on the lips one may note:

♣ Telangiectasia in Osler-Rendu-Weber syndrome.

Teeth

Lesions that may occur in relation to the teeth are:

♥ Poor oral health with resultant caries or lack of teeth would be a feature of self-neglect, which is common in patients who abuse alcohol and drugs.

♠ Supernumerary teeth may occur in Gardner's syndrome, which is a sub-type of familial adenomatous polyposis coli

Gums

Lesions that one may observe in the gums are the following:

♦ Gingivitis would be a reflection of poor oral health.

♣ A blue line may be seen in lead poisoning. Lead poisoning usually results in lethargy and abdominal discomfort. In more severe cases vomiting, constipation, abdominal pain, encephalopathy and peripheral motor neuropathy may develop.

♥ Gum hypertrophy may be seen in patients taking cyclosporin

295

Buccal Mucosa

Lesions that may be observed in the buccal mucosa are:

- ♠ Aphthous ulcers could occur in inflammatory bowel disease, coeliac disease.
- ♦ Lichen planus. This may be associated with oesophageal ulceration and stricture formation.
- ♣ Ulcers may be seen in Behcet's disease
- ♥ Pigmentation would be seen in Addison's disease

Tongue

When examining the tongue one may note changes in:

Size

A large tongue may be seen in:

- ♣ Amyloidosis

Surface

The abnormalities that may be detected on the surface of the tongue are:

- ♦ Furring occurs in mouth breathers, fever, liver failure
- ♣ Candidiasis occurs in patients who are:

  On steroids, being treated with antibiotics, immunosuppressed
- ♥ A dry tongue occurs in dehydration.
- ♠ Glossitis would be seen in iron or vitamin B_{12} deficiency.

Salivary Glands

Abnormalities that may occur are:

Unilateral Enlargement

Unilateral enlargement of the salivary glands may occur in:

- ♦ **Parotid Gland**

  Mixed parotid tumour
- ♣ **Submandibular Gland**

  Enlargement of the gland in relation to meals would signify a calculus in the duct.

Bilateral Enlargement

Bilateral enlargement of the parotid glands is a finding in patients with:

- ♥ Alcoholic liver disease, Sjogren's syndrome, sarcoidosis

Ears

Over the ears one may note:

- ♠ Dermatitis. This may occur in zinc deficiency

Upper Limbs

On general examination of the upper limbs one may note changes in the:

Dimensions

Changes that may occur are:

- ♦ Thin upper limbs in relation to the trunk may be seen in alcoholic pseudocushings
- ♣ Thin upper limbs would be a feature of nutritional failure

Abnormal Movements

Abnormal movements that may be noticed whilst examining the upper limbs are:

♥ Chorea may be observed in Wilson's disease

Hands

On examination of the hands one may note changes in the following:

Dimensions

The abnormalities that may occur are:

♠ Narrow fingers would be seen in systemic sclerosis

Dorsum of the Hands

When examining the dorsum of the hands one may observe abnormalities of the:

Nails

Abnormalities that may be observed in the nails are changes in:

Shape

Variations in the shape of the nails that would be significant are:

♦ **Clubbing**

Clubbing would be seen in:

Inflammatory bowel disease: Crohn's disease

Liver disease: cirrhosis of the liver

♣ **Koilonychia**

Koilonychia may occur in iron deficiency as a consequence of gastrointestinal blood loss.

Colour

Variations in the colour of the nails that occur in relation to gastrointestinal disease are the following:

♥ **White Nails**

Leuconychia may occur in liver disease.

♠ **Yellow Nails**

Yellow nails occur in the yellow nails syndrome.

♦ **Blue Lunulae**

Blue lunulae may be seen in Wilson's disease.

Skin

When examining the skin over the hands one may note:

♣ Taut skin and calcinosis may be seen in systemic sclerosis

♥ Porphyria cutanea tarda causes fragile skin, which blisters easily

♠ Cyanosis may occur in cirrhosis of the liver if there is marked intrapulmonary shunting

Palms

When examining the palms one may note changes in the:

Skin

The abnormalities that may be detected when examining the skin over the palms are:

♦ Tylosis or hyperkeratosis of the palms may occur in oesophageal cancer.

297

♣ Palmar erythema occurs in hepatocellular failure

Locomotor System

In the hands, lesions that may occur in relation to the locomotor system are:

♥ Dupuytren's contracture may reflect alcohol abuse.

♠ Pseudogout, which occurs in haemochromatosis, affects the second and third metacarpophalangeal joints

Radial Pulse

When examining the radial pulse one may note:

♦ Tachycardia, which would be a feature of acute decompensation of gastrointestinal disease.

Central Nervous System

Abnormalities that may occur in relation to the nervous system of the hands are:

♣ An exaggerated physiological tremor would be seen in acute alcohol withdrawal.

♥ A flapping tremor would be seen in hepatic encephalopathy.

Forearms

Abnormalities that may be noted in the forearms are:

♠ Grip strength is a good test of muscle function and this would be decreased in malnutrition.

♦ Hypertrophic pulmonary osteoarthropathy may occur in cirrhosis of the liver

♣ Lichen planus may be associated with primary biliary cirrhosis

Upper Arms

Abnormalities that may be noted when examining the upper arms are:

♥ Mid arm circumference and skin fold thickness would be decreased in malnutrition.

Shoulders

The abnormalities that could occur are:

♠ Squaring of the shoulders in nutritional failure

Axillae

The abnormalities that may be noted are:

♦ Acanthosis nigricans may occur in pancreatic cancer, gastric cancer

Neck

When examining the neck one may note changes in:

Dimensions

The abnormalities that may be detected when examining the dimensions of the neck are:

♠ A thin neck would be seen in nutritional failure

♥ Subcutaneous emphysema occurs in rupture of the oesophagus

Jugular Venous Pressure

Abnormalities that may be noted are:

♠ **Elevation of the Jugular Venous Pressure**

Elevation of the jugular venous pressure may occur in congestive cardiac failure, right ventricular failure, tricuspid regurgitation, constrictive pericarditis or cardiac tamponade. All these conditions may be associated with hepatomegaly and result in cirrhosis of the liver.

Confusion can occur as ascites may cause elevation of the jugular venous pressure because of its mechanical effects. However, in primary liver disease features of hepatocellular failure and portal hypertension are likely to be detected.

♦ **Absent Hepato-Jugular Reflux**

Absent hepato-jugular reflux would be a feature of Budd-Chiari syndrome

Lymph Nodes

The abnormalities that could occur are:

♣ An enlarged supra-clavicular node, the Virchow's node, may be felt in cancer of the stomach. This is known as Troisier's sign.

Chest Wall

On examination of the chest wall one may note abnormalities of the following:

Dimensions

One may note:

♥ A skeletal appearance in nutritional failure

Integument (Cover)

Abnormalities that may occur are as follows:

♠ Reduced chest and abdominal hair would occur in males with hepatocellular failure

♦ Cassal's necklace occurs in niacin deficiency. Niacin deficiency causes a dermatitis, which begins as redness of the skin in areas exposed to sunlight. It progresses to cause a cracked skin that may ulcerate. Later, chronic thickening, dryness and pigmentation develop. Cassal's necklace refers to these lesions occurring around the neck of women in whom the lesions occur in this area because of the clothes they wear.

♣ Spider naevi occur in hepatocellular failure. Spider naevi refer to telangiectasia with a central arteriole feeding radiating vessels. They blanch on pressure. This is best demonstrated by using an orange stick or pen to compress the central arteriole that feeds the naevus. More than 4-5 spider naevi should be present to be significant

♥ Central Venous Access

Evidence of ongoing or previous central venous access could signify that the patient has had total parenteral nutrition.

Breasts

Abnormalities that may be detected in relation to breast tissue are:

- Gynaecomastia in a male would be a feature of hepatocellular failure.

- Breast cancer should be considered as a cause of liver metastases

Respiratory System

Lesions of the respiratory system that may occur in relation to digestive diseases are:

- Pleural effusion may occur in cirrhosis of the liver (right-sided pleural effusion)

- Emphysema occurs in alpha$_1$ antitrypsin deficiency

- Bronchiectasis occurs in cystic fibrosis, which may result in pancreatic insufficiency or cirrhosis of the liver.

Cardiovascular System

Lesions of the cardiovascular system that are of relevance are:

- Tricuspid regurgitation, right heart failure, restrictive cardiomyopathy, constrictive pericarditis cause hepatomegaly and cardiac cirrhosis

- Cardiomyopathy may occur in haemochromatosis. This presents with cardiomegaly, cardiac failure or arrhythmias and is a more common presenting feature in younger patients.

Abdomen

Abnormalities may be noted of the:

- Abdominal Wall
- Contents of the Abdomen

Abdominal Wall

One may note abnormalities of the following:

- Dimensions
- Integument
- Consistency
- Tenderness
- Circulation
- Movement

Dimensions

On examination of the dimensions one may note changes in:

- Size
- Shape

Size

Variations in size could be:

- **Distension**

    Distension of the abdomen occurs in ascites, intestinal obstruction, severe organomegaly

Remember **fluid, fat, faeces, flatus, fibroid, foetus**

(Use fibroid to remind oneself of tumour and organomegaly)

- **Sunken Abdominal Wall**

    A sunken abdominal wall would occur in nutritional failure and cachexia

Shape

Variations in the shape of the abdominal wall that would be of significance are:

♥ **Global Distension**

The abdomen would be globally distended in ascites, intestinal obstruction

♠ **Localised Distension**

In organomegaly the distension may be localised as in:

Distension in the upper abdomen may occur due to enlargement of the gall bladder.

In a young female distension in the upper abdomen may occur due to a choledochal cyst

Upper abdominal distension occurs in hepatosplenomegaly.

Lumbar fullness would occur in bilateral renal enlargement

Enlargement of the bladder, ovaries and uterus causes supra-pubic distension

Flank fullness is seen in ascites

♦ **Scaphoid**

In nutritional failure the abdomen would be scaphoid

Integument

On examination of the skin over the abdomen one may note changes in:

Colour

Colour change would already have been noticed and changes such as jaundice and pigmentation would have been identified.

Surface

Abnormalities that may occur on the surface of the skin over the abdomen are:

♥ Decreased hair occurs in chronic hepatocellular failure (cirrhosis of the liver)

♠ Scars should be noted. If the scar is surgical, its position would be a clue to the operation that has been performed.

♦ Stoma like an ileostomy would indicate previous colectomy and give a clue to the cause of liver disease (primary sclerosing cholangitis as a complication of ulcerative colitis)

♣ Striae would occur in Cushing's syndrome

♥ Haemorrhage may occur in abdominal catastrophes.

Cullen's sign refers to peri-umbilical haemorrhage

Grey Turner's sign refers to haemorrhage in the loins. This occurs in retroperitoneal haemorrhage.

> **C**ullen's sign occurs in the **C**entre
>
> To see Grey **T**urner's sign one must **T**urn the patient

♠ *Erythema ab igne* (reticular erythema or pigmentation) would indicate the use of a hot water bottle to relieve pain caused by internal malignancy or chronic pancreatitis

Consistency of the Abdominal Wall

Changes in consistency are:

♦ Oedema of the abdominal wall occurs in conditions that cause generalised oedema.

♣ A doughy consistency occurs in severe malnutrition, typhoid fever

Tenderness

Tenderness and guarding reflect:

♥ Inflammation of the underlying organs or peritoneum

Circulation

When examining the blood vessels over the anterior abdominal wall one may observe:

♣ Distended veins may occur in portal hypertension, blood flow would be away from the umbilicus. Rarely caput medusae may be seen. Caput medusae refer to enlarged veins radiating away from the umbilicus, like the head of the Medusa in Greek mythology.

♦ Distended veins are also seen in inferior vena caval obstruction. The direction of blood flow in this instance would be from caudal to cephalic.

Movement

Abnormal movements of the abdominal wall may be:

♥ Respiratory

♣ Peristaltic

♦ Pulsation

Respiratory

The abnormalities are:

♣ Respiratory movement of the abdominal wall may be reversed in paradoxical respiration. This occurs in phrenic nerve palsy

♥ Decreased or absent respiratory movement indicates severe intra-abdominal inflammation like peritonitis

Peristaltic

Visible peristalsis reflects:

♣ Very thin abdominal musculature

♦ Intestinal obstruction

Pulsation

Pulsation may be seen if the abdominal wall is thin. Pulsation may be:

♣ Transmitted pulsation due to organomegaly

♥ Expansile pulsation in aneurysmal dilatation of the aorta. The presence of a clot within an aneurysm may result in transmitted pulsation rather than expansile pulsation.

Contents of the Abdomen

Abnormalities that may be detected are as follows:

Liver

On examination of the liver one may note abnormalities of:

Site

The liver is situated in the right hypochondrium. The very rare exception would be situs inversus. The upper margin is at the fifth, right intercostal space in the mid-clavicular line. The upper margin must be defined by percussion before a comment may be made about enlargement of the liver as displacement of the liver downwards by hyperinflated lungs pushing the diaphragm caudally could be mistaken for hepatomegaly.

Size

The degree of enlargement is traditionally defined as the number of finger breadths below the costal margin

Hepatomegaly

Hepatomegaly could be due to:

- ♣ **Inflammation**

  This would occur in:

  Viral hepatitis, glandular fever, leptospirosis, syphilis, amoebic liver disease, pyogenic liver abscess, hydatid cyst, autoimmune hepatitis, primary biliary cirrhosis, cirrhosis of the liver, sarcoidosis

- ♥ **Neoplasm**

  Hepatoma, secondary deposits, lymphoma

- ♠ **Congestion**

  Congestion may occur in the:

  IVC (Inferior Vena Cava): tricuspid regurgitation, congestive cardiac failure, right ventricular failure, restrictive cardiomyopathy, constrictive pericarditis

  Hepatic Veins: Budd-Chiari syndrome

- ♦ **Metabolic Conditions**

  Non-alcoholic fatty liver disease, haemochromatosis

- ♣ **Interstitial Infiltration**

  Amyloidosis

- ♥ **Developmental Disorders**

  Cysts, which may be part of polycystic disease, Riedl's lobe

Shape

The shape does not give much information but:

- ♠ A localised enlargement may represent a Riedl's lobe.

Margins

Define the margins or edge of the liver. This may be a:

- ♦ Well-defined sharp edge
- ♣ Rounded edge due to swelling of the liver in congestion
- ♥ Craggy edge in metastatic carcinoma

Surface

Note the surface of the liver.

- ♠ The surface of the liver is usually smooth.
- ♦ Nodularity of the liver may represent cirrhosis, metastatic deposits.

Consistency

One may note:

- ♣ The consistency of the liver is usually firm when enlarged.
- ♥ The consistency becomes hard in malignancy

Tenderness

Tenderness would indicate acute stretching of the liver capsule. Tenderness may occur in:

- ♠ Inflammation
- ♦ Congestion

Mobility

Note the mobility of the liver. The liver moves with respiration.

Pulsation

The liver is pulsatile in:

- ♣ Tricuspid regurgitation

Percussion Note

The percussion note over the liver is dull and this dullness is continuous with the normal hepatic dullness.

Auscultation of the Liver

On auscultation over the liver one may hear:

- ♥ Bruits
- ♠ Venous Hum
- ♦ Rub

Bruits

A bruit may occur in:

- ♣ Hepatoma, acute alcoholic hepatitis, metastatic cancer

Venous Hum

The Cruveilhier-Baumgarten syndrome refers to the presence of a venous hum over collaterals in the upper abdomen. This occurs in:

- ♥ Portal hypertension

Rub

A hepatic rub could indicate:

- ♠ Infection such as perihepatitis. The Fitz-Hugh-Curtis syndrome refers to perihepatitis caused by *Chlamydia trachomatis* tracking up the right paracolic gutter in women with salpingitis.
- ♦ Tumour invasion of the visceral peritoneum

Biliary Tract

Abnormalities that may be noted in relation to the biliary tract are:

- ♣ A choledochal cyst would present as an epigastric mass in a young female.
- ♥ The gall bladder may be swollen in obstructive jaundice caused by obstruction distal to the cystic duct

Spleen

Abnormalities of the spleen could be:

- ♠ The spleen would be enlarged in portal hypertension.
- ♦ In typhoid fever the spleen is enlarged and soft.
- ♣ A rub may be heard in splenic infarction.
- ♥ A bruit may occur over a large spleen but it is very rare.

Hepatosplenomegaly

Hepatosplenomegaly could occur in:

- ♠ **Inflammatory Disorders**

    Cirrhosis of the liver, hepatitis B and C, primary biliary cirrhosis, Weil's disease, schistosomiasis

♦ **Vascular Disorders**

Budd-Chiari syndrome

♣ **Developmental Disorders**

Polycystic disease

Other causes of hepatosplenomegaly are listed in the chapter on the haematological system

Cirrhosis of the Liver

The clinical diagnosis of cirrhosis of the liver rests on the demonstration of:

♥ Features of hepatocellular failure

♠ Features of portal hypertension

Features of Hepatocellular Failure

Features of hepatocellular failure are failure of:

♦ **Excretory Function**

Jaundice

♣ **Detoxification**

Spider naevi, palmar erythema, gynaecomastia, decreased body and facial hair, testicular atrophy, cyanosis, clubbing

♥ **Synthetic Function**

Bleeding (decreased coagulation factors), oedema (decreased albumin), leuconychia (associated with hypoalbuminaemia)

Features of Portal Hypertension

Features of portal hypertension are:

♣ Caput medusae (uncommon)

♥ Prominent abdominal-wall veins

♠ Venous hum (Cruveilhier-Baumgarten syndrome)

♦ Splenomegaly

♣ Ascites

♥ Foetor hepaticus

♠ Portosystemic encephalopathy

♦ Petechiae (thrombocytopaenia due to splenomegaly)

Causes of Cirrhosis of the Liver

Cirrhosis of the liver could be due to disorders of the:

♦ **Biliary Tract**

Primary sclerosing cholangitis, secondary sclerosing cholangitis, primary biliary cirrhosis

♣ **Hepatocellular Disorders**

Hepatocellular disorders, which may result in cirrhosis, are the following:

Biological Agents

Viruses: hepatitis B and C

Immune reactions: autoimmune hepatitis

Chemical Agents

Metabolic Disorders: haemochromatosis, Wilson's disease, $alpha_1$ antitrypsin deficiency

Toxins: alcohol

Drugs: methotrexate, amiodarone

♥ **Vascular Disorders**

Vascular disorders that may result in cirrhosis of the liver are those causing:

Venous Disease

Venous diseases that result in cirrhosis of the liver are conditions that cause congestion in the hepatic veins. They are the Budd-Chiari syndrome, tricuspid regurgitation, congestive cardiac failure, right heart failure, restrictive cardiomyopathy, constrictive pericarditis

305

Veno-occlusive disease is caused by injury to the hepatic veins and presents like the Budd-Chiari syndrome. It was originally described in Jamaica and was caused by ingestion of bush tea. It may occur as a complication of chemotherapy and total body irradiation.

Telangiectasia

Osler-Rendu-Weber syndrome

Clues to the Cause of Cirrhosis

Clues to the cause of cirrhosis that may be detected on clinical examination are:

- ♠ **Pigmentation**: haemochromatosis

- ♦ **Kayser Fleischer ring**: Wilson's disease

- ♣ **Xanthelasma**: primary biliary cirrhosis (female, scratch marks on skin)

- ♥ **Telangiectasia**: Osler-Rendu-Weber syndrome

- ♠ **Parotid enlargement and Dupuytren's contracture**: alcohol

- ♥ **Psoriasis, rheumatoid arthritis**: methotrexate

- ♠ **Elevated JVP**: cardiovascular cause

- ♦ **Absent hepatojugular reflux**: Budd-Chiari syndrome

- ♣ **Emphysema**: alpha$_1$ antitrypsin deficiency

- ♥ **Bronchiectasis**: cystic fibrosis

Pancreas

Lesions of the pancreas that may be noted clinically are:

- ♠ A pancreatic pseudocyst may result in a large mass.

- ♦ Pancreatic cancer is rarely palpable

Small Intestine

Clinical signs that may result from lesions of the small intestine are:

- ♣ Obstruction would cause distension of the abdomen and visible peristalsis.

- ♥ Thickened small bowel loops may be palpable in inflammatory bowel disease.

- ♠ A mass may occur due to matted loops of bowel together with inflammatory tissue.

Large Intestine

Clinical features that may result from lesions of the large intestine are:

- ♦ Obstruction of the large intestine causes abdominal distension.

- ♣ Cancer of the colon may result in a mass.

- ♥ An inflammatory mass may be due to inflammatory bowel disease or diverticular disease.

Difficulty may be encountered in distinguishing faecal masses from inflammatory or neoplastic lesions. Faecal masses are usually indentable or malleable and are not constant.

Epigastric Mass

An epigastric mass could be due to:

- ♠ Carcinoma of the stomach

- ♦ Carcinoma of the pancreas

Right Upper Quadrant

Masses in the right upper quadrant could be due to lesions in the:

- ♣ Liver
- ♥ Kidney
- ♠ Carcinoma of the colon
- ♦ Retroperitoneal sarcoma
- ♣ Lymphoma
- ♥ Diverticular mass

Left Upper Quadrant

Masses in the left upper quadrant could be due to lesions in the:

- ♠ Spleen
- ♦ Kidney
- ♣ Carcinoma of the colon
- ♥ Retroperitoneal sarcoma
- ♠ Lymphoma
- ♦ Diverticular mass

Right Iliac Fossa

Lumps in the right iliac fossa could be:

- ♣ Ileocaecal masses like a Crohn's mass
- ♥ Caecal cancer
- ♠ Transplanted kidney
- ♦ Appendicular mass
- ♣ Amoeboma would be a very rare cause of a mass in the right iliac fossa.

Left Iliac Fossa

Lumps in the left iliac fossa could be:

- ♥ Faecal masses
- ♠ Colon cancer

- ♦ Diverticular mass
- ♣ Transplanted kidney.

Ascites

To confirm the presence of ascites one should demonstrate:

- ♥ Flank dullness
- ♠ Horseshoe dullness
- ♦ Shifting dullness
- ♣ A fluid thrill may or may not be demonstrable.

Causes of Ascites

The causes of ascites have been discussed earlier

Succussion Splash

A succussion splash indicates gastric outlet obstruction due to:

- ♥ Peptic stricture
- ♠ Malignancy

Increased Bowel Sounds

Increased bowel sounds occur in:

- ♦ Small bowel obstruction

Silent Abdomen

A silent abdomen would signify:

- ♣ Paralytic ileus

Bruits

Bruits may occur in association with:

- ♥ Bowel ischaemia

Inguinal Lymph Nodes

Inguinal lymph nodes are usually enlarged on account of:

♠ Local disease

♦ Generalised lymphadenopathy.

Hernial Orifices

The abnormalities that may be detected are:

♣ The presence of a hernia would suggest the cause of intestinal obstruction

Genitals

The abnormalities that may be detected are:

♥ Decreased pubic hair, small testes would be features of cirrhosis of the liver

Perianal Region

Lesions that occur in the perianal region are:

♠ The surface may be affected by abscesses, fistulae in Crohn's disease

♦ Migratory necrolytic erythema occurs in glucagonoma.

Anus and Rectum

Lesions of the anus and rectum are:

♣ A mass may be felt in rectal cancer

♥ Fissure-in-ano may occur in Crohn's disease

Lower Limbs

On general examination of the lower limbs one may note changes in the:

Dimensions

Changes in the size of the lower limbs may occur due to:

♠ Nutritional failure where the lower limbs would be thin.

♦ Thin limbs in relation to the torso occur in pseudocushings

Knees

When examining the knees one may note the following:

♣ Pseudogout occurs in haemochromatosis

♥ Enteropathic arthropathy may affect the knees. It is commonly asymmetrical and affects the lower limb joints.

Lower Legs

Abnormalities that may be noted in the lower legs are:

♠ Pyoderma gangrenosum may occur in inflammatory bowel disease

♦ Erythema nodosum may occur in inflammatory bowel disease

♣ Corkscrew hairs, perifollicular haemorrhages occur in scurvy

♥ Oedema occurs in cirrhosis of the liver, nutritional failure

♠ Deep vein thrombosis may occur in pancreatic cancer, rectal cancer

Spine

Conditions that may affect the spine are:

♦ An axial arthropathy, which is very similar to ankylosing spondylitis, may occur in inflammatory bowel disease. It is commoner in males. The activity of the spinal disease is independent of the activity of the inflammatory bowel disease and symptoms may predate the development of bowel symptoms.

Gait

Abnormalities of gait that may occur in relation to bowel disease are:

♣ Foot drop may occur due to weight loss in nutritional failure. This is due to the loss of the protective pad of fat over the common peroneal nerve.

♥ Sensory neuropathy with resultant stamping gait may be seen in alcoholics and in malnutrition.

♠ A stamping gait may also occur in subacute combine degeneration of the cord complicating pernicious anaemia

Romberg's Sign

A positive Romberg's sign may be demonstrated in:

♦ Pernicious anaemia

309

Chapter 13

The Kidneys and Urinary System

In this system the kidneys and the urinary tract will be studied. In addition, clinical features of the causes and effects of diseases that involve the kidneys and urinary system but are reflected in other systems will also be studied.

History Taking

One should enquire about:

- ♥ Micturition
- ♠ The Act of Micturition
- ♦ Swelling of the Body
- ♣ Abdominal Pain

Micturition

Where micturition is concerned one should enquire about:

- ♥ **Frequency**

  The number of times the patient passes urine should be ascertained. Especially important is any nocturnal need to pass urine.

- ♠ **Quantity**

  Ascertain the quantity of urine passed by the patient per day. A rough idea would suffice. The most important feature is a change in the quantity of urine passed.

- ♦ **Quality**

  Ask if there has been a change in the colour of the urine, whether the patient has passed any blood or if the urine has become very smelly.

The Act of Micturition

Concerning the act of micturition, one should enquire about:

- ♦ Sensation of fullness of the bladder
- ♣ Initiation of micturition
- ♥ Straining
- ♠ Force of the urinary stream
- ♦ Interruption to the passage of urine
- ♣ Terminal dribble
- ♥ Sensation of incomplete emptying of the bladder
- ♠ Burning sensation on passage of urine

Following this one should perform a review of systems.

Physical Examination

Begin by performing a general examination and then proceed to perform regional examination.

General Examination

Note the posture of the patient. Assess the state of growth and development and the metabolic state of the patient. Weight and shape would be of particular importance in assessing the state of salt and water balance. Note any gross changes in the integument. Assess the body temperature if required. (Position, Height and Proportions, Weight and Shape, Integument, Body Temperature)

Regional Examination

Commence regional examination by examining the head. One may start with the hands if one wishes.

Head

Assess the mental state. Assess the dimensions of the head. Then examine the regions of the head, the nose, the eyes, the face (the scalp, the forehead, the malar region, the chin), the mouth (jaw, lips, teeth, gums, buccal mucosa, tongue, palate, fauces, salivary glands), the ears.

Upper Limbs

Perform a quick general examination of the upper limbs noting the dimensions and the state of the integument.

Hands

Assess the dimensions. Then examine the dorsum of the hands; the nails and skin, the bones, joints, tendons and muscles. Ask the patient to turn the hands over and examine the skin, the bones, joints, tendons and muscles. Palpate the hands and assess the state of the peripheral circulation and then examine the radial pulse. Ask the patient to stretch the arms out and look for tremors. Next, ask the patient to extend the wrists and spread the fingers apart and look for a flapping tremor. If the patient is unable to maintain this position, hold the patient's forearm, just above the wrist, with one hand. With one's other hand hold the patient's hand, wind it around a few times and push the patient's wrist into the dorsi-flexed position and maintain this position. If present, the flapping tremor will be felt against the examining hand.

Examine the nervous system and function of the locomotor system of the hands if required.

Forearms, Upper Arms, Shoulders and Axillae

Examine the forearms and upper arms. In the forearms note the presence or absence of an arterio-ovenous fistula. In the upper arms measure the blood pressure.

Examine the shoulders and the axillae.

In practice one should examine the locomotor system and the neurological system of the upper limbs if required.

Neck

Assess the dimensions. Note the state of the integument. Assess the jugular venous pulsation carefully. In practice one should examine the rest of the neck. In a professional examination it would be wise to mention to the examiners that one would do so. (Dimensions, integument, thyroid, sternocleidomastoid, jugular venous pressure, carotids, trachea, lymph nodes)

Chest

A quick inspection of the chest wall should be made. In practice one should examine the contents of the chest, the lungs and the heart, but in a professional examination this would not be required. In practice one should also examine the patient's back at this point but this would not be expected in a professional examination.

Back

Ask the patient to sit up, lean forward and examine the back of the patient. Examine the neck, the spine, the scapula, the back of the chest, the lower back and the sacrum. In the kidneys and urinary system the lower back would be of special importance.

Lower Back

Note the dimensions, look for any swelling of the loins. Assess the state of the integument. Tap on the loins and note if there is any tenderness.

Sacrum

Look for sacral oedema.

Abdomen

The procedure for examining the abdomen with respect to the kidneys and urinary system is the same as the procedure employed when examining the digestive system. The features that specifically relate to the kidneys and urinary system will be described here.

Kidneys

To examine the native kidneys one should palpate in the lumbar region. Deep palpation should be employed. After initial palpation with one's right hand, place one's left hand behind the patient, in the patient's loin, so that one may perform bimanual palpation. With the left hand gently push the kidney anteriorly. An enlarged kidney would be felt to move between the palpating hands. This is known as ballotment.

In the case of renal transplantation the transplanted kidney would be felt in the right or left iliac fossa.

Bladder

Remember to actively look for enlargement of the bladder, which presents as a lump arising from the pelvis.

Percussion

Percussion should be performed in the usual way. Define any lumps that are felt. Define the borders of the

313

intra-abdominal organs. Remember to demonstrate a resonant percussion note over enlarged kidneys. Percuss in the suprapubic region and demonstrate dullness over a distended bladder or a resonant percussion note if the bladder is not distended. Check for ascites using the method described in the previous chapter.

Auscultation

Remember to auscultate for a renal bruit.

The Kidneys

The features, that should be ascertained to confirm that a mass felt in the lumbar region is an enlarged kidney, are the following:

♥ The kidneys are felt on deep palpation

♠ The edge is rounded

♦ The upper border may be defined and the palpating fingers may be interposed between the upper border of the kidney and the costal margin. In other words it is possible to get above the kidney.

♣ The kidneys move with respiration.

♥ The kidneys are ballotable.

♠ The percussion note is resonant over the kidneys.

The remainder of the examination should be performed in practice and is included here for the sake of completeness and as a reminder. In a professional examination it would be wise to mention to the examiners that it is one's standard practice to complete this routine of examination.

Inguinal Region and the Genitalia

Remember that examination of the hernial orifices and the male genitalia is best performed with the patient standing.

Lower Limbs

Examine the dimensions then examine the hips, the thighs, the knees, the lower legs.

Feet

As for the hands, examine the dimensions and then examine the dorsum of the feet paying attention to the nails and skin, the bones joints, tendons and muscles. Look at the plantar aspect and examine the skin, the bones, the joints, the tendons and the muscles. Palpate the skin and assess the state of the peripheral circulation. Feel the dorsalis pedis and the posterior tibial pulses.

Examine active and passive movements of the lower limb and the nervous system only if required.

Buttocks, Perianal Region and Per Rectal Examination

This should be performed in practice but would not be required in a professional examination although it would be wise to mention to the examiners that one would examine these regions in practice.

Spine

Examine the patient's spine.

Gait, Romberg's Sign, Trendelenburg Test, Standing from a Seated or Squatting Position

These tests should be performed in practice if required but would not be required in a professional examination. This would conclude a full examination of the kidneys and urinary system.

Lesions of the Kidneys and Urinary System

Lesions of the kidneys and urinary system may be due to causes that are:

- ♠ Pre-Renal
- ♦ Renal
- ♣ Post-Renal

Pre-Renal Lesions

Pre-renal lesions refer to conditions that occur within the renal vasculature and may be conditions in the:

- ♥ **Lumen**

  Hypovolaemia, hypotension, hypertension, thromboembolism

- ♠ **Mural Factors**

  Renal artery stenosis, aneurysm of the renal artery, dissecting aneurysm of the aorta involving the renal arteries

Renal Lesions

Renal lesions may occur in the:

- ♦ Glomerulus
- ♣ Tubules
- ♥ Interstitium
- ♠ Renal Papilla

Glomerulus

Disorders affecting the glomerulus are:

- ♦ Glomerulonephritis
- ♣ Other Glomerular Disorders

Glomerulonephritis

Glomerulonephritis refers to a group of disorders characterised by primary abnormalities of the glomerulus. The suffix " itis" is loosely applied, as inflammation is not always a feature.

Glomerulonephritis may be:

- ♥ Non-Proliferative Glomerulonephritis
- ♠ Proliferative Glomerulonephritis

315

Non-Proliferative Glomerulonephritis

The main feature is leakage of the basement membrane with resultant proteinuria and nephrotic syndrome.

Proliferative Glomerulonephritis

The main feature is inflammation of the glomerulus with resultant haematuria, proteinuria, acute nephritic syndrome, nephrotic syndrome, progressive renal failure.

Non-Proliferative Glomerulonephritis

Non-Proliferative glomerulonephritis may be classified as:

- ◆ Minimal-Change Nephropathy
- ♣ Membranous Nephropathy
- ♥ Focal Segmental Glomerulosclerosis

Minimal-Change Nephropathy

Minimal-change nephropathy presents as the nephrotic syndrome. It may be:

- ♠ **Primary**

Or there may be:

- ◆ **Associated Conditions**

    Minimal change nephropathy may be associated with:

    Lymphoma usually Hodgkin's disease, solid tumours particularly benign and malignant thymoma

Membranous Nephropathy

Membranous nephropathy presents as the nephrotic syndrome. It may be:

- ♣ **Primary**

Or there may be:

- ♥ **Associated Conditions**

    Membranous nephropathy may be associated with conditions affecting the following:

    LMS systemic lupus erythematosus, rheumatoid arthritis

    E&M autoimmune thyroid disease, diabetes mellitus

    GIT hepatitis B, carcinoma of the stomach, carcinoma of the colon

    RAG syphilis, carcinoma of the prostate, carcinoma of the breast

    IS leprosy, filariasis

    RS carcinoma of the bronchus

    HS *Plasmodium malariae* infestation, rarely Hodgkin's and non-Hodgkin's lymphoma

    Drugs gold, penicillamine, captopril

Focal Segmental Glomerulosclerosis

Focal segmental glomerulosclerosis (FSGS) presents as the nephrotic syndrome. However, some patients may present with persistent proteinuria and some have haematuria as well. FSGS may be:

- ♠ **Primary**

Or there may be:

- ◆ **Associated Conditions**

    The conditions that may be associated with FSGS are those that affect the following systems:

    KUS Alport's syndrome, reduced renal mass in reflux nephropathy, remnant kidney, healed glomerulonephritis

    HS sickle cell disease

RAG HIV infection

GIT *Schistosoma mansoni* infection

Drugs heroin

Proliferative Glomerulonephritis

The main feature of proliferative glomerulonephritis may be:

- ♣ Proliferation of Mesangial Cells
- ♥ Endocapillary Proliferation
- ♠ Extracapillary Proliferation (crescent formation)
- ♦ Diffuse Proliferation (all the above elements, all glomeruli involved)
- ♣ Focal Segmental Proliferative Glomerulonephritis (some glomeruli involved, hence focal, parts of these glomeruli involved, hence segmental)
- ♥ Membranoproliferative (mesangiocapillary)

Mesangial Proliferative Glomerulonephritis

Mesangial proliferative glomerulonephritis presents with haematuria, proteinuria, impaired renal function or hypertension. The causes of mesangial proliferative glomerulonephritis are:

- ♥ Ig A nephropathy
- ♠ Ig M nephropathy
- ♦ Systemic Lupus Erythematosus
- ♣ Idiopathic

IgA Nephropathy

Ig A nephropathy is characterised by Ig A deposition in the basement membrane and mesangial prolifer-

ative glomerulonephritis. The presentation may be with:

- ♥ Macroscopic haematuria
- ♠ Asymptomatic haematuria/ proteinuria
- ♦ Nephrotic syndrome
- ♣ Acute renal failure
- ♥ Chronic renal failure

IgA nephropathy may be:

- ♠ **Primary**

Or there may be:

- ♦ **Associated Conditions**

  Conditions affecting the:

  GIT chronic liver disease (usually alcoholic), coeliac disease, dermatitis herpetiformis

  LMS rheumatoid arthritis, ankylosing spondylitis, Reiter's disease

  RAG HIV infection

Endocapillary Proliferation

Endocapillary proliferative glomerulonephritis usually presents as an acute nephritic syndrome. The causes are:

- ♣ **RS** post-streptococcal glomerulonephritis (pharyngitis)
- ♥ **CVS** infective endocarditis
- ♠ **IS** post-streptococcal (cellulitis, impetigo), leprosy

Extracapillary Proliferation (crescent formation)

Extracapillary proliferative glomerulonephritis presents with rapidly progressive glomerulonephritis and progressive renal failure. The causes are:

- ♦ **Idiopathic**

317

Or there may be:

♣ Associated Conditions

Those affecting the:

RS antiglomerular basement membrane disease, Wegener's granulomatosis, microscopic polyangiitis

LMS systemic lupus erythematosus

IS Henoch-Schonlein disease

Diffuse Proliferative Glomerulonephritis

Diffuse proliferative glomerulonephritis presents with haematuria, proteinuria, hypertension and renal insufficiency. Diffuse proliferative glomerulonephritis may be:

♥ Idiopathic

Or there may be:

♠ Associated Conditions

Systemic lupus erythematosus

Focal Segmental Proliferative Glomerulonephritis

Focal Segmental Proliferative Glomerulonephritis occurs in systemic lupus erythematosus but causes less severe disease.

Membranoproliferative Glomerulonephritis

Membranoproliferative glomerulonephritis presents with proteinuria sometimes sufficient to cause nephrotic syndrome. It may also cause haematuria, hypertension and renal impairment.

Three types of membranoproliferative glomerulonephritis occur depending on the pattern of complement activation.

Type I classical pathway

Type II alternative pathway

Type III terminal pathway

Conditions associated with membranoproliferative glomerulonephritis are those affecting the:

♦ **LMS** systemic lupus erythematosus

♣ **HS** cryoglobulinaemia

♥ **CVS** infective endocarditis

♠ **CNS** shunt nephritis

♦ **IS** partial lipodystrophy

Other Glomerular Disorders

Other disorders of the glomerulus that may occur are:

♣ Familial Conditions

Familial conditions that may be associated with glomerular disease are:

Alport's syndrome is a condition characterised by hereditary nephritis with haematuria and progressive renal failure and associated bilateral sensorineural deafness.

Thin Glomerular Basement Membrane Disease is an autosomal dominant inherited condition, which presents with microscopic haematuria.

♥ Systemic Conditions

Systemic conditions that may be associated with glomerular disease are those affecting the:

CVS hypertension

E&M diabetes mellitus

HS amyloidosis, haemolytic uraemic syndrome

LMS systemic sclerosis

IS nail patella syndrome

Tubular Disorders

Tubular disorders may be due to:

- ♠ Luminal Factors
- ♦ Mural Factors

Luminal Factors

Luminal factors that result in disorders of the tubules are:

- ♣ Pyelonephritis, myoglobinuria, multiple myeloma

Mural Factors

Mural factors may be associated with structural changes in the tubule or primarily present with functional changes. In short they may be associated with:

- ♥ Structural changes
- ♠ Functional changes

Structural Changes

Structural changes that could occur in the tubules are:

- ♣ Developmental Disorders
- ♥ Necrosis (acute tubular necrosis)

Developmental Disorders

Developmental disorders of the renal tubules are the following:

- ♠ Polycystic Disease
- ♦ Medullary sponge kidney
- ♣ Medullary cystic disease

Acute Tubular Necrosis

Acute tubular necrosis may be due to:

♥ **Shock**

Hypovolaemic, septic, cardiogenic

♠ **Direct Toxic Effect**

Tubular necrosis may be due to the direct toxic effect of the following:

Drugs amionoglycosides

Pigments myogolobin, haemoglobin

Functional Disorders of the Renal Tubules

Although these disorders present with functional problems ultimately they may progress to chronic renal failure. Functional disorders cause abnormalities of metabolism in relation to:

- ♦ Calcium
- ♣ Phosphate
- ♥ Potassium
- ♠ Magnesium
- ♦ Water
- ♣ Glucose
- ♥ Amino acids
- ♠ Hydrogen Ions

Calcium

Abnormalities of tubular handling of calcium may be:

- ♦ Increased Urinary Calcium Excretion
- ♣ Decreased Urinary Calcium Excretion

Increased Urinary Calcium Excretion

Increased urinary calcium excretion occurs in:

319

♥ **Idiopathic Hypercalciuria**

Idiopathic hypercalciuria results in calcium stone formation.

♠ **Hereditary hypercalciuric nephrolithiasis**

This refers to four rare disorders that present with low molecular weight proteinuria, hypercalciuria, nephrocalcinosis, renal stones, renal failure

Decreased Urinary Calcium Excretion

Decreased urinary calcium excretion occurs in:

♦ **Familial Hypocalciuric Hypercalcaemia (Benign Familial Hypercalcaemia)**

This presents with hypercalcaemia, hypocalciuria and hypermagesaemia. The PTH concentration is within the normal range but is inappropriately high in relation to the calcium concentration.

Phosphate

Excretion of phosphate may be:

♣ Increased

♥ Decreased

Increased Excretion

Increased excretion of phosphate occurs in:

♠ Hereditary hypophosphataemic rickets

♦ X-linked hypophosphataemic rickets

♣ Oncogenic rickets, which is an acquired disorder similar to X-linked hypophosphataemic

rickets. It occurs in association with mesenchymal tumours.

Reduced Excretion

Reduced excretion of phosphate occurs in:

♥ Hypoparathyroidism

♠ Pseudohypoparathyroidism

Potassium

Abnormalities of tubular handling of potassium are:

♦ Increased excretion

♣ Decreased excretion

Increased Excretion of Potassium

Increased excretion of potassium may be due to:

♥ **Renal Tubular Ion Transport Impairment**

Bartter's syndrome, Gitelman's syndrome, Magnesium depletion, diuretics

♠ **Apparent Mineralocorticoid Excess**

Liddle's syndrome

♦ **Mineralocorticoid Excess**

Decreased Excretion of Potassium

Decreased excretion of potassium may be due to:

♣ **Renal Tubular Ion Transport Impairment**

Renal tubular ion transport may be impaired due to:

Drugs potassium sparing diuretics, trimethoprim, calcineurin inhibitors like cyclosporin, tacrolimus

Pseudohypoaldosteronism, which is an inherited condition with mineralocorticoid resistance (Type I autosomal recessive presents in childhood and regresses spontaneously, type II presents in adolescence or young adults with hyperkalaemia and metabolic acidosis)

♥ **Mineralocorticoid deficiency**

Magnesium

Excretion of magnesium may be:

♠ Decreased

♦ Increased

Decreased Excretion

Decreased excretion of magnesium occurs in:

♣ Renal failure

Increased Excretion

Increased excretion of magnesium occurs in:

♥ Bartter's syndrome

♠ Tubulointerstitial nephropathies

♦ Hypercalcaemia

♣ Drugs: diuretics, aminoglycosides, cyclosporin, cisplatin

Water

Excretion of water may be:

♥ Increased

♠ Decreased

Increased Excretion

Increased excretion of water occurs in:

♦ Cranial diabetes insipidus

♣ Nephrogenic diabetes insipidus

♥ Primary polydypsia

Decreased Excretion

Decreased excretion of water occurs in:

♠ Syndrome of Inappropriate Anti Diuretic Hormone Secretion (SIADH)

Glucose

Increased Excretion

Increased excretion of glucose occurs in:

♦ Renal glycosuria (with normo-glycaemia)

♣ Diabetes mellitus (with hypergly-caemia)

Amino Acids

Aminoaciduria

Increased excretion of amino acids occurs in:

♣ Cystinosis, which causes renal stones

♥ Hartnup's disease, which causes pellagra

Hydrogen Ions

Reduced excretion of hydrogen ions occurs in renal tubular acidosis.

Types of Renal Tubular Acidosis:

♠ **Type 1** (Distal Renal Tubular Acidosis)

Failure of H^+ ion excretion in the distal tubule

♦ **Type 2** (Proximal Renal Tubular Acidosis)

Failure of HCO_3^- reabsorption in the proximal tubule

♣ **Type 3**

Combination of 1 & 2 (rare)

- ♥ **Type 4**

  Hyporeninaemic hypoaldosteronism

Distal Renal Tubular Acidosis

The causes are:

- ♠ **Genetic** autosomal dominant
- ♦ **KUS** obstructive uropathy, medullary sponge kidney, pyelonephritis, papillary necrosis, nephrocalcinosis
- ♣ **LMS** Sjogren's syndrome
- ♥ **RS** fibrosing alveolitis
- ♠ **HS** sickle-cell anaemia, hypergammaglobuinaemia, dysglobulinaemia
- ♦ **E&M** mineralocorticoid deficiency
- ♣ **Drugs** trimethoprim, amphotericin, analgesic nephropathy (papillary necrosis) amphotericin B

Proximal Renal Tubular Acidosis

Proximal renal tubular acidosis is often associated with other proximal tubular defects. The causes are:

- ♥ **Genetic** autosomal dominant
- ♠ **Carbonic anhydrase II deficiency**
- ♦ **Drugs** acetazolamide
- ♣ **Fanconi syndrome**
- ♥ **KUS** post-renal transplant, nephrotic syndrome
- ♠ **E&M** hyperparathyroidism, vitamin D deficiency
- ♦ **HS** multiple myeloma
- ♣ **Toxins** lead poisoning, copper, mercury, uranium, cadmium

Type 4 Renal Tubular Acidosis

(Hyporeninaemic Hypoaldosteronism)

The causes are:

- ♦ **KUS** chronic renal disorders such as diabetes mellitus, tubulointerstitial disease
- ♣ **Drugs** NSAIDS, ACE inhibitors, beta-blockers, potassium sparing diuretics, aldosterone antagonists
- ♥ **E&M** Addison's disease gives a similar picture

Fanconi Syndrome

The Fanconi syndrome refers to a disturbance of proximal tubular function that results in generalised aminoaciduria, phosphate wasting, metabolic bone disease, renal tubular acidosis and renal glycosuria. It may be:

- ♣ **Primary Idiopathic**

Or due to

- ♥ **Systemic Factors**

  Fanconi's syndrome occurs in conditions affecting the:

  E&M cystinosis, tyrosinaemia, Wilson's disease, Lowes syndrome, galactosaemia, hereditary fructose intolerance

  Hyperparathyroidism either primary or secondary

  KUS acute tubular necrosis, hypokalaemic nephropathy, transplant rejection

  HS myeloma

  LMS Sjogren's syndrome

  Toxins heavy metals

  Drugs 6-mercaptopurine

Interstitial Lesions

Interstitial lesions of the kidneys (interstitial nephritis) may be due to:

Biological Agents

- **Bacterial Infections**: strepto-cocci, typhoid fever, brucella, legionella, mycoplasma, leptospira, syphilis, tuberculosis
- **Viruses**: cytomegalovirus, HIV, Epstein-Barr
- **Parasites**: toxoplasma, leish-mania
- **Transplant Rejection**

Chemical Agents

- **Drugs**: NSAIDS, anticonvulsants, antibacterials
- **Heavy Metals**: lead, cadmium

Physical Agents

- **Irradiation**

Systemic Disease

- **Secondary to Systemic Disease**

  Interstitial nephritis may be secondary to conditions affecting the:

  E&M oxalate crystals, uric acid crystals, hypercalcaemia, diabetes mellitus

  HS multiple myeloma, sickle cell disease

  LMS Sjogren's syndrome

Papillary Necrosis

Papillary necrosis may occur as a result of:

- Diabetes mellitus

- Sickle cell disease
- Analgesic use

Post-Renal Disorders

Post-renal conditions that result in disease may be due to:

- **Luminal Factors**

  Stones, blood clot, sloughed papilla

- **Mural Factors**

  Pelvi-ureteric junction obstruction, stricture, urothelial tumours, chronic interstitial cystitis, posterior urethral valves, prostate enlargement, pinhole urethral meatus, phimosis

- **External Factors**

  Retroperitoneal tumours, retroperitoneal fibrosis, gynaeco-logical malignancies, gynaeco-logical surgery

- **Systemic Factors**

  Post-renal kidney disorders may be consequent on conditions affecting the:

  CNS sacral plexus lesions, cauda equina lesions, lesions of the spinal cord

Tumours of the Kidneys and Urinary System

Tumours of the kidneys and urinary system may be:

- Renal Tumours
- Urothelial Tumours
- Prostate Tumours

323

Renal Tumours

Tumours of the kidneys are:

- ♥ Renal Cell Carcinoma (Hypernephroma)
- ♠ Renal Cell Adenoma
- ♦ Oncocytoma
- ♣ Angiomyolipoma

Urothelial Tumours

Urothelial tumours may occur in the:

- ♥ Renal pelvis
- ♠ Bladder

Prostate Tumours

Lesions of the prostate are:

- ♦ Benign prostatic hyperplasia
- ♣ Carcinoma

Presentation of Renal Disease

Renal disease may present to the clinician in a wide variety of manners. They are as follows:

- ♥ **Acute Renal Failure**

  Acute renal failure refers to a sudden loss of excretory renal function and includes disturbances of glomerular and tubular function.

- ♠ **Chronic Renal Failure**

  Chronic renal failure refers to irreversible impairment of renal function, the evidence being a reduced glomerular filtration rate.

- ♦ **Acute Nephritic Syndrome**

  Acute nephritic syndrome is a syndrome characterised by haematuria, proteinuria, hypertension, oedema, oliguria and uraemia.

- ♣ **Nephrotic Syndrome**

  Nephrotic syndrome refers to a syndrome characterised by heavy proteinuria, hypoalbuminaemia and oedema. Hypercholesterolaemia is almost always present.

- ♥ **Proteinuria**

  Detection of proteins in the urine on routine testing.

- ♠ **Haematuria**

  Haematuria may be macroscopic or microscopic.

- ♦ **Urinary Tract Infection**

  Urinary tract infection presents with increased frequency of micturition, dysuria, pain, discolouration of urine, smelly urine, fever

- ♣ **Ureteric Colic**

  Ureteric colic classically presents as a severe pain radiating from the loin to the groin.

- ♥ **Retention of Urine**

  Retention of urine may be acute or chronic

- ♠ **Tubular Dysfunction**

  Tubular dysfunction presents as abnormalities of growth, abnormalities of development or metabolic disturbances.

Findings on History

The findings that may be obtained on taking a history are as follows:

Polyuria

Polyuria, or passage of large volumes of urine, is caused by a failure to concentrate the glomerular filtrate. It may be due to:

♦ **Luminal Factors**

Osmotic effects due to glycosuria, chronic renal failure

♣ **Mural Factors**

Resolving acute tubular necrosis, nephrogenic diabetes insipidus

♥ **Systemic Factors**

Conditions affecting the:

CNS cranial diabetes insipidus, hysterical polydypsia

E&M hypercalcaemia

Drugs diuretics

Oliguria

Oliguria or passage of small volumes of urine (<400ml /day) may be due to:

♣ **Pre-Renal Causes**

Oliguria occurs in conditions where both renal arteries are involved:

Severe hypertension, hypotension, hypovolaemia, dissecting aneurysm

♦ **Renal Causes**

Glomerulonephritis, acute tubular necrosis, interstitial nephritis

♣ **Post-Renal Causes**

Oliguria occurs in conditions where both ureters are involved by:

Retroperitoneal fibrosis, stones, blood clot, gynaecological malignancy

Anuria

Anuria (no urine) is usually due to:

♥ Bladder outflow obstruction

♠ Obstruction to drainage of both kidneys and or ureters

Increased Frequency of Micturition

Increased frequency of micturition may be due to:

♦ **Luminal Factors**

This refers to conditions where the bladder lining is irritated by:

Infection, calculi, blood, urothelial tumour

♣ **Mural Factors**

Increased frequency of micturition occurs in conditions where filling of the bladder is restricted. This may be due to a contracted bladder, chronic interstitial cystitis, a pelvic tumour

♥ **External Factors**

This refers to conditions that prevent complete emptying of the bladder:

Prostatic enlargement in the male

Utero-vaginal prolapse in the female

Retention of Urine

Retention of urine may be due to:

♠ **Luminal Factors**

Stone, blood clot

♦ **Mural Factors**

Stricture, enlargement of the prostate gland, posterior urethral valves, pinhole urethral meatus

♣ **Systemic Factors**

Conditions affecting the:

CNS sacral plexus lesions, cauda equina lesions, spinal cord lesions

Incontinence

Incontinence may be classified as:

♥ **Continuous Incontinence (Total)**

Continuous incontinence refers to continuous leakage of urine due to urinary tract fistulae such as vesico-vaginal fistula, ectopic ureter.

♠ **Stress Incontinence**

Stress incontinence refers to urinary leakage with increased intra-abdominal pressure.

Females: in females it is caused by weakening of the pelvic floor muscles

Males: in males it is caused by damage to the external urethral sphincter following prostatectomy

♦ **Urge Incontinence**

Urge incontinence is the inability to control voiding when the patient has an urge to pass urine. It may be caused by:

Cystitis, neurogenic bladder, which is caused by detrusor hyperreflexia, advanced bladder outflow obstruction

♣ **Overflow Incontinence**

Overflow incontinence refers to urinary retention with overflow. It may be caused by chronic urinary outflow obstruction, autonomous bladder and sensory bladder.

Enuresis

Enuresis refers to incontinence that occurs during sleep

Pain

In relation to the kidneys and the urinary system, pain may be felt as:

♥ **Loin Pain**

Loin pain could be due to:

Renal Causes: pyelonephritis, renal vein thrombosis, renal infarction. It may also occur in acute glomerulonephritis and exacerbations of IgA nephropathy.

Post-Renal Causes: obstruction to urinary outflow

♠ **Ureteric Colic**

Ureteric colic may be caused by passage of a calculus and more rarely passage of a blood clot or a sloughed papilla

♦ **Bladder and Urethra**

Pain may be due to obstruction or more rarely chronic interstitial cystitis

Haematuria

Haematuria (passage of blood in the urine) may be due to:

♣ Renal Causes

♥ Post-Renal Causes

Renal Causes

Renal causes of haematuria are:

♠ Glomerulonephritis

♦ Renal carcinoma

Post-Renal Causes

Post-renal causes of haematuria are:

♣ **Luminal Factors**

Calculi

♥ **Mural Factors**

Urothelial tumours, schistosomiasis, bacterial infections, tuberculosis

Pneumaturia

Pneumaturia refers to passage of air in the urine.

♠ Pneumaturia would suggest entero-vesical or colo-vesical fistulae

Faeces in the Urine

The presence of faeces in the urine would suggest:

♦ A colo-vesical fistula

Findings on Examination

The abnormalities that may be detected on clinical examination of the patient are as follows:

General Examination

On general examination of the patient one may note changes in the:

♥ Dimensions

♠ Integument

♦ Body temperature

Dimensions

On examination of the dimensions one may detect abnormalities of:

♣ Height

♥ Weight

♠ Shape

Height

Variations in height may be:

♣ **Short Stature**

Short stature would indicate chronic renal impairment from childhood.

Weight

Variations in weight could be:

♥ **Increased Weight**

Increased weight would suggest salt and water overload

♠ **Decreased Weight**

Emaciation is a feature of chronic renal failure

Shape

Variations in shape that may be of significance are:

◆ Renal oedema affects the face preferentially.

♣ Partial lipodystrophy (asymmetric loss of subcutaneous fat from the face, trunk and arms, the legs appear fatter than normal) is associated with mesangiocapillary (membranoproliferative) glomerulonephritis

♥ A Cushingoid appearance would be due to treatment with steroids

Integument

When examining the integument one would note:

♠ Colour

◆ Surface

Colour

Changes in colour that may be noted are:

♠ **Pigmentation**

Increased photosensitive pigmentation is a feature of chronic renal failure

◆ **Pallor**

The skin would be pale and lack lustre in chronic renal impairment. Anaemia would be a feature of chronic renal failure

♣ **Suffusion** (Plethora)

Diffuse reddening may occur in polycythaemia, which could be due to renal causes

Surface

Abnormalities that may be noted on the surface of the skin are:

♣ Scratch marks occur if the patient has pruritus due to chronic renal failure

♥ Angiokeratoma occur in alpha galactosidase deficiency (Anderson-Fabry disease) where renal failure occurs

♠ Dermatitis. Pellagra may occur in aminoaciduria (Hartnup's disease)

◆ The skin would be dry and flaky in chronic renal failure

♣ Easy bruising would occur due to platelet dysfunction as a result of chronic renal failure

Body Temperature

Fever could indicate:

♠ Kidney infections

◆ Transplant rejection

♣ Infective endocarditis

Regional Examination

Abnormalities that may be detected on regional examination are as follows:

Head

On examination of the head one may detect changes in the:

♥ Mental state

♠ Dimensions

Mental State

The level of consciousness is important as drowsiness may occur in advanced renal failure. Irritability would be a feature and fits may occur.

Dimensions

When assessing the dimensions of the head one may note changes in:

Shape

Variations in the shape of the head that would be significant are:

- ♠ **Swelling**

  In renal oedema swelling of the face would occur.

- ♦ **Skeletal Appearance**

  A skeletal appearance may be due to cachexia or partial lipodystrophy. In partial lipodystrophy loss of fat occurs in the face and upper part of the body. These patients may develop mesangiocapillary glomerulonephritis and hypocomplementaemia

- ♣ **Moon Face**

  A moon face would occur in:

  Iatrogenic Cushing's syndrome

Nose

On examination of the nose one may note abnormalities of:

- ♥ Shape
- ♠ Internal aspect
- ♦ Smell

Shape

Variations in the shape of the nose that may be significant are:

- ♥ A beak like nose occurs in scleroderma
- ♠ A saddle shaped nose occurs in Wegener's granulomatosis

Internal Aspect

On examination of the internal aspect of the nose one may note:

- ♣ Ulceration and septal perforation may occur in Wegener's granulomatosis

Smell

Whilst examining the patient one may notice:

- ♥ Uraemic foetor, an ammoniacal smell, may occur in chronic renal failure

Eyes

On examination of the eyes one may detect abnormalities of the following:

Eyeballs

When examining the eyeballs one may note changes in:

Position

The position of the eyeballs may be abnormal.

- ♠ Proptosis can occur due to granulomatous vasculitis forming a pseudotumour

329

Eyelids

Lesions that may occur in the eyelids are:

♦ Xanthelasma may be seen in the nephrotic syndrome

♣ Periorbital oedema occurs in the nephrotic syndrome

Conjunctiva

Lesions that may be seen in the conjunctiva are:

♥ A red eye occurs in uraemia. This is due to high phosphate levels.

♠ Conjunctivitis may occur in leptospirosis, Wegener's granulomatosis

Sclera

Abnormalities that may be seen in the sclera are:

♦ Icterus would be seen in conditions affecting the:

GIT leptospirosis, hepato-renal syndrome

HS haemolytic uraemic syndrome, incompatible blood transfusion

♣ Scleritis can occur in Wegener's granulomatosis

Cornea

In the cornea one may note:

♥ Calcification, which occurs in the lateral margins of the cornea in hyperparathyroidism

Anterior Chamber

In the anterior chamber one may note:

♠ Hypopyon in iritis

♦ Hyphaema can occur in rubeosis iridis, which may complicate diabetes mellitus.

Iris

Lesions that may occur in the iris are:

♣ Uveitis can occur in Wegener's granulomatosis

♥ Rubeosis iridis may occur in diabetes mellitus

Fundus

Lesions that may occur in the fundus are:

♠ Hypertensive Retinopathy

♦ Diabetic Retinopathy

♣ Retinal haemangioblastoma occur in von Hippel-Lindau disease in which renal carcinoma may occur

Eye Movements

When examining eye movements one may detect:

♥ A 3rd nerve lesion due to a berry aneurysm which may be associated with polycystic kidneys

Face

On examination of the face one may detect abnormalities of the following:

Scalp

In the scalp one may note:

♠ Alopecia. This may occur in systemic lupus erythematosus.

Forehead

On inspection of the forehead one may notice:

- ♦ Uraemic frost. Rarely, uraemic frost may be seen on the forehead. It is crystallisation of urea in sweat

Malar Region

Lesions that may occur in the malar region are:

- ♣ A malar rash may occur in systemic lupus erythematosus
- ♥ Telangiectasia may occur in systemic sclerosis
- ♠ Adenoma sebaceum occurs in tuberose sclerosis, which may be associated with renal cysts

Mouth

On examination of the mouth one may detect abnormalities of the following:

Lips

On inspection of the lips one may note:

- ♦ A small mouth in scleroderma

Gums

Abnormalities that may be noted in the gums are:

- ♣ Gum hypertrophy may be caused by treatment with cyclosporin

Tongue

Abnormalities that may be seen in the tongue are:

- ♥ A large tongue occurs in amyloidosis
- ♠ An ulcerated tongue may occur in Wegener's granulomatosis

Ears

On examination of the ears, the abnormalities that may be detected are:

- ♦ Tophi may be seen in chronic tophaceous gout.
- ♣ Deafness occurs in Alport's syndrome

Hands

When examining the hands one may note abnormalities of the:

Dimensions

The main deviation from the normal dimensions would be a change in the shape of the hands.

Shape

Abnormalities in the shape of the hands that may be noted are:

- ♥ Apparently contracted and tapered hands in scleroderma
- ♠ Short fourth and or fifth finger in pseudohypoparathyroidism

Nails

When examining the nails one may note abnormalities of:

Shape

Abnormalities in the shape of the nails that may be observed are the following:

- In the nail patella syndrome split deformed nails would be observed. The other features are a rudimentary patella, iliac horns, chronic glomerulonephritis. Autosomal dominant inheritance.

- Pseudoclubbing would be seen in hyperparathyroidism.
  Pseudoclubbing refers to the shape seen due to resorption of the terminal phalanx causing the nail to slope downwards.

Colour

Variations that may occur in the colour of the nails are:

- Muehrcke's lines are two white lines parallel to the nail fold. This indicates hypoalbuminaemia.

- Mee's lines are multiple white lines parallel to the nail fold. This is seen in chemotherapy for cancer, cardiac or renal failure, Hodgkin's disease. They are also seen in poisoning by arsenic and thallium.

- Lindsay's nails are nails in which the proximal half of the nail is white whilst the distal half is brown or pink or red. This is seen in chronic renal failure

Circulation

Abnormalities that one may note in relation to the blood vessels of the nails are:

- Periungual infarcts indicate vasculitis

- Splinter haemorrhages could indicate bacterial endocarditis

Skin

On examination of the skin one may note:

- Infected scabies. This would indicate the cause of glomerulonephritis

Peripheral Circulation and Radial Pulse

No specific abnormalities occur in relation to the kidneys and urinary system but abnormalities that occur in association with circulatory and metabolic disturbances would be noted

Nervous System

When examining the nervous system of the hands one may detect:

- A flapping tremor (asterixis) may occur in uraemia

- Fasiculation may be seen in uraemia.

- Carpal tunnel syndrome may occur in association with haemodialysis

Locomotor System

On examination of the locomotor system of the hands one may detect:

- Deformity of arthritis. This would suggest associated renal disease or disease as a consequence of the treatment used in arthritis.

- A polyarthropathy may occur in association with dialysis.

Forearms

On examination of the forearms one may note:

- ♣ A fistula would be seen in patients who have been on haemodialysis
- ♥ A thrill would signify patency of the fistula

Upper Arms

In the upper arm one may note:

- ♠ Elevation of the blood pressure in renal disease.

Neck

On examination of the neck one may note changes in the:

Integument

The abnormalities that may occur are:

- ♦ A parathyroidectomy scar may be seen

JVP

On examination of the JVP one may note:

- ♣ An elevated jugular venous pressure could indicate salt and water overload.
- ♥ An elevated JVP may be seen in constrictive pericarditis complicating chronic renal failure

Chest Wall

The skin over the sternum could be used to assess the state of salt and water balance.

- ♠ Decreased skin elasticity would indicate loss of salt and water.

Respiratory System

Abnormalities that may be detected in the respiratory system in renal disease are:

- ♦ Deep sighing respiration would indicate acidosis
- ♣ Rapid shallow breathing would suggest fluid overload
- ♥ Hiccoughs occur in advanced renal failure
- ♠ Basal crepitations would indicate salt and water overload
- ♦ Pleural effusions occur in the nephrotic syndrome

Cardiovascular System

Abnormalities that may be detected in the cardiovascular system in renal disease are:

- ♣ A heaving apex occurs in hypertension
- ♥ Mitral valve prolapse may be associated with polycystic kidneys
- ♠ Pericarditis occurs in renal failure
- ♦ Constrictive pericarditis may occur in renal failure
- ♣ Subacute bacterial endocarditis may cause haematuria as a result of glomerulonephritis or as a

333

result of emboli causing infarction of the kidney

Back

On examination of the back one may detect abnormalities of the following:

Loins

Abnormalities that may occur are:

- ♥ Loss of the concavity of the flank and fullness in the loins may be due to enlargement of the kidney or perinephric infection.

Sacrum

One may note:

- ♠ Oedema in fluid overload

Abdomen

On examination of the abdomen one may detect abnormalities of the following:

Abdominal Wall

Abnormalities that may be detected in the abdominal wall are:

- ♦ Scars would be seen if the patient has had a renal transplant.
- ♣ A peritoneal dialysis catheter may be observed.
- ♥ Peritoneal dialysis scars may be observed

Contents of the Abdomen

Abnormalities that may be detected are as follows:

Kidneys

On examination of the kidneys, abnormalities that may be detected are:

- ♠ **Bilateral Enlargement**

  Bilateral enlargement of the kidneys occurs in polcystic kidneys, amyloidosis, bilateral hydronephrosis, von Hippel Lindau disease, tuberose sclerosis

- ♦ **Unilateral Enlargement**

  Unilateral enlargement of a kidney could indicate unilateral hydronephrosis or tumour. Unilateral enlargement may also be due to hypertrophy of a solitary kidney, contralateral kidney in renal artery stenosis, carcinoma, single polycystic kidney

- ♠ **Transplanted Kidney**

  A transplanted kidney would be felt in the right or left iliac fossa.

- ♥ **Graft Tenderness**

  Graft tenderness would indicate rejection

Aortic Aneurysm

An aortic aneurysm may:

- ♠ Involve the renal arteries.

Bladder

Distension of the bladder could indicate:

- ♦ Acute or chronic urinary outflow obstruction

Liver

The liver may be enlarged in:

- ♣ Hepato-renal syndrome
- ♥ Polycystic renal disease
- ♠ Non-alcoholic steato hepatitis due to diabetes mellitus
- ♦ Leptospirosis

Spleen

The spleen may be enlarged in:

- ♣ The hepato-renal syndrome
- ♥ Subacute bacterial endocarditis

Ascites

Ascites occurs in:

- ♠ The nephrotic syndrome

Bruit

A bruit would indicate:

- ♦ Renal artery stenosis

Male Genitalia

The abnormalities that may be detected on examination of the male genitalia are:

- ♣ Developmental abnormalities could account for recurrent urinary infection
- ♥ Phimosis or a pinhole urethral meatus may be observed

Female Genitalia and Pelvic Organs

Conditions that may present with problems of micturition and renal dysfunction are:

- ♠ Utero-vaginal prolapse
- ♦ Carcinoma of the cervix

- ♣ Uterine enlargement
- ♥ Ovarian tumours.

Rectum

The abnormalities that may occur are:

- ♠ Enlargement of the prostate in the male causes urinary outflow obstruction

Lower Limbs

Lesions that may be detected on general examination of the lower limbs are:

Dimensions

Abnormalities of shape would be observed in:

- ♦ Renal rickets.

Integument

The abnormality that may occur is:

- ♣ Henoch-Schonlein purpura commonly occurs in the lower limbs.

Hips

Proximal myopathy may be associated with:

- ♥ Renal osteodystrophy

Knees

One may note:

- ♠ An absent patella in the nail patella syndrome

335

Lower Leg

Abnormalities that may be noted are:

- ◆ Ankle oedema may occur as a result of salt and water overload

Feet

Lesions that may be detected are:

- ♣ The manifestations of gout may be observed in the foot
- ♥ Peripheral vascular disease may occur in association with diabetic nephropathy, renal artery stenosis

Gait

Abnormalities of gait that may occur in relation to renal disease are:

- ♠ Peripheral neuropathy may occur in chronic renal failure
- ◆ Proximal myopathy may occur in renal osteodystrophy

Standing from a Seated or Squatting Position

Lesions that may occur in relation to renal disease are:

- ♣ Proximal myopathy may occur in renal osteodystrophy

Chapter 14

The Reproductive and Genital System

In this system one will study the genitalia and the reproductive system. Clinical features of conditions that involve the genitalia and the reproductive system will be studied together with the clinical features of the causes and effects of these conditions that are reflected in other systems.

History Taking

The important points in history taking in relation to the reproductive and genital system are as follows:

Males

One should enquire about:

- ♥ Erectile function
- ♠ Ejaculation
- ♦ Pain in the genitalia
- ♣ Swelling of the genitalia
- ♥ Rash
- ♠ Ulceration
- ♦ Discharge

Females

One should enquire about:

- ♣ Menstrual periods:

  Frequency

  Number of days the period lasts

  Quantity of menstrual flow

  Pain during menstruation
- ♥ Vaginal discharge

- ♠ Pain
- ♦ Irritation
- ♣ Rash
- ♥ Ulceration
- ♠ Dyspaerunia. This refers to pain or discomfort during sexual intercourse

Obstetric History

One should enquire about:

- ♦ Number of pregnancies
- ♣ Number of deliveries
- ♥ Types of delivery
- ♠ Complications of pregnancy, labour and puerperium

Sexual History (Males and Females)

One should enquire about:

- ♦ Partners
- ♣ Contraception

One should then perform a review of systems.

Physical Examination

One should commence with a general examination and then proceed to perform regional examination.

General Examination

Note the posture of the patient. Assess the state of growth and development and the metabolic state of the patient. Note the height and weight. Pay particular attention to the overall shape of the patient. Assess the state of the integument. In particular note the quantity and distribution of hair, both scalp hair and body hair. Note whether the hair has a masculine or feminine distribution. Assess the body temperature. (Position, Height and Proportions, Weight and Shape, Integument, Body Temperature)

Of particular importance in general examination, in relation to the reproductive and genital system, is to define whether the overall appearance of the patient is masculine, feminine or eunuchoid.

Regional Examination

Commence regional examination by examining the head. One may start with the hands if one prefers.

Head

Note the mental state. Assess the dimensions of the head. Examine the regions of the head, the nose, the eyes, the face (scalp, forehead, malar region, chin) the mouth (jaw, lips, teeth, gums, buccal mucosa, tongue, palate, fauces, salivary glands), the ears. In particular, importance should be placed on defining the quantity and distribution of scalp and facial hair.

Upper Limbs

Perform a quick general examination of the upper limbs noting the dimensions and the state of the integument.

Hands

Assess the dimensions. Then examine the dorsum of the hands; the nails and skin, the bones, joints, tendons and muscles. Ask the patient to turn the hands over and examine the palmar aspect; the skin, the bones, the joints, the tendons and the muscles. Examine the peripheral circulation and the radial pulse. Look for tremors. Examine the functions of the nervous system and the locomotor system of the hands if required.

Forearms and Upper Arms

Examine the forearms and the upper arms. Note the carrying angle

Shoulders and Axillae

Examine the shoulders and the axillae.

If required one should assess active and passive movements of the upper limbs and perform neurological examination of the upper limbs.

Neck

Neck examination should be performed in the usual manner (dimensions, integument, thyroid, sternocleidomastoid, jugular venous pressure, carotids, trachea, lymph nodes)

Chest

Examine the chest wall and if required the contents of the chest; the lungs and the heart. When examining the chest wall, emphasis should be placed on defining the quantity and distribution of any hair on the chest and the state of development of any breast tissue.

A detailed description of examination of the female breast is outside the scope of this book. Only a brief outline will be included.

Breasts

The breasts should be inspected with the patient in a seated position. After initial inspection, ask the patient to clasp her hands behind her head whilst inspection is continued and finally request the patient to rest her hands on her hips until inspection is concluded. Next, ask the patient to lie down. Commence palpation. Initially, examine the nipple area and then examine each quadrant of the breast. Finally, carefully palpate the axilla.

Back

In practice one should examine the patient's back at this juncture

Abdomen

Examine the abdominal wall and the contents of the abdomen in the usual manner

Inguinal Region and Genitals

Although examination of these regions is not required in professional examinations, for the sake of completeness a short description follows.

Male Genitalia

The male genitalia are best examined with the patient standing. However, one should refrain from requesting to examine the patient in the erect position!

The distribution of pubic hair should be noted.

Make an overall assessment of the genitalia. Examine the characteristics of the pubic hair.

Note the structure of the penis, look for any deformity. Retract the prepuce and examine the glans. Remember to draw the prepuce back to cover the glans after examination is completed.

Examine the scrotum. Note the dimensions of the testes, gently palpate and perform transillumination if a swelling is noted. Next, examine the epididymis and the spermatic cord. Examine the inguinal lymph nodes.

Female Genitalia

A short description of examination of the female genitalia will be included for the sake of completeness. For a detailed description one should refer to a textbook of gynaecology

The patient should assume the supine position with the knees bent.

Assess the quantity, distribution and characteristics of the pubic hair. Examine the labia majora and minora, the clitoris, the urethral orifice and the vaginal outlet. Perform digital examination and note the state of the walls of the vagina, the cervix and the fornices. Note any abnormality in the pouch of Douglas. Perform speculum examination.

Buttocks, Perianal Region and Per Rectal Examination

Per rectal examination is of importance in assessing the prostate in the male and the pelvic organs in the female.

Lower Limbs

Perform a general examination and then proceed to examine the hips, the thighs, the knees, the lower legs and the feet. Examine the locomotor system and perform neurological examination if required.

Spine

Examine the spine if required.

Gait, Romberg's Sign, Trendelenburg test, Standing from a Seated or Squatting Position

Perform these tests if required

Lesions of the Genitalia and Reproductive System

The lesions that may occur are as follows:

Disorders of Sexual Development

Disorders of sexual development may be classified as disorders of:

♥ Primary Sexual Development

♠ Disorders of Secondary Sexual Development

Primary Sexual Development

Development of the genitalia and the organs of reproduction depend upon:

♦ Genotype

♣ Gonadal development

♥ Hormone sensitivity (receptor defects)

♠ Hormonal environment

Disorders of Primary Sexual Development in the Male

Disorders of primary sexual development in the male may be due to:

♦ **Genetic Disorders**

Klinefelter's syndrome XXY, XX male (male phenotype, sparse facial hair, gynaecomastia, small genitalia, hypospadias, absent spermatogenesis), XXXY disorder, XXXXY disorder, XYY disorder, Noonan's syndrome (XY autosomal dominant)

♣ **Testicular Disorders**

Cryptorchidism, testicular agenesis, mixed gonadal dysgenesis (testis on one side, streak gonad on the other side), dysgenetic male pseudohaemophroditism (persistent Mullerian structures, bilateral dysgenetic testes, cryptorchidism, external genitalia poorly virilised)

♥ **Androgen Receptor Defects**

Androgen receptor defects may be expressed as male phenotypes or female phenotypes:

Female Phenotypes

Complete testicular feminisation syndrome (female phenotype, normal breasts, blind ending vagina, gonads show Leydig cell hyperplasia with no spermatogenesis)

Incomplete testicular feminisation (dominant feminisation with some virilisation, clitoral enlargement and fusion of labia)

Male Phenotypes

Reifenstein syndrome (male phenotype, severe perineal hypospadias, incomplete virilisation at puberty with associated gynaecomastia)

Infertile male syndrome (male phenotype, small penis and testes, possible gynaecomastia, oligospermia and infertility)

♠ **Hormone Imbalances**

Leydig cell hypoplasia, inborn errors of testosterone biosynthesis, iatrogenic male pseudohaemophroditism

Disorders of Primary Sexual Development in the Female

Disorders of primary sexual development in the female may be due to:

♦ **Genetic Conditions**

Turner's syndrome (XO)

♣ **Gonadal Disorders**

Gonadal dysgenesis (female external genitalia, streak gonads, clitoromegaly sometimes), absent or anomalous genitalia

♥ **Hormonal Imbalances**

Hormonal imbalances in the female may cause foetal virilisation. This may be due to:

Foetal Hormonal Imbalances

Congenital adrenal hyperplasia, which may be:

17-hydroxylase deficiency

21-hydroxylase deficiency

11-hydroxylase deficiency

Foetal adrenal adenoma

Maternal Hormonal Imbalances

Maternal ovarian tumour or adrenal tumour, iatrogenic

True Hermaphroditism

True hermaphroditism is rare and refers to the presence of both testicular and ovarian tissue. The presenting feature is an abnormal appearance of the external genitalia.

Disorders of Secondary Sexual Development

One should consider:

- ♣ Secondary Sexual Development in the Male
- ♥ Secondary Sexual Development in the Female

Disorders of Secondary Sexual Development in the Male

Disorders of secondary sexual development in the male are the following:

- ♠ Precocious Puberty in the Male
- ♦ Hypogonadism in the Male

Precocious Puberty in the Male

Precocious puberty may be:

- ♣ True Precocious Puberty
- ♥ Pseudo Precocious Puberty

True Precocious Puberty

True precocious puberty is associated with a pubertal response to gonadotrophin releasing factors

True precocious puberty may be:

- ♠ **Idiopathic**

Or it may be due to conditions affecting the:

- ♦ **CNS** hydrocephalus, irradiation, surgery, infection, hypothalamic hamartoma, glioma, pinealoma

- ♣ **E&M** hypothyroidism

Pseudo Precocious Puberty

Pseudo precocious puberty is independent of pituitary gonadotrophins.

Pseudo precocious puberty may be due to conditions affecting the:

- ♥ **E&M** adrenal tumours, congenital adrenal hyperplasia
- ♠ **RAG** testoxicosis, teratoma, Leydig cell tumour
- ♦ **GIT** hepatoblastoma

Hypogonadism in the Male

Hypogonadism in the male may be due to:

- ♣ **Hypothalamic Lesions**

  Isolated gonadotrophin releasing hormone deficiency, Kallman's syndrome, male anorexia nervosa

- ♥ **Pituitary Lesions**

  Craniopharyngioma, pituitary adenoma, hyperprolactinaemia, cranial irradiation, haemochromatosis, transfusion siderosis, granulomatous destruction due to tuberculosis, histiocytosis X

- ♠ **Testicular Disorders**

  Klinefelter's syndrome, testicular agenesis, torsion, trauma

- ♦ **Systemic Disease**

  Conditions affecting the:

  CNS Prader-Willi syndrome, Laurence-Moon-Biedl syndrome, familial cerebellar degeneration

  GIT cirrhosis of the liver

  E&M thyrotoxicosis

  KUS chronic renal failure

Any other chronic debilitating illness

Failure of Spermatogenesis

Failure of spermatogenesis may be due to:

♣ **Failure of Production**

Failure of production of sperm may be caused by:

Idiopathic hypospermatogenesis, varicocoele, cryptorchidism, orchitis, irradiation

♥ **Failure of Passage of Sperm**

Failure of passage of sperm may be due to:

Sperm antibodies, Kartagener's syndrome, immotile cilia, agenesis of the epididymis and vas, obstruction due to infection, retrograde ejaculation, accessory gland infection

♠ **Systemic Factors**

Systemic factors that result in failure of spermatogenesis may be conditions involving the:

CNS dystrophia myotonica, spinal cord injury

Drugs cytotoxic chemotherapy, sulphasalazine, anticonvulsants

Toxins ethanol, opiates, cannabis, heavy metals, pesticides

Disorders of Secondary Sexual Development in the Female

Disorders of secondary sexual development in the female are the following:

♦ Precocious Puberty in the Female

♣ Female Hypogonadism

♥ Virilisation in the Female

Precocious Puberty in the Female

Precocious puberty in the female may be:

♠ True Precocious Puberty

♦ Pseudo Precocious Puberty

True Precocious Puberty

True precocious puberty is dependent on pituitary gonadotrophins.

True precocious puberty could be:

♣ Idiopathic either sporadic or familial

Or secondary to conditions affecting the:

♥ **CNS** hydrocephalus, irradiation, surgery, infection, hypothalamic hamartoma, glioma, pinealoma

♠ **E&M** hypothyroidism

Pseudo Precocious Puberty

Pseudo precocious puberty is independent of pituitary gonadotrophins

Pseudo precocious puberty could be due to conditions affecting the:

♦ **E&M** congenital adrenal hyperplasia, adrenal adenoma, carcinoma

♣ **RAG** ovarian cyst, ovarian tumour, dysgerminoma, teratoma

♥ **LMS** polyostotic fibrous dysplasia

♠ **GIT** hepatoblastoma

♦ **Drugs** sex hormones

Female Hypogonadism

Female hypogonadism may be due to:

♣ **Hypothalamic Lesions**

343

Isolated hypogonadotrophic hypogonadism, Kallman's syndrome

Weight related amenorrhoea following loss of weight due to:

Voluntary or involuntary starvation

Nutritional failure

Exercise related weight loss (following strenuous exercise regimes)

Sarcoidosis, tuberculosis

♥ **Pituitary Lesions**

Prolactinoma, craniopharyngioma

♠ **Gonadal Lesions**

Gonadal dysgenesis (the commonest cause is Turner's syndrome), primary ovarian failure due to autoimmune damage

Virilisation in the Female

Virilisation may be due to:

♦ **Ovarian Lesions**

Polycystic ovarian syndrome, masculinising tumours

♣ **Adrenal Lesions**

Cushing's syndrome, adrenal tumours, congenital adrenal hyperplasia

♥ **Systemic Factors**

Conditions affecting the:

RS bronchial carcinoma

Drugs anabolic steroids, glucocorticoids, phenytoin

Hirsutes

Hirsutes refers to the growth of coarse, androgen dependent hair in women

Hypertrichosis Lanuginosa

Hypertrichosis lanuginosa refers to a condition in which hair growth is observed where normally no hair would occur for example the forehead. This is seen in bronchial carcinoma (and in carcinoma of the colon, uterus and in lymphoma), porphyria cutanea tarda and with the use of drugs such as minoxidil, diazoxide, phenytoin, cyclosporin, PUVA, prednisolone, streptomycin, acetazolamide, penicillamine, fenoterol.

Other lesions that may occur in the reproductive and genital system are the sexually transmitted infections and malignancies of the reproductive and genital system.

Findings on History

The findings that may be obtained on history taking are as follows:

Males

The abnormalities that may occur in males are as follows:

Impotence

Impotence may be due to:

♠ Vascular disease involving the pelvic vessels

♦ Neurological disease such as autonomic neuropathy, multiple sclerosis, spinal injuries

♣ **Systemic Factors**

Conditions affecting the:

E&M androgen deficiency, hyper-prolactinaemia

CNS depression, psychogenic impotence

Severe systemic disease

Surgery retroperitoneal and bladder neck surgery

Toxins alcohol abuse

Drugs beta-blockers

Decreased Libido

Decreased libido could be due to:

♥ Androgen deficiency

♣ Hyperprolactinaemia

♦ Severe systemic disease

Ejaculation

Problems with ejaculation are usually associated with erectile failure

Pain in the Genitalia

Pain in the genitalia is usually due to infection

Swelling of the Genitalia

Swelling of the genitalia may be due to:

♣ Tumour

♥ Hydrocoele

♠ Oedema

Females

The abnormalities that may occur in females are as follows:

Menstrual Periods

Disorders of menstruation are the following:

♦ Amenorrhoea

♣ Oligomenorrhoea

♥ Menorrhagia

Amenorrhoea

Amenorrhoea refers to the absence of menstrual periods for more than six months. Amenorrhoea may be due to conditions affecting the:

♠ **RAG** pregnancy, genital tract abnormalities (imperforate hymen, Mullerian agenesis, transverse vaginal septum, cervical stenosis, intrauterine adhesions), gonadal dysgenesis, premature ovarian failure, resistant ovary syndrome

♦ **E&M** hypogonadism, hyperthyroidism

♣ **Severe Illness**

♥ **Drugs** use of hormonal contraceptives

Oligomenorrhoea

Oligomenorrhoea refers to the interval between menstrual periods being greater than six weeks but less than six months.

Oligomenorrhoea occurs in:

♠ Polycystic ovarian syndrome

Menorrhagia

Menorrhagia or excessive menstrual flow may be due to conditions affecting the:

♦ **RAG** disorders of the uterus

♣ **E&M** hypothyroidism

Disorders of fertility and the consequences of pregnancy are beyond the scope of this book and will not be discussed.

Findings on Examination

The abnormalities that may be detected on clinical examination of the patient are as follows:

General Examination

On general examination one may note abnormalities of the:

♦ Dimensions

♣ Integument

Dimensions

Abnormalities of the dimensions may affect:

♠ Height

♦ Weight

♣ Shape

Height

Variations in height are as follows:

Males

Variations in height in males may be:

♥ **Tall Stature**

In males, tall stature is associated with lack of androgens as fusion of the epiphyses is dependent on androgens. Tall stature would be seen in conditions like Klinefelter's syndrome. Eunuchoid proportions would be observed.

♠ **Short Stature**

In males short stature may be due to early, excessive production of androgens causing premature fusion of the epiphyses (precocious puberty).

Females

In females variations in height that may be of significance are:

♦ **Short Stature**

Short stature is associated with decreased production of hormones in Turner's syndrome.

Turner's Syndrome

The features are:

Female phenotype, amenorrhoea, short stature, low hairline, high arched palate, short metacarpals (fourth), cubitus valgus, webbed neck, shield chest with widely spaced nipples, left sided heart lesions. Lymphoedema, multiple pigmented naevi and hearing loss commonly occur.

Noonan's Syndrome

The features are:

Mild mental retardation, triangular micrognathic facies, hypertelorism, low set ears with posterior angulation, webbed neck, shield chest, pectus excavatum, cubitus valgus, right sided heart lesions

Klinefelter's Syndrome

The features are:

Tall stature, gynaecomastia, small testes, sparse pubic and body hair, small penis, fine wrinkling of the skin later in life. Decreased potency occurs and these patients are invariably sterile.

Weight

Abnormalities that one may note are:

Obesity

The causes of obesity are:

♣ **Males**

In males, obesity of the female type would occur in the Prader-Willi syndrome, Laurence-Moon-Biedl syndrome

♥ **Female**

In females, obesity of the male type would occur in polycystic ovarian syndrome, Cushing's syndrome, alcoholic pseudo-cushings.

Decreased Weight

Decreased weight could be due to:

♠ Anorexia nervosa

♦ Other causes of nutritional failure

♣ Exercise related

Shape

Variations in the overall shape of the patient that would be of significance are:

♦ A masculine shape with broad shoulders and narrow hips in a female would indicate a virilising syndrome

♣ A feminine shape with wide hips and narrow shoulders in a male would indicate a feminising syndrome

♥ Lipoatrophy may be seen following antiretroviral treatment in AIDS

Integument

On examination of the integument one may note abnormalities of the following:

Hair

Variations in the distribution of hair are:

♠ Hair distribution would be masculine with facial hair and hair on the torso in virilising syndromes

♦ Feminine hair distribution with lack of facial hair and lack of hair on the torso occurs in feminising syndromes

Skin

On examination of the skin one may note abnormalities of the following:

Surface

The abnormalities that one may detect on the surface of the skin are as follows:

Rash

A rash would suggest the presence of sexually transmitted disease

- ♣ A pustular rash occurs in gonococcal septicaemia
- ♥ A papular rash occurs in secondary syphilis
- ♠ Tinea and pityriasis verscicolor may indicate HIV infection

Ulcer

Detection of an ulcer on the surface of the skin would suggest:

- ♣ Cutaneous gumma. Gumma start out as a painless nodule that breaks down into a punched out ulcer

Circulation

One may note abnormal circulatory changes in the skin.

- ♥ Flushing may be due to polycythaemia, which may occur in the presence of a large uterine fibroid

Regional Examination

The abnormalities that one may detect on regional examination are as follows:

Head

On examination of the head one may note abnormalities of:

- ♠ Mental state
- ♦ Shape

Mental State

Abnormalities that one may note are:

- ♠ Mental deterioration may occur in GPI (General Paralysis of the Insane in tertiary syphilis), AIDS encephalopathy
- ♦ Encephalitis may occur in HIV infection
- ♣ CNS lymphoma can occur in HIV infection

Shape

Abnormalities that may be detected are:

- ♥ A moon face may be seen in Cushing's syndrome

Nose

Abnormalities that may be detected on examination of the nose are:

- ♦ A saddle shaped nose occurs in congenital syphilis
- ♣ Anosmia occurs in Kallman's syndrome

Eyes

When examining the eyes one may note changes in the:

Orbits

Abnormalities that may be detected are:

- ♠ Hypertelorism occurs in Turner's syndrome and Noonan's syndrome

Eyelids

Lesions that may be detected are:

♦ Ptosis occurs in Turner's syndrome

♣ Bilateral ptosis may occur in tabes dorsalis and this contributes to the tabetic facies.

Iris

One may note:

♥ Iritis in secondary syphilis, Reiter's syndrome

Cornea

Lesions that may be detected are:

♠ Interstitial keratitis occurs in late congenital syphilis

Fundus

Lesions that may be detected in the fundus are the following:

♦ Optic atrophy is seen in late congenital syphilis, tabes dorsalis

♣ Papilloedema may occur in meningovascular syphilis

♥ Retinitis pigmentosa is seen in the Laurence-Moon-Biedl syndrome

♠ Acute cytomegalovirus choroidoretinitis is seen as a yellow discolouration of the retina with haemorrhages. It is seen in immunosuppression in AIDS.

♦ Chronic choroidoretinitis shows a salt and pepper appearance. This may be seen in late congenital syphilis

3rd, 4th and 6th Nerves

On testing eye movements one may detect:

♣ Strabismus in Turner's syndrome

♥ 3rd and 6th nerve palsies may occur in meningovascular syphilis

Pupils

One may detect:

♠ Argyll Robertson pupil, which occurs in tabes dorsalis

Face

When examining the face one may note abnormalities of the:

Scalp

Abnormalities that may be noted are:

♦ Alopecia may occur in secondary syphilis

♣ A male pattern of balding occurs in virilising syndromes

♥ A low hairline is seen in Turner's syndrome

Forehead

On inspection of the forehead one may detect:

♦ Seborrheic dermatitis which occurs in HIV infection

Malar Region

In the malar region one may note:

♣ In congenital syphilis, the maxilla would be underdeveloped and the jaw prominent resulting in a bulldog-like appearance

♥ Chloasma or pigmentation of the malar region and forehead occurs in pregnancy and in usage of the oral contraceptive pill

Chin

Over the chin one may note abnormalities of:

Hair Distribution

Hair distribution over the chin would be:

♠ Increased in masculinising syndromes

♦ Decreased in feminising syndromes

Facial Nerve

Abnormalities that one may detect when examining the facial nerve are:

♣ 7th nerve lesions may occur in meningovascular syphilis

Mouth

On examination of the mouth one may note abnormalities of the:

Lips

Lesions that could occur are:

♥ Rhagades refer to white, linear scars around the lips. They extend into the mouth. They occur in congenital syphilis

Teeth

Lesions that may occur are:

♠ Hutchison's teeth occur in congenital syphilis. The features are:

The two permanent upper central incisors are notched and rounded in section

♦ Moon's molars refer to dome shaped first molars. They occur in congenital syphilis.

Buccal Mucosa

Lesions that may be detected on the buccal mucosa are:

♣ Hairy Leukoplakia. This refers to a painless, poorly demarcated, white patch with a corrugated or hairy surface. This is seen in HIV infection

♥ Chancre occurs in primary syphilis

♠ Snail track ulcers occur in secondary syphilis

Palate

Abnormalities that one may note are:

♦ Gumma occur in tertiary syphilis. They may cause perforation of the hard palate.

♣ A high arched palate may be seen in Turner's syndrome

Ears

On examination of the ears one may note:

♥ Nerve deafness in late congenital syphilis, meningovascular syphilis

♠ Deafness occurs in Kallman's syndrome which refers to hypogaonadotrophic hypogonadism with other defects like anosmia, cleft lip or palate, renal agenesis, nerve deafness, cryptorchidism, syndactyly, short fourth metacarpal, craniofacial asymmetry. Anosmia is the defining feature.

Upper Limbs

Dimensions

Abnormalities that may occur are:

♦ A long arm span would be a feature of eunuchoid proportions

Hands

On examination of the hands one may note abnormalities of the:

Dimensions

Variations that may be of significance are:

♣ A short fourth metacarpal occurs in Turner's syndrome

♥ Polydactyly occurs in the Laurence-Moon-Biedl syndrome

♠ Sausage shaped digits occur in Reiter's syndrome

Skin on the Dorsum of the Hands

One may note:

♦ Scabies in patients infected with HIV especially Norwegian scabies, the severe crusted variety

Palms

Over the palms one may note:

♣ Palmar erythema in pregnancy

♥ A rash in secondary syphilis. It is a pinkish-brown, maculopapular rash with fine scales.

Locomotor System

Lesions that may occur in relation to the locomotor system of the hands are:

♠ Gonococcal tenosynovitis causes swelling and erythema over the tendons

♦ Gonococcal arthritis may occur in the hand

Elbow

On examination of the elbow one may note:

♣ An increased carrying angle occurs in Turner's syndrome

♥ An enlarged epitrochlear lymph node occurs in secondary syphilis

Shoulders

The shoulders would be:

♠ Wide in masculinising syndromes

♦ Narrow in feminising syndromes (Eunuchoid appearance)

Nervous System

Lesions that may be detected in relation to the nervous system of the upper limbs are:

♣ Wrist drop occurs in chronic meningovascular neurosyphilis

♥ Asymmetric wasting of the arm and neck extensors may be seen in amyotrophic meningomyelitis, which occurs as a result of cervical leptomeningitis (syphilitic)

Neck

In the neck one may note:

- ♠ Generalised lymphadenopathy occurs in secondary syphilis, AIDS
- ♦ A buffalo hump may occur in patients on antiretroviral treatment for AIDS

Chest

In the chest one may note:

- ♣ A shield chest with widely spaced nipples occurs in Turner's syndrome and in Noonan's syndrome

Female Breast

Abnormalities that may occur are:

- ♥ The position of the nipples is important. Retraction could indicate carcinoma or fibrosis.
- ♠ Dimpling of the surface of the breast would indicate underlying malignancy.
- ♦ An orange peel or *peau d' orange* effect indicates malignancy resulting in lymphatic blockage causing localised lymphoedema.

Lump in the Breast

Any lump should be examined carefully and defined. Lumps in the breast could be:

- ♣ Carcinoma
- ♥ Fibroadenoma

- ♠ Traumatic fat necrosis

Temperature

Abnormalities that may occur are:

- ♦ Abscess or mastitis would cause an increase in temperature.

Mobility

If a lump is found in the breast, defining the mobility of the lump is important.

- ♣ Tethering to the underlying muscle or overlying skin would indicate carcinoma.

Male Breast

Enlargement of the male breast, gynaecomastia, is usually obvious on inspection and easily confirmed on palpation.

Gynaecomastia

The cause of gynaecomastia is either decreased production or decreased action of testosterone or increased production of oestrogen. It may be physiological in the newborn, in adolescence and in ageing.

Decreased Testosterone

Decreased testosterone may be due to lesions in the:

- ♥ **Testes**

  Klinefelter's syndrome, congenital anorchia, orchitis, trauma

- ♠ **Systemic Conditions**

  Conditions affecting the:

CNS myotonia dystrophica, spinal cord lesions, bulbospinal muscular atrophy

KUS renal failure

Decreased Action of Testosterone

Decreased action of testosterone may be due to:

♦ **Androgen Receptor Defects**

Reifenstein syndrome, infertile male syndrome

♣ **Drugs**

Cyproterone acetate, flutamide, cimetidine

Increased Oestrogen

Increased oestrogen may be due to lesions in the:

♥ **Testes**

Leydig cell tumour, Sertoli cell tumour, which produce androgens and oestrogen autonomously

True hermaphroditism in which oestrogen is produced by the ovotestis

♠ **Systemic Factors**

Conditions affecting the:

E&M adrenal disorders like congenital adrenal hyperplasia, adrenal cancer, Addison's disease. Thyrotoxicosis

GIT cirrhosis of the liver

RS bronchial cancer

Drugs digitalis

Galactorrhoea

The function of the breast is production of milk, lactation. This is physiological following pregnancy but at any other time it is pathological and is known as galactorrhoea.

Galactorrhoea may be due to conditions affecting the:

♦ **E&M**

Pituitary disorders: hyperprolactinaemia

Adrenal disorders: Cushing's syndrome

Thyroid disease

♣ **Drugs** oral contraceptives, phenothiazines, tricyclic antidepressants, methyldopa

Cardiovascular System

Lesions that could occur in the cardiovascular system are:

♥ Aortic aneurysm and aortic regurgitation occur in syphilitic aortitis

Abdomen

On examination of the abdomen one may detect the following abnormalities:

Abdominal Wall

Abnormalities that may be noted are:

♠ Hair distribution on the abdomen should be noted. The pattern would vary with increased hair in masculinising syndromes and decreased hair in feminising syndromes.

♦ Striae gravidarum would be seen in pregnancy, striae may also occur in Cushing's syndrome.

Contents of the Abdomen

The following abnormalities may be detected:

Uterus

The uterus may be enlarged due to:

♣ Fibroids

♥ Pregnancy

Ovary

The ovary may be enlarged due to:

♠ Tumour

♦ Cyst

♣ Tubo-ovarian mass

Hepatosplenomegaly

Hepatosplenomegaly may occur in:

♥ Secondary syphilis

Bladder

Abnormalities that may be detected are:

♠ A large bladder occurs in tabes dorsalis

Ascites

Ascites occurs in:

♦ Meig's syndrome, which is an ovarian fibroma with ascites

Pubic Hair

Abnormalities that may be noted are:

♣ The shape of the escutcheon would be either female with the apex of the triangular escutcheon pointing downward or male with the apex of the triangle pointing upwards. This would be a defining feature in feminising and masculinising syndromes

♥ *Phthyrus pubis* may be seen on the hair shaft when infestation occurs

Genitals

The abnormalities that may be detected are as follows:

Male Genitalia

Abnormalities of the male genitalia may affect the following:

Urethra

Abnormalities that occur are:

♠ Urethral discharge may occur in gonorrhoea, Reiter's syndrome

Glans

Lesions that may occur are the following:

♦ Circinate balanitis refers to superficial lesions that present as a circle of erythema with a pale centre. The edge is slightly raised and adjacent lesions may coalesce. It occurs in Reiter's syndrome

♣ Ulcers may occur in Behcet's disease

♥ Lichen planus may occur on the glans penis

♠ Chancre occurs in primary syphilis. A chancre begins as a small, painless papule that rapidly ulcerates to give a solitary, round or oval, painless, indurated ulcer.

♦ Condylomata lata are seen in secondary syphilis. They present as highly infectious, pink or grey discs.

♣ Condylomata acuminata may be seen on the penis

♥ Chancroid causes multiple, painful, non-indurated ulcers. It is caused by *Haemophilus ducreyi*

♠ Balanoposthitis may be caused by candida infections. Balanitis refers to inflammation of the glans, posthitis refers to inflammation of the prepuce.

Shaft

Lesions that may occur on the shaft of the penis are:

♦ Periurethral abscesses occur in gonococcal infection

Testes

Lesions of the testes may cause:

♠ Small testes

♦ Enlarged testes

Small Testes

Small testes may occur in:

♣ Laurence-Moon-Biedl syndrome, Klinefelter's syndrome

♥ Atrophic testes occur as a consequence of mumps orchitis

Enlarged Testes

Enlargement of the testes may be:

♠ Painless Enlargement

♦ Painful enlargement

♣ Lump

♥ Hydrocoele

Painless Enlargement

Painless enlargement of the testes may occur in:

♠ Tertiary syphilis. In this condition gummatous infiltration and fibrosis produce smooth, painless enlargement of the testis

Painful Enlargement

Painful enlargement of the testes may be due to:

♦ Acute epididymo-orchitis (mumps, following prostatitis, following urethral instrumentation)

Lump

A lump in the testes could indicate:

♠ Testicular cancer

Hydrocoele

A hydrocoele causes an apparent swelling of the testes. It presents as a fluctuant enlargement that may be transilluminated.

Epididymis

The epididymis may be affected by:

♣ Bacterial epididymorchitis

♥ Tuberculous epididymorchitis

♠ Filarial epididymorchitis

Female Genitalia

The lesions that may occur in the female genitalia are:

- ♦ Chancre in primary syphilis
- ♣ Chancroid which presents as multiple painful ulcers
- ♥ Ulcers may also be seen in Behcet's disease
- ♠ Condylomata lata occur in secondary syphilis
- ♦ Condylomata acuminata occur in human papilloma virus infection. They present as multiple, soft, fleshy, vascular lesions that may coalesce to form large masses.

Vaginosis

Vaginosis could be:

- ♣ Non-specific bacterial
- ♥ Trichomoniasis
- ♠ Candidiasis

Endocervicitis

Endocervicitis may be caused by:

- ♦ Gonococcus
- ♣ Chlamydiae
- ♥ Chancre

Inguinal Region

Inguinal lymphadenopathy may be due to:

- ♠ Syphilis
- ♦ Lymphogranuloma venereum which is caused by *Chlamydia trachomatis*

- ♣ Granuloma inguinale which is caused by *Calymmatobacterium granulomatis*

Perianal Region

Lesions that may occur in the perianal region are:

- ♥ Chancre in primary syphilis
- ♠ Condylomata lata in secondary syphilis
- ♦ Herpes simplex causes multiple painful ulcers
- ♣ Condylomata acuminata

Per Rectum

On rectal examination one may detect:

- ♥ Prostatitis, which causes swelling and tenderness of the prostate gland

Lower Limbs

On examination of the lower limbs in general one may detect abnormalities of the:

Dimensions

One may note:

- ♠ The lower limbs would be long in relation to the trunk in eunuchoid proportions

Hips

Abnormalities that may be noted are:

♦ The hips would be narrow in masculinising syndromes

♣ The hips would be wide in feminising syndromes

♥ Sacro-ileitis occurs in Reiter's syndrome

Knees

Lesions that may be detected are the following:

♠ Charcot's joints occur in tertiary syphilis

♦ Gonococcal arthritis can cause acute inflammation of the knee joint

♣ Clutton's joints refer to a painless chronic arthropathy that occurs in the second decade in congenital syphilis. It causes effusion but no bony change.

Lower Legs

Abnormalities that may be seen are:

♥ Sabre tibia occurs in congenital syphilis

Ankles

Lesions that may be detected are:

♠ Charcot's joints may occur at the ankle

♦ Achilles tendonitis occurs in Reiter's syndrome

Feet

On examination of the feet one may note:

♣ Keratoderma blenorrhagica. This occurs in Reiter's syndrome

♥ Kaposi's sarcoma is seen as purple-brown macules or plaques or nodules around the toes

Nervous System

Abnormalities that one may note in relation to the nervous system are:

♠ Spastic paraparesis may occur in meningovascular syphilis. It is slowly progressive with little sensory loss

♦ Paraparesis can occur in HIV infection as a result of:

Acute transverse myelitis, myelopathy due to infection by herpes simplex or zoster or cytomegalovirus, lymphoma

♣ Tabes dorsalis causes an up going plantar response with reduced ankle jerks

♥ HIV can cause a mononeuropathy, mononeuritis multiplex, peripheral neuropathy

Spine

When examining the spine one may detect:

♠ Meningitis in meningovascular syphilis

♦ Aseptic meningitis may occur in primary HIV infection

♣ Cryptococcal meningitis may complicate HIV infection

♥ Sciatica may occur in meningovascular syphilis

Gait

Abnormalities that may be detected when examining the patient's gait are the following:

♥ A broad based stamping gait may occur in tabes dorsalis

♠ Foot drop may occur in meningo-vascular syphilis

♦ Cerebellar syndrome may occur in AIDS

Chapter 15

The Haematological System

In the haematological system one studies the corpuscles of the blood, haemostasis, immunoglobulins, lymph nodes, the liver and spleen and the bone marrow. That is, the blood and the tissues and organs concerned with production and destruction of blood. The clinical features of conditions that affect the haematological system will be studied. In addition one will study the clinical features that are reflected in other systems but result from the causes and effects of conditions that affect the haematological system.

History Taking

History taking is conveniently divided into analysis of the red cells, the white cells, the platelets and haemostatic factors, the lymph nodes, the liver and spleen and the bone marrow. This is done by asking about:

- ♥ Breathlessness
- ♠ Lack of energy
- ♦ Recurrent infections
- ♣ Bleeding tendency
- ♥ Swelling of lymph nodes
- ♠ Swelling of the abdomen
- ♦ Bone pain

A review of systems should then be performed.

Physical Examination

Commence physical examination by performing a general examination and then proceed to perform regional examination.

General Examination

Make a note of the patient's posture, state of growth and development and the metabolic state. Note the state of the integument. Note the body temperature. (Position, Height and Proportions, Weight and Shape, Integument, Body Temperature)

Regional Examination

Examination is performed in the usual manner. Special emphasis should be placed on certain areas and these areas will be highlighted.

Head

Assess the mental state. Examine the dimensions of the head and the integument. Examine the regions of the head, the nose, the eyes, the face (scalp, forehead, malar region, chin) the mouth (jaw, lips, teeth, gums, buccal mucosa, tongue, palate, fauces, salivary glands), the ears.

Upper Limbs

Commence examination in the usual fashion starting off with a general assessment of the upper limbs. Then examine the hands, forearms and upper arms, the shoulders and the axillae.

Hands

Note the dimensions. Examine the dorsum of the hands; the nails and skin, the bones, joints, tendons and muscles. Ask the patient to turn the hands over and examine the skin, the bones, the joints, the tendons and the muscles. Palpate the hands and note the state of the peripheral circulation and examine the radial pulse. Look for involuntary movements and examine the functions of the nervous system and locomotor system of the hands if required.

Forearms, Elbows, Upper Arms

Examine the forearms, the elbows and the upper arms.

Hess' test

In this test one should inflate a blood pressure cuff to between systolic and diastolic blood pressure and maintain this state of mid-inflation for a period of five minutes. Upon release one should look at a previously marked circle of diameter 5 cms drawn on the patient's antecubital fossa. More than five purpuric spots appearing within this circle in the antecubital fossa will denote a positive test and this indicates thrombocytopaenia or platelet dysfunction. This test is rarely used now.

Shoulders and Axillae

Next examine the shoulders and the axillae.

Lymph Nodes in the Axillae

Examine the lymph nodes in the axillae.

For the patient's right axilla use one's left hand to examine the axilla. Place the palpating fingers of one's left hand in the patient's right axilla. The patient's right forearm should rest on the examiner's left forearm. The examiner's right hand should be placed on the patient's right shoulder to discourage the patient from pulling the arm away. Repeat the process for the left axilla using the fingers of one's right hand for palpation of the axilla and one's left hand to steady the patient's shoulder. Examine the apex of the axilla, the anterior axillary fold, the medial wall, the posterior axillary fold and the lateral wall.

In practice, if required, examine active and passive movements of the upper limbs and perform neurological examination of the upper limbs. This would not be expected in professional examinations.

Neck

Next, examine the patient's neck. The usual method is followed for the anterior aspect of the neck. That is, note the dimensions, assess the state of the integument, inspect the thyroid gland, the sternocleido-mastoid muscle and the jugular venous pressure. Examine the carotid arteries and the trachea. The lymph nodes should be examined when the patient is asked to sit up to examine the back of the patient.

Chest

Examine the chest wall. Look for deformities and examine the integument. Feel for tenderness over the sternum. In practice one should examine the contents of the chest; the heart and the lungs.

Back

One should now ask the patient to sit up and examine the patient from the back. Note the dimensions of the spine and proceed to examine the neck from behind.

Neck (from behind)

The principal examination carried out is palpation of the cervical lymph nodes.

Palpation of the Lymph Nodes of the Neck

To examine the cervical lymph nodes, palpate the neck from behind the patient. Place one's thumbs at the back of the patient's neck and use one's fingers for palpation. Palpate the lymph nodes in a sequence from the occipital region to the submental region following the horizontal ring of lymph nodes that occur in this position. That is, the occipital, the retro-auricular, pre-auricular, sub-mandibular and sub-mental lymph nodes. Then palpate the lymph nodes that are distributed vertically along the carotid artery. Finally, palpate the lymph nodes in the posterior triangle.

In practice one should complete examination of the back by examining the spine, the scapula, the back of the chest, the lower back and the sacrum.

Abdomen

Examine the abdomen in the manner described in the section on the gastrointestinal tract. In particular look for enlargement of the liver, the spleen and the para-aortic lymph nodes.

Examination of the Aorta and Para-Aortic Lymph Nodes

The aorta is not easy to palpate. When palpable it may be felt in a position a little above the umbilicus and to the left of it. One should use the tips of one's fingers for palpation and employ deep palpation.

Achieving deep palpation will be made easier by placing one's left hand over the palpating right hand. Define the aorta.

If the aorta is palpable, test whether the pulsation felt is transmitted or expansile. Place the tips of the index fingers of both hands on either side of the aorta and watch the movement of the fingers. In transmitted pulsation the distance between the fingers will remain the same with each pulsation. In expansile pulsation the fingers will move apart in systole and return to the starting position in diastole.

Para-aortic nodes would be palpable only if they are considerably enlarged. They would be felt along the border of the aorta. Para-aortic nodes present as rounded, firm masses that are immobile.

Inguinal Region and Genitals

Examine the inguinal region looking in particular for enlarged inguinal lymph nodes. Examine the genitals if required.

Lower Limbs

In practice one should examine the lower limbs. Examine the lower limbs in general then examine the hips, the thighs, the knees, the lower legs and the feet. One should examine the locomotor system and perform neurological examination if required.

Buttocks, Perianal Region and Per Rectal Examination

For the sake of completeness one should remember examination of the buttocks, perianal region and per rectal examination.

Spine

Ideally one should examine the spine.

Gait, Romberg's Sign, Trendelenburg test, Standing from a Seated or Squatting Position

In practice one should examine the patient's gait and perform these tests if required.

Lesions of the Haematological System

The study of the haematological system is a study of the corpuscles of the blood and some of the plasma proteins. This lends itself to a simple classification of conditions that affect the haematological system. Basically, they may be divided into conditions that affect the components of the corpuscles, the production of corpuscles and destruction of corpuscles. For plasma proteins this will be conditions that affect the structure of the plasma proteins, the production of plasma proteins and destruction of plasma proteins.

Aide Memoire

The aide memoire **PIPES** *may be used with the modification that the second* **P** *would stand for production and* **E** *for extinction. It would be* **P**onder the **I**nternal, **P**roduction, **E**xtinction and **S**ystemic.

Red Cells

Conditions that affect the red cells would be:

- ♣ Internal Abnormalities of Red Cells
- ♥ Anaemia
- ♠ Polycythaemia

Internal Abnormalities of Red Cells

Internal abnormalities of the red cells could be:

- ♦ High Oxygen Affinity Haemoglobin Variants
- ♣ Methaemoglobinaemia
- ♥ Sulphaemoglobinaemia

High Oxygen Affinity Haemoglobin Variants

In these patients, haemoglobin does not readily give up oxygen to the tissues; the resultant tissue hypoxia leads to an increased production of erythropoietin with consequent polycythaemia.

Methaemoglobinaemia

Methaemoglobinaemia is a condition caused by oxidation of haemoglobin; this may be due to a deficiency of red cell NADH-diaphorase or to an abnormality of either the alpha or beta globin chains of haemoglobin. Abnormal haemoglobin variants that are associated with genetic methaemoglobinaemia are called Haemoglobin M. Several types are known and these are further identified by their place of discovery; an example being Haemoglobin M Boston.

Acquired methaemoglobinaemia may be caused by drugs such as nitrites, primaquine, sulphonamides.

Sulphaemoglobinaemia

Sulphaemoglobinaemia is a condition similar to that caused by the action of hydrogen sulphide on haemoglobin in vitro. It can be caused by drugs such as sulphonamides and phenacetin. It may also occur in chronic constipation or malabsorption.

Anaemia

Anaemia could be due to:

- ♠ Internal abnormalities of red cells
- ♦ Decreased production of red cells
- ♣ Increased destruction of red cells

Internal Abnormalities of Red Cells

Internal abnormalities of the red cells that result in anaemia are those that interfere with the production of haemoglobin. These are conditions that affect:

- ♥ Production of haem
- ♠ Production of globin chains

Haem Production

Haem production may be reduced due to:

- ♦ **Genetic Defects**: congenital (erythropoietic) porphyria (Gunther's disease)
- ♣ **Toxins**: lead poisoning, alcohol ingestion

Globin Synthesis

Globin synthesis may be reduced because of:

- ♥ **Genetic Defects**: thalassaemia, haemoglobinopathies such as sickle cell disease, haemoglobin C, haemoglobin D, haemoglobin E

Decreased Production of Red Cells

Decreased production of red cells could be due to:

- ♠ **Internal Factors (abnormalities of bone marrow)**

  Decreased precursor cells. This could be either aplastic anaemia or pure red cell aplasia

  Marrow replacement

  Myelodysplasia

  Defective red cell maturation

- ♦ **Systemic Factors**

  Deficiency anaemia

  Secondary anaemia or anaemia secondary to chronic disease

Aplastic Anaemia

Aplastic anaemia refers to stem cell failure not related to nutrient deficiencies and associated with marrow hypoplasia with no fibrosis of the marrow or infiltration. It may be due to:

- ♣ Genetic Conditions
- ♥ Acquired Aplastic Anaemia

Genetic Conditions

Genetic conditions that cause marrow aplasia are:

- ♠ Fanconi's anaemia where there are associated features such as short stature, hyperpigmentation of the skin, mental retardation, deafness, skeletal defects, renal defects, cryptorchidism in males
- ♦ Non-Fanconi anaemia
- ♣ Dyskeratosis congenita where there is abnormal skin, nails and hair

Acquired Aplastic Anaemia

Acquired aplastic anaemia could be:

- ♥ Idiopathic

Or due to:

Chemical Agents

- ♠ **Drugs**: phenylbutazone, chloramphenicol, gold, sulphonamides, antithyroid drugs
- ♦ **Cytotoxics**: busulphan, cyclophosphamide
- ♣ **Toxins**: insecticides, benzene

Physical Agents

- ♥ Irradiation

Biological Agents

- **Infections**: viral hepatitis, EBV, HIV, parvovirus, tuberculosis

Pure Red Cell Aplasia

Pure red cell aplasia refers to a condition where there is anaemia with a reduction of reticulocytes but neutrophils and platelets are normal. It may be:

- Congenital
- Acquired

Congenital

Congenital red cell aplasia occurs in the:

- Diamond-Blackfan syndrome in which there are associated skeletal defects.

Acquired

Acquired causes of red cell aplasia are:

- Idiopathic
- Associated with thymoma or lymphoma
- Parvovirus infection
- Drugs: penillamine, phenytoin, chlorpropamide, chloramphenicol

Marrow Replacement

Marrow replacement may be due to:

- Secondary deposits from the breast, lung, kidney, thyroid, prostate, less commonly stomach, pancreas, colorectal
- Leukaemia
- Lymphoma
- Myeloma

- Myelofibrosis
- Mast cells in systemic mastocytosis
- Granulomata in sarcoid, tuberculosis
- Infections: kala azar
- Amyloid
- Osteopetrosis

Myelodysplasia

Myelodysplasia refers to acquired disorders of haemopoiesis that affect clones of cells and are characterised by cytopaenias and abnormal morphology of cells. There are several different types of myelodysplasia. Some progress to leukaemia. The types of myelodysplasia are:

- Refractory anaemia (RA)
- Refractory anaemia with ringed sideroblasts (RARS)
- Refractory anaemia with an excess of blasts (RAEB)
- Refractory anaemia with an excess of blasts in transformation (RAEB-T)
- Chronic myelomonocytic anaemia (CMML)

Defective Red Cell Maturation

Defective red cell maturation is caused by defective production of haemoglobin due to hereditary or acquired causes.

Sideroblastic Anaemia

Sideroblastic anaemia refers to a group of disorders that are characterised by severe dyserythropoieses, marked iron loading of red cell precursors and in some cases widespread haemosiderosis. It is a condition in which ring sideroblasts are found in the bone marrow. Sideroblastic anaemia may be due to:

♣ **Internal Factors (abnormalities of the bone marrow)**

Hereditary Causes: X-linked or autosomal recessive

Acquired Causes: myelodysplasia (refractory anaemia with ring sideroblasts)

♥ **External Factors**

Irradiation

♣ **Systemic Factors**

Toxins: alcohol

Drugs: chloramphenicol, isoniazid, pyrazinamide, cancer chemotherapy

Nutrients: zinc overload, copper deficiency

Deficiency Anaemia

Deficiency anaemia refers to anaemia caused by deficiency of haematinics chiefly:

♦ Iron

♣ Vitamin B_{12}

♥ Folic acid

Iron Deficiency

Iron deficiency may be due to:

♠ Decreased Absorption

♦ Increased Loss

Decreased Absorption

Decreased absorption of iron may be due to factors affecting the gut:

♣ **Luminal Factors (gut)**

Dietary failure

♥ **Mural Factors (gut)**

Gastrectomy, small bowel disease (coeliac disease)

Increased Loss

Increased loss of iron could be due to factors primarily affecting the gut:

♠ **Luminal Factors (gut)**

Hookworm infestation (*Necator americanus, Ankylostaoma duodenale*)

♦ **Mural Factors (gut)**

Inflammatory bowel disease, ulcers, which may be benign (acid peptic, NSAID induced) or malignant, vascular abnormalities (telangiectasia, angiodysplasia), colorectal malignancy, small bowel tumours (rarely)

♣ **Systemic Factors**

Conditions affecting the:

RAG increased menstrual loss

Vitamin B_{12} Deficiency

Deficiency of vitamin B_{12} may be due to factors affecting the gut:

♥ **Luminal Factors (gut)**

Dietary failure in vegans, bacterial overgrowth in the small bowel in blind loop syndrome, diverticulae, infestation with *Diphyllobothrium latum*

♠ **Mural Factors (gut)**

Those involving the:

Stomach: pernicious anaemia, gastrectomy

Ileum: ileal resection, Crohn's disease

Folic Acid Deficiency

Deficiency of folic acid may be due to:

- ♦ Decreased Absorption
- ♣ Increased Demand

Decreased Absorption

Decreased absorption of folate may be due to factors affecting the gut:

- ♥ **Luminal Factors (gut)**

  Dietary failure

- ♠ **Mural Factors (gut)**

  Coeliac disease, tropical sprue

Increased Demand

Increased demand for folic acid may be due to conditions affecting the following:

- ♦ **RAG** pregnancy and lactation
- ♣ **HS** haemolytic anaemia
- ♥ **KUS** haemodialysis, peritoneal dialysis
- ♠ **Drugs** anticonvulsants, methotrexate, trimethoprim

Secondary Anaemia (anaemia of chronic disease)

Secondary anaemia refers to anaemia caused by systemic disease. These may be conditions involving the:

- ♦ **GIT** liver failure
- ♣ **KUS** renal failure
- ♥ **LMS** connective tissue disorders

Increased Extinction of Red Cells

Increased extinction of red cells may be due to:

- ♠ Haemolysis
- ♦ Blood Loss

Haemolysis

The causes of haemolytic anaemia may be classified as:

- ♣ Internal Factors or factors within red cells
- ♥ Membrane Defects
- ♠ External Factors
- ♦ Systemic Factors

Internal Factors

Internal factors that cause haemolysis are conditions affecting:

- ♦ Haemoglobin
- ♣ Intracellular enzymes
- ♥ Parasites

Haemoglobin

The defects in haemoglobin that result in haemolytic anaemia are those that affect the following:

- ♠ Haem Production
- ♦ Globin Production
- ♣ Unstable Haemoglobins
- ♥ Methaemoglobinaemia with haemolysis

Haem Production

Abnormalities of haem production that result in haemolysis occur in:

- ♠ Congenital (erythropoietic) porphyria

Globin Production

Abnormalities of globin synthesis that result in haemolysis are:

- ♦ Thalassaemia

♣ Haemoglobinopathies (Haemoglobin S, Haemoglobin C, Haemoglobin D, Haemoglobin E)

Unstable Haemoglobins

Unstable haemoglobins are rare inherited haemolytic anaemias where intracellular precipitation of haemoglobin occurs with formation of Heinz bodies. This is due to a structural abnormality of haemoglobin.

Methaemoglobinaemia with haemolysis

Chronic methaemoglobinaemia with haemolytic anaemia which shows Heinz body formation occurs in patients treated with sulphasalazine, dapsone

Enzyme Deficiency

Enzyme deficiencies that result in haemolytic anaemia are:

♦ Glucose-6-phosphate dehydrogenase deficiency

♣ Pyruvate kinase deficiency

♥ Other enzymes: pyrimidine-5-nucleotidase, adenylate kinase, hexokinase, glucose phosphate isomerase, glutathione peroxidase, glutathione reductase (rare)

Parasites

Intracellular parasites that cause haemolytic anaemia are:

♠ Malaria parasites

Membrane Defects

Membrane defects that cause haemolytic anaemia are:

♦ Genetic Defects

♣ Acquired Defects

Genetic Defects

Genetic defects in the red cell membrane that may result in haemolytic anaemia are:

♥ Hereditary Spherocytosis

♠ Hereditary Elliptocytosis

♦ Hereditary Spherocytic Elliptocytosis

♣ Hereditary Stomatocytosis

♥ Hereditary Pyropoikilocytosis

♠ Hereditary Xerocytosis

Acquired Defects

Acquired defects of the red cell membrane that may result in haemolytic anaemia are:

♦ Acanthocytosis

Acanthocytes are red cells with many projections (spur cells). They occur in:

Severe liver disease, Abetalipoproteinaemia

♣ Paroxysmal nocturnal haemoglobinuria

External Factors

External factors that cause haemolysis may be classified as:

♥ Antibody mediated (Immune Haemolysis)

♠ Drug induced haemolysis

♦ Hypersplenism

♣ Red cell fragmentation syndromes

♥ Venoms and toxins

Immune Haemolysis

Immune haemolysis may be due to:

- ♦ Warm antibodies
- ♣ Cold antibodies
- ♥ Isoantibodies

Warm Antibodies

Warm antibodies that cause haemolysis may be:

- ♠ Idiopathic

Or secondary to:

- ♦ Systemic lupus erythematosus
- ♣ Other connective tissue disorders
- ♥ Chronic lymphocytic leukaemia
- ♠ Lymphoma
- ♦ Ulcerative colitis
- ♣ Ovarian teratoma
- ♥ Drugs like methyldopa

Cold Antibodies

Cold antibodies may be due to:

- ♠ Mycoplasma pneumonia
- ♦ Infectious mononucleosis
- ♣ Lymphoma
- ♥ Paroxysmal cold haemoglobinuria

Isoimmune Haemolysis

Isoimmune haemolysis may be due to:

- ♠ Incompatible blood transfusion
- ♦ Haemolytic disease of the newborn

Drug Induced Haemolysis

Drug induced haemolysis may be due to glucose-6-phosphate dehydrogenase deficiency (G-6-PD) or due to drug-induced antibodies. Examples of drugs that induce haemolysis are:

- ♣ Penicillin, phenacetin, methyldopa, sulphonamide, phenothiazines

Hypersplenism

A large spleen due to any cause may increase destruction of red cells.

Red Cell Fragmentation

Red cell fragmentation may be caused by:

- ♠ Artificial heart valves
- ♦ Thrombotic thrombocytopaenic purpura
- ♣ Microangiopathic haemolytic anaemia in disseminated intravascular coagulation, malignant hypertension
- ♥ March haemoglobinuria

Venoms and Toxins

Venoms and toxins that cause haemolysis are:

- ♠ Snake venom
- ♦ Clostridial toxins

Systemic Factors

Systemic diseases that result in haemolysis are conditions affecting the:

- ♣ **KUS** renal failure
- ♥ **GIT** liver failure, Wilson's disease, Zieve's syndrome
- ♠ **CVS** cardiopulmonary bypass
- ♦ **E&M** vitamin E deficiency

Polycythaemia

Polycythaemia is caused by increased production of red cells and may be:

- ♣ Primary

♥ Secondary

Primary Polycythaemia

Primary polycythaemia is due to:

♠ Polycythaemia Rubra Vera

Secondary Polycythaemia

Secondary polycythaemia is the result of conditions affecting the:

♦ **RS** smoking, chronic respiratory disease

♣ **CVS** right to left shunts

♥ **KUS** hypernephroma, hydronephrosis, renal artery stenosis, Bartter's syndrome, renal cysts

♠ **RAG** fibroid

♦ **CNS** cerebellar haemangioma

♣ **GIT** hepatocellular carcinoma

♥ **E&M** phaeochromocytoma, aldosterone-secreting adenoma

♠ **HS** high oxygen affinity haemo-globin variants

White Cells

Diseases of the white cells may affect:

♦ Neutrophils

♣ Eosinophils

♥ Basophils

♠ Lymphocytes

♦ Plasma cells

♣ Monocytes

Neutrophils

Problems that affect the neutrophils are:

♥ Internal abnormalities or functional defects

♠ Neutropaenia

♦ Neutrophilia

Internal Abnormalities

Internal abnormalities that affect the neutrophils are the inability of the neutrophils to perform their function of killing bacteria. This may be due to:

♠ **Leucocyte Adhesion Deficiency**

An inherited disorder of leucocyte adhesion

♥ **Chronic Granulomatous Disease**

This is a disorder in which cells are unable to generate superoxide

♠ **Myeloperoxidase Deficiency**

An autosomal recessive disorder in which the cells cannot form myeloperoxidase

♦ **Chediak-Higashi Syndrome**

In this disorder the cells contain giant granules that show impaired degranulation and impaired fusion with phagosomes. Defective chemotaxis also occurs.

♣ **Specific Granule Deficiency**

In this condition neutrophil specific granules are absent or empty.

Neutropaenia

Neutropaenia refers to a neutrophil count less than 1.5×10^9/l. Neutropaenia may be due to:

♠ Internal abnormalities affecting neutrophils

◆ Decreased production of neutrophils

♣ Increased extinction of neutrophils

Internal Abnormalities Affecting Neutrophils

Internal abnormalities of the neutrophils may be caused by:

♥ Congenital disorders. Congenital agranulocytosis (Kostman's syndrome)

♣ Cyclic neutropaenia. This is a condition in which neutropaenia, along with a reduction in numbers of the other blood cells, occur in 3 to 4 weekly cycles.

Decreased Production (Marrow disorders)

Decreased production of neutrophils occurs due to disorders of the bone marrow. They are:

◆ **Internal Factors**

Internal factors affecting the bone marrow are:

Marrow aplasia

Marrow infiltration

Myelodysplasia

♣ **External Factors**

External factors that affect the bone marrow are:

Irradiation

♥ **Systemic Factors**

Systemic factors, that result in decreased production of neutrophils by the bone marrow, are conditions affecting the:

HS large granular lymphocytosis (a form of T-cell lymphoma that occurs in the elderly)

Drugs induce decreased production of neutrophils by the bone marrow. This is caused by cytotoxics, immunosuppressive agents, antithyroid agents. Many other drugs cause decreased production of neutrophils as a result of idiosyncratic reactions.

Viral infections: influenza, hepatitis, rubella, infectious mononucleosis

Bacterial infections: *Salmonella typhi*, mycobacteria, severe sepsis

E&M: nutritional deficiency, deficiency of vitamin B_{12}, folate, copper

Increased Extinction of Neutrophils

Increased extinction of neutrophils may be due to:

♣ Hypersplenism

◆ Autoimmune destruction

Apparent Neutropaenia

An apparent neutropaenia may be caused by an increase in the marginating pool of neutrophils. This may occur in:

♣ Severe sepsis

♥ Haemodialysis

♣ Adult respiratory distress syndrome

Neutrophilia

Neutrophilia refers to a neutrophil count greater than $7.5 \times 10^9/l$. Neutrophilia may be:

♦ Hereditary

♣ Reactive, the most severe form being a leukaemoid reaction

♥ Neoplastic increase

♠ Decreased extinction

Hereditary Neutrophilias

The hereditary neutrophilias are:

♦ Hereditary Neutrophilia

This is a dominantly inherited syndrome. The manifestations are leucocytosis, splenomegaly and widened diploe of the skull is.

♣ Chronic Idiopathic Neutrophilia

In this condition the white cell count is between 11,000 to 40,000 with neutrophils predominant. It is benign. The occurrence is sporadic.

♥ Leucocyte Adhesion Deficiency

Reactive Neutrophilia

A reactive increase in neutrophils could be in response to:

♠ Bacterial infections

♦ Tissue injury

♣ Drugs: steroids, beta agonists

♥ Severe haemorrhage

♠ Stress: exercise, seizures

Leukaemoid Reaction

A leukaemoid reaction refers to an excessive leucocytosis, including the presence of immature forms, in response to severe infections, haemorrhage, metastatic cancer, severe haemolysis

Neoplastic Increase in Neutrophils

A neoplastic increase in neutrophils occurs in:

♦ Acute myeloid leukaemia

♣ Chronic myeloid leukaemia

Decreased Extinction of Neutrophils

Decreased extinction of white cells occurs in:

♥ Hyposplenism

♠ Splenectomy

Leucoerythroblastic Reaction

A leucoerythroblastic reaction refers to the presence of immature red and white cells in the peripheral blood and occurs in bone marrow infiltration

Eosinophils

Eosinophils may be affected in disease states and result in:

♣ Eosinophilia

♥ Eosinopaenia

Eosinophilia

Eosinophilia refers to an eosinophil count greater than $0.4 \times 10^9/l$. Eosinophilia may be:

♣ Congenital

♥ Reactive

♠ Neoplastic increase

Congenital Eosinophilia

Congenital eosinophilia occurs in:

♦ Job's Syndrome (hyper Ig E syndrome). This is a syndrome, which is characterised by recurrent cold abscesses, eczema and coarse facies. The other features are high levels of Ig E and impaired neutrophil locomotion.

Reactive Eosinophilia

A reactive increase in eosinophils may be in response to:

♣ Allergies

♥ Parasitic infestation

♠ **Systemic Disorders**

Conditions affecting the:

IS eczema, psoriasis, dermatitis herpetiformis, erythema multiforme

RS tropical pulmonary eosinophilia, worm infestations (pulmonary phase), allergic bronchopulmonary aspergillosis, eosinophilic pneumonia, Churg-Strauss syndrome

GIT eosinophilic gastroenteritis, inflammatory bowel disease

LMS eosinophilic granuloma, rheumatoid arthritis

CVS vasculitis, cholesterol embolism

E&M hypoadrenalism (as a consequence of reduced steroids)

Idiopathic Hypereosinophilic Syndrome

The idiopathic hypereosinophilic syndrome is one characterised by eosinophil counts greater than 1.5 $x10^9/l$ for more than six months and damage to organs such as the heart, lungs, CNS, GIT, skin due to eosinophilic infiltration. There should be no other cause to explain the eosinophilia.

Neoplastic Increase in Eosinophils

A neoplastic increase in eosinophils may occur in:

♦ Eosinophilic leukaemia

♣ Hodgkin's disease

♥ Chronic Myelogenous Leukaemia

Eosinopaenia

Eosinopaenia occurs in response to:

♠ Increased cortisol levels; either endogenous or exogenous.

Basophils

An increase in the number of basophils may occur in disease states (Basophilia).

Basophilia

Basophilia may be:

♦ Reactive

♣ Neoplastic increase

Reactive Basophilia

A reactive increase in basophils may be in response to inflammatory conditions such as:

♥ **IS** chicken pox, smallpox

♠ **GIT** ulcerative colitis

♦ **E&M** myxoedema

Neoplastic Increase

A neoplastic increase in basophils may occur in:

- ♣ Chronic myelogenous leukaemia, polycythaemia rubra vera, mast cell leukaemia
- ♥ Basophilia also occurs in systemic mastocytosis and in urticaria pigmentosa.
- ♠ Basophilia occurs rarely in mast cell leukaemia.

Lymphocytes

Disorders of lymphocytes may manifest as:

- ♦ Disorders of function
- ♣ Disorders of the number of lymphocytes

Disorders of Lymphocyte Function

Disorders of lymphocyte function result in immunodeficiency, which may be classified as:

- ♥ Primary Immunodeficiency
- ♠ Secondary Immunodeficiency

Primary Immunodeficiency

Primary immunodeficiency may affect:

- ♦ B cells
- ♣ T cells
- ♥ Combined; affecting both B and T cells

B Cell Disorders (causing Antibody Deficiency)

B cell disorders, which result in antibody deficiency, are:

- ♠ Common variable immunodeficiency

- ♦ X-linked agammaglobulinaemia
- ♣ Thymoma with hypogammaglobulinaemia
- ♥ Selective Ig A deficiency
- ♠ Selective Ig G subclass deficiency
- ♦ Autosomal recessive hyper-IgM
- ♣ Autosomal recessive agammaglobulinaemia

T Cell Deficiency (resulting in decreased Cell Mediated Immunity)

T cell disorders, which result in decreased cell mediated immunity, are:

- ♥ Thymic aplasia
- ♠ Purine nucleoside phosphorylase deficiency
- ♦ CD 3-complex defects

Mixed T and B Cell Deficiency

Mixed T and B cell deficiency occurs in:

- ♣ Severe combined immunodeficiency:

  Adenosine deaminase deficiency, Purine nucleoside phosphorylase deficiency, Non-expression of MHC class II, Reticular dysgenesis

- ♥ Ataxia telangiectasia
- ♠ Wiskott-Aldrich syndrome
- ♦ Transporter for antigen presentation (TAP) deficiency
- ♣ X-linked lymphoproliferative syndrome
- ♥ Ligase 1 deficiency

Secondary Immunodeficiency

Secondary immunodeficiency may be due to:

- ♠ Decreased production of antibodies
- ♦ Increased extinction or loss of antibodies
- ♣ T cell deficiency
- ♥ Combined B and T cell deficiency

Decreased Production of Antibodies

Decreased production of antibodies occurs in:

- ♠ **Systemic Disorders**

  Conditions affecting the:

  HS chronic lymphatic leukaemia, myeloma

  E&M deficiency of vitamin A, transcobolamin 2 deficiency

  Viral Infections rubella

  Drugs gold, penicillamine, phenytoin, valproate, carbamazepine, sulphasalazine

  IS burns

Increased Extinction or Loss of Immunoglobulins

Loss of immunoglobulins occurs in conditions affecting the:

- ♦ **KUS** nephrotic syndrome
- ♣ **GIT** protein losing enteropathy such as intestinal lymphangiectasia, inflammatory bowel disease
- ♥ **CNS** dystrophia myotonica

T Cell Deficiency

T cell deficiency occurs in:

- ♠ **Viral Infections** AIDS, measles
- ♦ **Drugs** azathioprine, methotrexate, cyclosporin, corticosteroids
- ♣ **E&M** selenium deficiency, zinc deficiency

Combined B and T cell deficiency

Combined B and T cell deficiency occurs in conditions affecting the:

- ♥ **E&M** protein-calorie malnutrition, biotin dependent carboxylase deficiency
- ♠ **KUS** renal failure
- ♦ **GIT** liver failure
- ♣ **Trauma**

Disorders of Lymphocyte Numbers

Disorders of lymphocyte numbers may result in:

- ♥ Lymphopaenia
- ♠ Lymphocytosis

Lymphopaenia

Lymphopaenia is uncommon. It may be associated with conditions affecting the:

- ♥ **HS** marrow failure
- ♠ **Drugs** steroids and immunosuppressive treatment
- ♦ **LMS** autoimmune disease in particular systemic lupus erythematosus
- ♣ **RAG** HIV infection.

Lymphocytosis

Lymphocytosis could be either:

- ♥ Reactive

♠ Neoplastic

Reactive Lymphocytosis

A reactive increase in lymphocytes may be due to:

- ♦ **Viral infections**: infectious mononucleosis, cytomegalovirus, rubella, viral hepatitis, acute HIV infection
- ♣ **Bacterial infections**: brucellosis, tuberculosis
- ♥ **Parasitic infestations**: *Toxoplasma gondii*

Neoplastic Proliferation of Lymphocytes

Neoplastic proliferation of lymphocytes may present as an increase in the number of lymphocytes in the:

- ♥ Blood
- ♠ Lymph nodes
- ♦ Jaw
- ♣ Skin

Blood

Neoplastic proliferation of lymphocytes, presenting as an increased number of lymphocytes in the blood, occurs in:

- ♥ Acute Lymphoblastic Leukaemia
- ♠ Chronic Lymphocytic Leukaemia

Lymph Nodes

Neoplastic proliferation of lymphocytes, presenting as an increased number of lymphocytes in the lymph nodes, occurs in:

- ♦ Hodgkin's lymphoma
- ♣ Non-Hodgkin's lymphoma

Jaw Lesions

Neoplastic proliferation of lymphocytes, presenting as an increased number of lymphocytes in the jaw, occurs in:

- ♥ Burkitt's lymphoma, which also causes abdominal lesions and in females ovarian lesions. It may also involve the breast, the testes, the cranium and the spinal cord.

Skin

Neoplastic proliferation of lymphocytes, presenting as an increased number of lymphocytes in the skin, occurs in:

- ♠ Mycosis fungoides where discrete areas are involved
- ♦ Sezary syndrome where diffuse involvement of the skin occurs

Plasma Cells

Function of the B cells has already been dealt with. An increase in number is usually due to neoplastic proliferation.

Neoplastic Proliferation of Plasma Cells

Neoplastic proliferation of plasma cells may be either:

- ♣ Generalised
- ♥ Localised

Generalised

A generalised proliferation of plasma cells occurs in:

- ♠ Multiple myeloma

Localised

A localised proliferation of lympho-cytes occurs in:

- Plasmacytoma which may occur in bone or soft tissue

Monocytes

Disease states may result in an increase in the number of monocytes (Monocytosis).

Monocytosis

An increase in the number of monocytes may be due to a:

- ♣ Reactive increase
- ♥ Neoplastic proliferation

Reactive Increase in Monocytes

A reactive increase in monocytes may be in response to infections, infestations or inflammation involving the:

- ♣ **RS** tuberculosis, sarcoidosis
- ♦ **HS** brucellosis, kala-azar
- ♣ **CVS** infective endocarditis
- ♥ **RAG** syphilis
- ♠ **LMS** systemic lupus erythe-matosus, rheumatoid arthritis
- ♦ **GIT** inflammatory bowel disease

Neoplastic Proliferation of Monocytes

Neoplastic proliferation of monocytes/macrophages results in histiocytoses. Histiocytoses may be classified into three subclasses:

- ♣ Class I Disorders of Dendritic Cells
- ♥ Class II Disorders of Macrophages
- ♠ Class III Malignant Histiocyte Disorders

These are rare disorders. They may present with involvement of:

- ♦ Blood
- ♣ Tissues

Blood

Neoplastic proliferation of monocytes with an increase in the number of monocytes in the blood occurs in:

- ♥ Monocytic leukaemia

Tissues

Neoplastic proliferation of monocytes with involvement of tissues may result in either localised or generalised disease. Examples of these diseases are:

- ♠ Langerhan's cell histiocytosis, which presents with single system or multisystem disease
- ♦ Haemophagocytic lymphohistio-cytosis, which presents with hepatosplenomegaly, lymphadenopathy, pancy-topaenia, fever, liver and CNS involvement
- ♣ Sinus histiocytosis with massive lymphadenopathy, which presents with lymphadenopathy and sometimes extranodal disease

Platelets

Problems affecting the platelets may be:

♥ Internal problems resulting in functional abnormalities

♠ Problems affecting the number of platelets in circulation either an increase or a decrease in number

Functional Abnormalities

Internal problems result in functional abnormalities of the platelets. These may be:

♦ Inherited

♣ Acquired

Inherited Disorders of Platelet Function

Inherited conditions that result in functional abnormalities of the platelets are:

♥ **Disorders of Platelet Aggregation and Adhesion**

   Bernard-Soulier syndrome, Glanzmann's thrombasthenia

♠ **Disorders of Platelet Secretion**

   Grey platelet syndrome (alpha granules decreased or absent), dense granule deficiency, alpha delta storage pool deficiency (deficiency of both alpha and dense granules)

♦ **Disorders of Platelet Procoagulant Activity**

   Phospholipids on the platelet membrane are important for coagulation reactions. In the Scott syndrome an abnormal platelet membrane impairs its procoagulant activity.

Acquired Disorders of Platelet Function

Acquired disorders of platelet function may be due to conditions affecting the:

♣ **HS** chronic myelogenous leukaemia, essential thrombocythaemia, polycythaemia rubra vera, myelodysplasia, dysproteinaemia

♥ **KUS** uraemia

♠ **Drugs** aspirin, NSAIDs, dipyridamole, clopidrogel

♦ **CVS** extra-corporeal circulation, dacron aortic grafts

♣ **GIT** chronic liver disease

Platelet Numbers

Problems affecting the number of platelets in circulation may be:

♥ Increased Number of Platelets (Thrombocytosis > 600 x10^9/l)

♠ Decreased Platelets (Thrombocytopaenia)

Increased Number of Platelets

Thrombocytosis refers to a platelet count greater than 600 x10^9/l. Thrombocytosis may be:

♦ Reactive

♣ Neoplastic

Reactive Thrombocytosis

A reactive increase in platelet numbers may be due to:

♥ **Inflammatory disorders**: infections, rheumatoid arthritis, inflammatory bowel disease

♠ **Malignancy**

♦ **Hyposplenism**

Neoplastic Thrombocytosis (Thrombocythaemia)

Neoplastic proliferation of platelets occurs in:

♣ Essential Thrombocythaemia, which is a myeloproliferative disorder

Decreased Platelets

A decrease in the number of platelets in circulation may be due to:

♦ Decreased production

♣ Increased extinction

Decreased Production

Decreased production of platelets may be due to disorders involving the:

♣ Megakaryocytes

♥ Bone marrow

Megakaryocytes

Disorders that affect the megakaryocytes and result in a decreased number of platelets are the following:

♣ **Congenital Disorders**

Thrombocytopaenia with absent radii

Other rare congenital disorders that cause decreased platelet production are Wiskott -Aldrich syndrome, May-Hegglin anomaly, Sebastian platelet syndrome,

Fechtner's syndrome, Epstein's syndrome, congenital amegakaryocytic thrombocytopaenia

♥ **Acquired Disorders**

Acquired amegakaryocytic thrombocytopaenic purpura. This is a rare disorder that may progress to aplastic anaemia. It is usually idiopathic but may be secondary to infection, toxins or drugs.

Marrow

Disorders that affect the bone marrow and result in thrombocytopaenia are the following:

♣ **Internal Factors**

Marrow aplasia

Marrow infiltration

Myelodysplasia

♥ **External Factors**

Irradiation

♠ **Systemic Factors**

Drugs chemotherapy (cancer), chloramphenicol, NSAIDs, gold, anticonvulsants

Toxins alcohol

E&M nutritional deficiency such as vitamin B_{12} and folic acid deficiency

Increased Extinction of Platelets

Increased extinction of platelets occurs in conditions affecting the:

♦ **HS**

Idiopathic thrombocytopaenic purpura, disseminated intravascular coagulation, thrombotic thrombocytopaenic purpura

Post transfusion purpura

Haemophagocytic syndrome. This refers to phagocytosis of haematological cells by macrophages. It is associated with Epstein Barr virus, T cell lymphoma, histiocytosis, systemic lupus erythematosus, Still's disease

- ♣ **RAG** HIV
- ♥ **GIT** hypersplenism
- ♠ **Drugs** heparin, sulphonamides, gold
- ♦ **CVS** extracorporeal circulation
- ♣ **E&M** hypothermia

Plasma Proteins

When studying the plasma proteins one should consider disorders affecting:

- ♥ Gamma Globulins
- ♠ Complement
- ♦ Coagulation Factors

Gamma Globulins

Problems related to the gamma globulins may be an:

- ♠ Increase in gamma globulins
- ♥ Decrease in gamma globulins

Increased Gamma Globulins

An increase in gamma globulins occurs due to increased production and is seen in:

- ♦ Multiple Myeloma
- ♣ Waldenstrom's macroglobuli- naemia

- ♥ Heavy chain disease
- ♠ Primary amyloidosis
- ♦ Benign monoclonal gammopathy

Decreased Gammaglobulins

The causes of decreased gamma-globulins have been discussed under immunodeficiency

Complement

Disorders affecting the complement system may be:

- ♥ Hereditary Disorders
- ♠ Acquired Disorders

Hereditary Disorders

Hereditary disorders may result in abnormalities of the complement system. They may present as:

- ♦ **Complement Deficiency and Infection**

    Complement deficiency may result in an increased suscepti-bility to pyogenic infections

- ♣ **Complement Deficiency and Autoimmune Disease**

    Complement deficiency may result in an increased suscepti-bility to autoimmune disease

- ♥ **Abnormalities of Complement Regulation**

    C1 Esterase inhibitor deficiency (Hereditary angioedema)

    Unregulated C3 activation

    Factor I and Factor H deficiency results in unregulated C3 activation (increased suscepti-bility to infection, inherited mesangiocapillary glomeru-lonephritis)

Acquired Disorders

Acquired disorders of complement are caused by autoantibodies against complement components:

- ♠ C3 Nephritic Factor causes mesangiocapillary glomeru-lonephritis
- ♦ Anti C1 q antibody occurs in systemic lupus erythematosus
- ♣ Anti C1 inhibitor antibody results in a late onset picture similar to hereditary angioedema.

Coagulation Factors

When considering abnormalities of the coagulation factors one should consider:

- ♥ Coagulation Defects
- ♠ Thrombophilia

Coagulation Defects

Coagulation defects may be due to:

- ♦ Decreased production of coagu-lation factors
- ♣ Increased loss of coagulation factors
- ♥ Coagulation Factor Inhibitors
- ♠ Excessive Fibrinolysis

Decreased Production of Coagulation Factors

Decreased production of coagu-lation factors may be due to:

- ♦ Genetic disorders
- ♣ Acquired conditions

Genetic Disorders

Genetic disorders that affect coagu-lation factors are:

- ♥ Haemophilia A (factor VIII deficiency)
- ♠ Haemophilia B (factor IX deficiency)
- ♦ Von Willebrands disease
- ♣ Rarely deficiencies of other factors may occur

Acquired Disorders

Failure to produce coagulation factors may be due to:

- ♥ Liver disease
- ♠ Deficiency disorders such as vitamin K deficiency
- ♦ Drugs: warfarin

Increased Loss of Coagulation Factors

Increased loss of coagulation factors may occur in:

- ♣ Disseminated intravascular coagulation
- ♥ Nephrotic syndrome

Coagulation Factor Inhibitors

Rarely Ig G antibodies that bind to specific coagulation factors may be formed in some patients

Excessive Fibrinolysis

Rarely, excessive fibrinloysis may occur as a secondary phenomenon in disseminated intravascular coagu-lation.

Vascular Disorders that Result in Bleeding

Vascular disorders that result in bleeding are:

♥ **Congenital Disorders**: Osler-Rendu-Weber syndrome, Ehlers-Danlos syndrome, Pseudoxanthoma elasticum, Marfan's syndrome, osteogenesis imperfecta

♠ **Inflammatory Disorders**: systemic lupus erythematosus, rheumatoid arthritis, septicaemia

♦ **Metabolic disorders**: scurvy

♣ **Degenerative disorders**: senile purpura

♥ **Drugs**: steroids

Thrombophilia

An increased tendency to clotting may occur in:

♠ Genetic Disorders

♦ Acquired Disorders

Genetic Disorders

Genetic disorders that result in an increased tendency to clotting are:

♣ Factor V Leiden

♥ Prothrombin variant

♠ Antithrombin deficiency

♦ Protein C deficiency

♣ Protein S deficiency

Acquired Disorders

Acquired disorders that result in an increased tendency to clotting are:

♥ Antipholipid syndrome

♠ Antithrombin deficiency (Acquired antithrombin deficiency may occur in severe proteinuria)

Findings on History

The findings that one may obtain on history taking are as follows:

Breathlessness

In relation to the haematological system:

♠ Breathlessness would be due to anaemia.

Recurrent Infections

Recurrent infections may be due to:

♦ A decreased number of neutrophils

♣ Inadequate functioning of neutrophils

♥ Immunodeficiency

Bleeding Tendency

It is usually possible to differentiate the types of bleeding tendency.

♠ If bleeding involves the skin or mucous membranes it is more likely to be a platelet or capillary defect.

♦ If bleeding involves deeper tissues and causes larger haematomas it is more likely to indicate a coagulation disorder.

Bone Pain

Bone pain would indicate involvement of the bone marrow by a neoplastic process either of:

♣ Hamopoietic tissue

♥ Secondary deposits

Findings on Examination

The abnormalities that one may detect on clinical examination of the patient are as follows:

General Examination

On general examination one may note abnormalities of the following:

♠ Dimensions

♦ Integument

♣ Body Temperature

Dimensions

The abnormalities that may be detected are those in relation to:

♥ Height

♠ Weight

Height

Variations in height that may be noted are:

Short Stature

Short stature would indicate chronic disease from childhood. This would usually mean a genetic abnormality affecting the haematological system. This could involve the:

♠ **Red Cells**

Inherited haemolytic anaemia like thalassaemia

♦ **White Cells**

Neutrophil dysfunction giving chronic or recurrent infections, Immunodeficiency syndromes

Weight

In relation to the haematological system, decreased weight would either indicate:

♣ Malabsorption resulting in weight loss and anaemia

♥ Cachexia consequent on malignant disease, immune deficiency

Integument

On examination of the skin one may note changes in:

♣ Colour

♥ Surface

Colour of the Skin

Change in colour may be:

♠ **Pigmentation**

Pigmentation may be increased in folic acid and vitamin B_{12} deficiency. It could also be increased in iron overload.

♦ **Lemon-Yellow Colour**

A lemon-yellow colour occurs in megaloblastic anaemia

♣ **Pallor**

Pallor would indicate anaemia.

♥ **Suffusion (Plethora)**

The skin would appear plethoric (diffuse reddening) in

polycythaemia rubra vera. This would be associated with cyanosis of the nose, lips ears, hands and feet.

Surface of the Skin

Abnormalities that one may note on the surface of the skin are:

Excoriations

Scratch marks may be due to:

♠ Pruritus which occurs in polycythaemia rubra vera

Rash

Rashes that may be observed are the following:

♦ An erythematous maculopapular rash occurs in infectious mononucleosis, graft versus host disease

♣ Erythema and pruritus followed by vesicle and bullae formation is seen in congenital (erythropoietic) porphyria

♥ A blistering rash occurs in dermatitis herpetiformis

♠ Skin infiltrates occur in monoblastic leukaemia, chronic granulocytic leukaemia, mycosis fungoides

♦ A diffuse erythematous rash occurs in the Sezary syndrome

♣ Skin infections and cellulitis occur in acute myeloid leukaemia

♥ Bleeding:

Petechiae occur in capillary and platelet disorders

Larger haematomas occur in haemophilia A and B

Body Temperature

Fevers could be due to:

♠ Lymphoma

♦ Infection

Regional Examination

The abnormalities that may be detected on regional examination are as follows:

Head

On examination of the head one may detect abnormalities of the:

Dimensions

Abnormalities that may be noted are:

♣ Frontal and parietal bossing occur as a result of marrow hyperplasia in hereditary haemolytic anaemias such as thalassaemia and sickle cell disease.

♥ Localised deformity may occur due to bone deposits in myeloma and in the histiocytoses

♠ Swelling of the head may occur in obstruction of the superior vena cava

Integument

Abnormalities that may be noted are:

♦ Generalised erythema of the face, *l' homme rouge*. This would be seen in polycythaemia rubra vera

♣ The skin may be darker and suffused in obstruction of the superior vena cava

Nose

On examination of the nose one may note:

♠ A sunken bridge of the nose occurs in the Diamond-Blackfan syndrome

♦ Lupus pernio occurs in sarcoidosis

Eyes

When examining the eyes one may observe abnormalities of the:

Dimensions

Changes that may occur are:

♣ Proptosis due to bone deposits

Eyelids

In the eyelids:

♥ Lacrimal gland swelling occurs in lymphoma, leukaemia

Conjunctiva

On examination of the conjunctiva one may observe:

♠ Pallor in anaemia

♦ Haemorrhages in leukaemia

Sclera

Abnormalities that may be detected in the sclera are:

♣ Jaundice would be seen in haemolytic anaemia.

♥ Remember that obstructive jaundice may occur due to pigment stone formation in haemolytic anaemia

Anterior Chamber

In the anterior chamber of the eye one may note:

♠ Leukaemic infiltrates in acute lymphoblastic leukaemia.

Fundus

Lesions that could occur in the fundus are the following:

♦ Papilloedema may be caused by meningeal deposits in acute lymphoblastic leukaemia

♣ Engorged retinal veins with a dark background occur in polycythaemia rubra vera

♥ Engorged retinal veins with beading occur in the hyperviscosity syndrome

♠ Retinal haemorrhage occurs in aplastic anaemia, iron deficiency anaemia

♦ Choroidoretinitis due to cytomegalovirus (CMV) occurs in immunocompromised individuals

♣ Infiltrates may be seen in chronic granulocytic leukaemia, Hodgkin's disease.

Eye Movements

When examining eye movements one may detect:

♥ Lesions of the 3rd, 4th and 6th nerves which may occur in acute lymphoblastic leukaemia

Face

On examination of the face one may note abnormalities of the following:

Scalp

In the scalp abnormalities that may be detected are:

- Loss of hair would most often reflect the effects of chemotherapy.
- White hair would be seen in vitamin B_{12} deficiency

Forehead

On examination of the forehead one may note:

- Frontal bossing, which occurs in thalassaemia, sickle cell disease

Facial Nerve

On examination of the facial nerve one may note:

- Facial nerve palsy, due to meningeal involvement, in acute lymphoblastic leukaemia

Mouth

On examination of the mouth one may note abnormalities of the following:

Lips

In the lips one may note:

- Telangiectases in the Osler-Rendu-Weber syndrome
- Stomatitis in iron, vitamin B_{12} deficiency
- Angular chelosis in vitamin B_{12} deficiency

Teeth

Abnormalities that may be of significance are:

- Protruding splayed teeth occur in thalassaemia
- Teeth would be irregular in size and shape in dyskeratosis congenita

Gums

Lesions that may occur in the gums are the following:

- Swelling and bleeding occur in scurvy
- Bleeding gums occur in thrombocytopaenia
- Phenytoin use can cause gum changes and also result in folic acid deficiency
- A blue line may be seen in lead poisoning
- Bleeding and infection occur in acute monocytic leukaemia
- Gum expansion can occur due to leukaemic infiltrates. This may cause thickening of the gums which may then partially cover the teeth

Tongue

Abnormalities that may occur in the tongue are:

- A large tongue would be seen in amyloidosis
- Glossitis occurs in iron, vitamin B_{12} and folate deficiency

Buccal Mucosa

Lesions that may occur on the buccal mucosa are:

♣ Lichen planus like lesions occur in graft versus host disease.

♥ Thrush occurs in immunodeficiency

♠ Ulceration may occur due to neutropaenia

Fauces

In the fauces one may note:

♦ Ulceration. This occurs in leukaemia, aplastic anaemia

♣ The tonsils may be enlarged in infectious mononucleosis, chronic lymphocytic leukaemia, lymphoma

Salivary Glands

Lesions that can occur in the salivary glands are:

♥ Unilateral or bilateral enlargement occurs in lymphoma

♣ Mikulicz syndrome refers to enlargement of the salivary and lacrimal glands. The causes are sarcoidosis, lymphoma, tuberculosis

Ears

When examining the ears one may note:

♦ Tophi, which may be seen in gout. Gout may occur in polycythaemia rubra vera

Hands

On examination of the hands one may note abnormalities of the following:

Dimensions

Variations that may be of note are:

♣ Scleroderma like hands occur in graft versus host disease

♥ The thumbs look like fingers in Fanconi's anaemia

♠ Short fingers may be caused by dactylitis affecting the epiphyses in sickle cell anaemia

Nails

Abnormalities that may be noted in the nails are:

♦ Koilonychia occurs in iron deficiency

♣ Abnormal nails are seen in dyskeratosis congenita

Skin

On examination of the skin of the hands one may note:

♥ Abnormal hair in dyskeratosis congenita

♠ Raynaud's phenomenon occurs in cold agglutinin disease

Locomotor System

Lesions of the locomotor system of the hands that may occur in relation to the haematological system are:

♦ Dactylitis (swollen, tender, sausage-shaped fingers) occurs in haemoglobinopathies such as sickle cell disease

♣ Rheumatoid arthritis could be associated with Felty's syndrome (rheumatoid arthritis, splenomegaly, leucopaenia), anaemia of chronic disease, NSAID induced gastrointestinal blood loss, myelosuppression due to drugs

Axillae

On examination of the axillae one may note:

♥ Lymphadenopathy. This may be due to pathology within the field of regional drainage or it may be part of a generalised lymphadenopathy.

Neck

On examination of the neck one may note abnormalities of the following:

Dimensions

One may note:

♠ Swelling of the neck in superior vena cava obstruction. This may occur in Hodgkin's disease.

Lymph Nodes

Cervical lymphadenopathy may be due to:

♦ Pathology within the field of regional drainage such as pyogenic infection, tuberculosis or malignancy

♣ Generalised lymphadenopathy

Generalised Lymphadenopathy

Generalised lymphadenopathy may occur in:

♥ **Neoplastic Disorders**

Lymphoma, chronic lymphocytic leukaemia

♠ **Inflammatory Disorders**

Brucellosis, toxoplasmosis, infectious mononucleosis, cytomegalovirus infection, HIV, sarcoidosis

♦ **Metabolic Conditions**

Thyrotoxicosis

Chest Wall

Abnormalities that may be noted are:

♣ Sternal tenderness may occur in acute leukaemia

♥ Fractures of the ribs and sternum may occur in myeloma

Respiratory System

Lesions that may occur in the respiratory system in relation to the haematological system are:

♠ Pneumonia may occur in immunocompromised individuals

♦ Bruits may occur due to pulmonary arteriovenous fistulae in hereditary haemorrhagic telangiectasia

Cardiovascular System

Lesions that may occur in the cardiovascular system in relation to the haematological system are:

♣ A flow murmur may occur due to anaemia

♥ Valvular lesions may indicate the cause of anaemia either related to:

Bacterial endocarditis

Haemolysis caused by a prosthetic valve

Abdominal Wall

Abnormalities that may be noted are:

- Scars could indicate the cause of anaemia:

  Gastrectomy (iron deficiency)

  Ileal resection (vitamin B_{12} deficiency)

- Scars could be the result of anaemia:

  Splenectomy in haemolytic anaemia

Splenomegaly

Enlargement of the spleen may be due to:

- **Neoplastic Disorders**

  Chronic myeloid leukaemia, polycythaemia rubra vera, chronic lymphocytic leukaemia, lymphoma, myeloma

- **Inflammatory Disorders**

  Infectious mononucleosis, brucella, septicaemia, typhoid, tuberculosis, sarcoid, rheumatoid arthritis (Felty's syndrome)

- **Extramedullary Erythropoiesis**

  Myelofibrosis, thalassaemia

- **Hypertrophy**

  Haemolytic anaemia (Hereditary spherocytosis), idiopathic thrombocytopaenic purpura

- **Congestion**

  Malaria (acute phase in the chronic phase hyperplasia occurs)

- **Portal Hypertension**

Cirrhosis of the liver, portal vein thrombosis

Hyposplenism

Hyposplenism cannot be detected clinically. It may be caused by:

- Coeliac disease
- Sickle cell disease
- Surgery

Hepatosplenomegaly

Hepatosplenomegaly may be due to:

- **Neoplastic Disorders**

  Myeloproliferative disease (chronic myeloid leukaemia)

  Lymphoproliferative disease (lymphoma, chronic lymphocytic leukaemia)

- **Inflammatory Disorders**

  Cytomegalovirus, malaria, kala azar, tuberculosis, brucella, toxoplasmosis

- **Extramedullary Erythropoiesis**

  Extramedullary erythropoiesis occurs in:

  Myelofibrosis, thalassaemia

- **Venous Congestion**

  Venous congestion occurs in:

  Malaria

- **Lysosomal Storage Diseases**

  Lysosomal storage diseases are a group of disorders caused by inherited deficiencies of individual enzymes within lysosomes. Patients with Niemann-Pick disease, Gaucher disease have hepatosplenomegaly.

389

♠ **Interstitial Infiltration**

Amyloidosis

Hepatosplenomegaly and Palpable Lymph Nodes

Hepatosplenomegaly and palpable lymph nodes may be due to:

♦ **Neoplastic Conditions**

Chronic lymphocytic leukaemia, lymphoma

♣ **Inflammatory Disorders**

Infectious mononucleosis, sarcoidosis

Para-Aortic Lymph Nodes

If para-aortic lymph nodes are palpable consider:

♥ Generalised Lymphadenopathy. Para-aortic lymphadenopathy may be part of a generalised lymphadenopathy

♠ Remember the drainage of the lymph nodes in particular testicular tumours in a male

Kidneys

Abnormalities that may be noted in relation to the kidneys are:

♦ Renal failure may result in anaemia

♣ Polycythaemia could be due to hydronephrosis, renal cysts, polycystic kidneys, hyper-nephroma

Right Iliac Fossa

An ileocaecal mass in a patient presenting with anaemia could be:

♥ Crohn's disease

♠ Colon cancer

Colon

Lesions in the colon that may present with disease in relation to the haematological system are:

♦ Colon cancer may present as anaemia

Uterus

Lesions of the uterus that may present with disease in relation to the haematological system are:

♣ Fibroids cause iron deficiency anaemia

♥ Uterine fibroids could cause polycythaemia

Hepatic Bruit

The presence of a hepatic bruit could indicate:

♠ Shunts from the hepatic artery to the hepatic vein in hereditary haemorrhagic telangiectasia. This may result in high output cardiac failure

Inguinal Lymph Nodes

On examination of the inguinal lymph nodes one may note enlarged inguinal lymph nodes, which could be due to:

- Generalised lymphadenopathy
- Pathology within the field of regional drainage

Genitalia

On examination of the genitalia one may note:

- The testes may be infiltrated in acute lymphoblastic leukaemia, lymphoma

Per Rectal Examination

Rectal examination may reveal:

- Carcinoma rectum may present as anaemia

Lower Limbs

On general examination of the lower limbs one may note abnormalities of the:

Dimensions

One may note:

- Swollen limbs due to inguinal and pelvic lymph node involvement in lymphoma

Hips

Lesions that may occur are:

- Avascular necrosis of the hips occurs in sickle cell disease

Knees

Lesions that may occur are:

- Osteoarthrosis may be caused by recurrent haemarthroses in haemophilia

Lower Legs

In the lower legs one may note:

- Leg ulcers in hereditary haemolytic anaemia
- Deep vein thrombosis may be a feature of paroxysmal nocturnal haemoglobinuria, polycythaemia
- Erythema nodosum occurs in sarcoidosis

Feet

In the feet one may note:

- Peripheral vascular disease, which occurs in hyperviscosity syndromes
- Gout may be due to polycythaemia rubra vera, acute myeloid leukaemia
- Erythema and exfoliation of the soles of the feet occur in graft versus host disease

Spine

Abnormalities that may occur in the spine are:

- Wedging and collapse of the vertebrae may occur in myeloma

Gait

Abnormalities of gait that may occur in relation to the haematological system are:

♥ Cerebrovascular disease may be secondary to polycythaemia

♠ Cerebellar signs would occur in cerebellar haemangioblastoma which can cause polycythaemia

♦ A broad based stamping gait occurs in vitamin B_{12} deficiency

Romberg's Sign

Romberg's sign may be positive in patients who have:

♣ Vitamin B_{12} deficiency

Chapter 16

The Central Nervous System

In the central nervous system one will study the sensory elements that detect changes in the environment, both external and internal, the central organisation that processes this information and determines the appropriate response and the efferent aspect that implements this response.

The nervous system has a somatic component that deals mainly with the organism's responses to changes in the external environment and an autonomic component that deals mainly with changes in the internal environment. This is not an exclusive division as under certain conditions both the somatic and autonomic components come into play, the striking example of this being the response to danger. Both the somatic and autonomic components should be studied.

In addition one should study the clinical features that result from the causes and effects of conditions that affect the nervous system but are reflected in other systems.

History Taking

This is an instance where history taking and examination are inextricably linked. When taking a history, in addition to obtaining a description of the disease process, one is evaluating speech and the higher functions of the cerebral hemispheres.

To make history taking easier it would be wise to start cranially and work caudally.

Aide Memoire

One could conveniently divide history taking into questions regarding the cortex, the cranium, the cranial nerves, the cord (spinal cord) and its connections (the connections are motor, sensory and autonomic), and the canal (referring to the spine as the canal through which the spinal cord runs).

One should begin with:

♥ **Speech**

Evaluate speech. Although strictly speaking this is part of examination of the cerebral hemispheres, if an abnormality is detected at this stage it should be defined, as history taking will probably not be possible in full. Evaluation of speech is discussed in detail later.

Then one should ask about the:

♠ **Cortex** (Cerebral Hemispheres)

Enquire about the following:

Dominant side (whether the patient is right or left handed)

Fits

Loss of consciousness

Mood

Sleep

♦ **Cranium**

Assess the cranium and the coverings of the brain (meninges) by asking about:

Headaches

♣ **Cranial Nerves**

Enquire about the following:

Nose

Changes in the sense of smell

Eyes

Visual disturbances

Face

Weakness

Sensory disturbance

Mouth

Speech

Swallowing

Taste

Ears

Vertigo

Hearing (deafness, hyperacusis, tinnitus)

♥ **Cord and Connections** (the connections are motor, sensory and autonomic)

Enquire about:

Abnormal movements

Weakness

Incoordination

Sensory disturbance

Gait

Bowel function

Bladder function

♠ **Canal** (spine)

Ask about:

Backache

Next, perform a review of systems.

Physical Examination

Most students and junior doctors consider examination of the nervous system the most difficult system to master. This often leads to avoidance of performing neurological examinations and this compounds the problem. Neurological examination is easy if basic principles are learned and adhered to.

To begin with one must have a sound knowledge of basic neuro-anatomy and neuro-physiology. This cannot be overemphasised.

The basic principles of examination of the nervous system are no different from any other system. Examination involves examination of structure and function and assessment of any pathological and aetiological features that may be present.

Commence examination by observing the way the patient is dressed and then proceed with the physical examination.

Dress

In neurological examination an assessment of the way the patient is dressed would give important clues to the underlying mental state.

General Examination

Begin by noting the position of the patient.

Position

A very important feature to note in examination of the nervous system is the site or position of the patient. The position adopted by the patient would give important clues to the presence of an underlying neurological deficit. Note the direction of gaze of the patient and the position of the patient's head in relation to the trunk. Also note the position of the patient's limbs in relation to the trunk.

One should then make a quick note of the patient's state of growth and development and the metabolic state of the patient. A quick assessment should be made of any gross changes in the integument. Body temperature should be noted. (Position, Height and Proportions, Weight and Shape, Integument, Body Temperature)

Regional Examination

One should proceed in a cephalo-caudal direction. Usually one examines structure and then function but in examination of the head this may be reversed in certain instances for ease of examination.

Cortex (Cerebral Hemispheres)

Examination of the cortex refers to examination of the cerebral hemispheres.

Examination of the Cerebral Hemispheres

Evaluate function of the cerebral hemispheres by assessing the following:

♦ Level of Consciousness

♣ Speech

♥ Higher Functions

Level of Consciousness

Start off by evaluating the patient's level of consciousness. The patient may be:

♣ **Conscious and Alert**

In a normal alert state

♦ **Conscious but Drowsy (Stupor)**

The patient appears sleepy but is rousable. Responds to verbal commands.

♣ **Unconscious (Coma)**

The patient does not respond to verbal commands but may respond to pain. If the patient responds to pain the type of response should be noted that is withdrawal, flexion or extension.

The **Glasgow Coma Scale** may be used as an objective assessment of the level of consciousness.

Speech

Speech is of crucial importance. The remainder of the examination of the cerebral hemispheres will depend upon whether there is an impairment of speech.

The function of speech may be divided into a:

♥ Sensory aspect

♠ Motor aspect

Sensory Aspect

The sensory aspect is the ability to understand the spoken word. The ability to understand the spoken word should be evaluated on the basis of an intact sensory system. The inability to understand the spoken word in the presence of an intact sensory system is termed **Sensory Aphasia.**

Motor Aspect

The motor aspect is the ability to produce or utter the spoken word. This ability may be broken down into:

♦ The ability to choose the correct words. The inability to do so is termed **Motor Aphasia**

♣ The ability to produce the sound required or phonation.

The inability to produce sound is termed **Aphonia**

Abnormal production of sound is termed **Dysphonia**

♥ The ability to articulate the words. The inability to do so is termed **Dysarthria**

Evaluation of Speech

In formal evaluation of speech one should:

♠ Ask the patient a few simple questions

♦ Give the patient a few simple commands to test comprehension

Without gestures (first)

With gestures (if the patient fails to comprehend without gestures)

♣ Ask the patient to say a few long words to test articulation (the words should be in the patient's native tongue)

♥ Ask the patient to repeat a given phrase or sentence

♠ Ask the patient to identify some common objects

Aide Memoire

When evaluating speech, test the patient's ability to **P**olitely **CARIE** *(carry) on a conversation. Here* **P**olitely *stands for* **P**honation, **CARIE** *stands for* **C**omprehension, **A**rticulation, **R**epetition, **I**dentification, **E**xpression

Now move on to evaluate the higher functions of the brain.

Higher Functions

For convenience one may divide examination of the higher functions of the brain into examination of the higher functions of the:

♠ Frontal Lobe

♦ Temporal Lobe

♣ Dominant Parietal Lobe

♥ Non-Dominant Parietal Lobe

♠ Occipital Lobe

The main motor and sensory functions of these lobes will be discussed later.

Frontal Lobe

One should assess the higher functions of the frontal lobe by testing:

- ◆ Orientation
- ♣ Attention or concentration
- ♥ Thoughts

Aide Memoire

FLOAT *stands for* **F**rontal **L**obe **O**rientation, **A**ttention, **T**houghts

Orientation

Assess the patient's orientation in:

- ♣ Place
- ◆ Time
- ♣ Person

This should have been done when taking the history if not it may be formally tested by asking the patient where they are, the date and time and by asking them to identify themselves.

Concentration

Note whether the patient has normal powers of attention or concentration. The power of attention may be formally tested by asking the patient to remember a set of numbers both forwards and backwards. Usually people can remember seven numbers forwards and five backwards.

Thoughts

Next one should analyse the patient's thought process. That is whether they follow a normal orderly fashion or whether there are abnormalities of the thought process such as:

♥ Flight of Ideas

Flight of ideas is where there is flitting from one thought to another but there is some connection.

♠ Thought Disorder

Thought disorder is where one idea follows the next without any connection.

◆ Perseveration

Perseveration is where the patient keeps repeating the question or his or her own remarks.

♣ Neologisms

Neologisms refer to the use of strange words.

♥ Word Salad

Word salad refers to actual words but strung together incorrectly.

Note any:

♠ Delusions

Delusions are false, unshakeable beliefs

◆ Hallucinations

Hallucinations refer to the patient having a sensory perception without the appropriate stimulus

Temporal Lobe

In evaluating the temporal lobe one should assess:

- ♣ Memory
- ♥ Mood

Memory

Both short-term and long-term memory should be tested.

Mood

A note should be made of the patient's mood.

Dominant Parietal Lobe

The dominant parietal lobe is usually the left in right-handed people and the right in left-handed individuals. The dominant parietal lobe subserves the functions of:

♠ Calculation

♦ Writing

♣ Identification or recognition

Abnormalities of these functions would be detected by demon-strating:

♥ Acalculia

♠ Agraphia

♦ Agnosia

Acalculia

The ability to perform mathematical calculations that is simple mental arithmetic may be tested. The inability to do this is known as acalculia.

Agraphia

The ability to write may be tested. The inability to write is known as agraphia.

Agnosia

Left-right disorientation should be tested by asking the patient to identify his or her right or left hand.

The patient's ability to identify his or her fingers may be tested. Inability to do this is known as finger agnosia

Non-Dominant Parietal Lobe

The non-dominant parietal lobe subserves the functions of:

♣ Spatial orientation

♥ Bodily perception

These functions should be assessed by testing for:

♠ **Visual and Sensory Inattention**

This will be discussed later.

♦ **Spatial Neglect**

Spatial neglect is unawareness of one side of the body. This is usually associated with a left hemiplegia.

♣ **Dressing Apraxia**

Test for dressing apraxia by asking the patient to put on an item of clothing that has been turned inside out

♥ **Constructional Apraxia**

Test for constructional apraxia by asking the patient to draw an object, usually a five-pointed star.

Remember that these tests may be performed only if gross motor and sensory functions are intact. Hence, it would not be possible to perform these tests until the end of the examination of the nervous system. However, unless one bears these tests in mind at this stage, they would tend to be forgotten.

Occipital Lobe

Lesions of the higher functions of the occipital lobe result in:

♠ Visual agnosia

Visual Agnosia

Visual agnosia refers to the failure to recognise objects or people visually although vision is intact. Recognition may be possible using another sensory modality such as touch or hearing. Again this may be tested only after demonstrating intact vision. Hence, this will be discussed later.

Limbic Lobes

The limbic lobes are not usually assessed in practice. They are concerned with the function of olfaction but in addition they subserve the function of emotions such as fear and rage, motivation, sexual behaviour. In addition stimulation of the limbic lobes may produce autonomic effects. In summary the limbic lobes subserve the functions of:

♦ Olfaction

♣ Emotions

   Fear, Rage, Motivation, Sexual behaviour

♥ Autonomic effects

Mental Score

A mental score may be performed in an attempt to objectively assess the higher functions of the cerebral hemispheres. One of the many available may be used.

Cranium

Make a quick note of any structural abnormalities of the head.

Next, move on to examine the cranial nerves.

Cranial Nerves

The cranial nerves are best tested with the patient seated, if possible.

Nose

Make a note of any structural abnormality of the nose.

Olfactory Nerve

Begin examination of the cranial nerves with the first, the olfactory nerve. A detailed examination is not usually required. It should be sufficient to enquire from the patient whether he or she has perceived any change in his or her sense of smell and perform formal examination only if the answer is affirmative. If so each nostril should be tested separately with the bottles that would be provided. In practice one may use substances like fruit, soap or perfume that may be available at the bedside. Use the fingers of one hand to close one nostril of the patient and test smell in the other nostril. Repeat for the other side. Remember to use the same finger to close the other nostril so that smell is not transmitted to the nostril that has already been tested by the finger that was holding the substance being tested

Eyes

One should examine:

♠ Structure

♦ Function

Structure

Make a note of any structural abnormality of the eyes.

Function

Examine the functions of the:

♦ Optic nerve

♣ 3rd, 4th and 6th Nerves

Optic Nerve

Proceed to examine the second cranial nerve, the optic nerve. One should examine:

♠ Visual acuity

♦ Visual fields

♣ Sensory inattention

♥ Visual agnosia (if required)

♠ Fundus

Visual Acuity

Begin by testing visual acuity. At the bedside ask the patient whether he or she can identify an object at a distance and ask them to read small text from a paper or book. The testing of visual acuity with formal charts will not be dealt with in this book. Formal testing would also require testing of colour vision but this will not be dealt with in bedside examination.

Visual Fields

Next, examine the visual fields using confrontation perimetry. Stand or sit directly in front of the patient approximately an arms length away.

The examiner's eyes and the patient's eyes should be at the same horizontal level. The examiner should shut one eye. The patient should be asked to shut the corresponding eye. The patient may use his or her hand but one should be able to shut an eye without the use of a hand. Now lift up one hand so that it is just outside the upper, temporal quadrant of the field of vision about mid-way between the patient and oneself. Keep the index finger relatively straight and partially curl up the other fingers and the thumb so that the index finger stands out from the rest. The patient should be asked to look at the examiner's forehead or nose and not at the hand. Move the hand from the periphery into the field of vision, shaking the index finger all the time. The movement of the hand should be in a radial direction. Ask the patient to say when he or she can see the moving finger. The patient's field of vision should be compared to one's own field of vision. Repeat the procedure for all four quadrants of the field of vision. For the patient's left eye use one's right hand for the temporal aspect of the patient's visual field and one's left hand for the nasal aspect. The converse would apply for the patient's right eye. Repeat the procedure for the other eye.

Ideally, a white hatpin should be used for visual fields and a red hatpin to look for central scotoma.

Central Scotoma

For detecting central scotoma a red hatpin should be used. It should be moved from the temporal periphery, across the centre of the field of vision, to the nasal periphery and its disappearance and reappearance documented.

Sensory Inattention

Now hold up both hands with one's fingers at the opposite ends of the periphery of the patient's field of vision. The patient should have both eyes open. Shake the index finger of one hand and ask the patient whether it can be seen. Next, shake the index finger of the other hand and ask the patient whether it can be seen. Now shake both index fingers simultaneously and ask the patient whether he or she can see them shaking. The patient should be able to identify that both fingers are shaking simultaneously. If not the patient has sensory inattention.

Bedfast Patients

For bedfast patients, one may modify the technique of testing visual fields. Turn the patient's head to a side and test the eye that does not have its field of vision hindered by the bedclothes. One should start with the left eye, as examination is conducted from the right-hand side of the bed. Then move over to the left-hand side of the bed, turn the patient's head so that the right eye is uppermost and test the field of vision in that eye.

Menace Reflex

If a patient is unable to cooperate with testing one may use the menace reflex to obtain a rough idea of a visual field defect. This is performed by bringing one's index finger towards the patient's eye from the different quadrants. The finger should point directly at the patient's eye as it is brought towards the patient. If the field of vision in the quadrant being tested is intact the patient will blink. Care should be taken not to be too forceful, as a fanning effect may cause blinking of the eyes by stimulating the corneal reflex.

Visual Agnosia

If required test for visual agnosia. Show the patient some common objects and ask the patient whether he or she can recognise them by sight alone. If not he or she may be able to recognise them by using another sensory modality.

The ability to recognise people's faces or photographs may also be tested if required.

Fundus

Perform examination of the eyes using an ophthalmoscope. To examine the patient's right eye use one's right hand to hold the ophthalmoscope and use one's right eye to visualise the fundus. The converse applies when examining the patient's left eye.

Hold the ophthalmoscope with the thumb, fourth and fifth finger. Use the second finger to change the focus of the ophthalmoscope. Straighten the middle finger, maintain it in that position so that when one moves close to the patient the extended middle finger will rest on the patient's cheek and prevent one's face bumping into the patient's face.

Ask the patient to look straight ahead and ask him or her to try and focus on an object in the distance. Begin examination from the temporal aspect of the patient a short distance away. Look at the pupil; note the red reflex, then move closer to the patient. Note any abnormality of the cornea, the anterior chamber, the iris, the lens and the vitreous as one gets closer. As the fundus comes into view one should be able to see the optic disc. If not, follow a blood vessel medially until the optic disc is reached. Define the optic cup. Following this carefully examine the optic disc and then the blood vessels, the four quadrants of the retina, including the periphery, and finally the macula.

In summary:

- ♠ Optic cup
- ♦ Optic disc
- ♣ Blood vessels
- ♥ Four quadrants
- ♠ Macula

Third, Fourth and Sixth Nerves (Occulomotor, Trochlear, Abducent)

Next proceed to examine the third, fourth and sixth nerves. Examine the following aspects:

- ♦ Position
- ♣ Eye movements
- ♥ Pupils

Position

Note the position of the:

- ♠ Eyelids
- ♦ Eyeballs

Eyelids

Note any:

- ♣ Ptosis

Eyeballs

Look at the position of the eyes at rest. Note any:

- ♥ Proptosis
- ♠ Enophthalmos
- ♦ Strabismus

Cover Test

Ask the patient to fix his or her gaze on an object. Cover one of the patient's eyes and then uncover it whilst the patient keeps his or her gaze fixed on the object. If the eye has to correct, as it is uncovered, this eye has a latent strabismus. Repeat for the other side.

Eye Movements

Steady the patient's head with one's left hand across the patient's forehead. Hold the right hand, with the index finger extended, in front of the patient's eyes. Ask the patient to keep looking at the finger and move it first up and down and then in a H shaped pattern. Next, bring the finger directly in front of the patient's eyes, ask the patient to look straight ahead and note the movement of the eyes. Then ask the patient to look at the finger and move it up against the patient's nose. This will test convergence. When performing these tests note whether the patient has a full range of eye movements and note any nystagmus. When testing convergence, observe whether the pupils constrict during convergence.

In summary when testing eye movements one should note the following:

- ♣ Range of movement
- ♥ Nystagmus
- ♠ Pupillary constriction during convergence

Pupils

When examining the pupils note:

- ♥ Structure of the iris
- ♠ Function of the pupil

Structure of the Iris

Assess any structural abnormalities of the iris and note the colour of the iris

Function of the Pupil

Note the following:

- ♣ Size
- ♥ Shape
- ♠ Pupillary Light Reflexes
- ♦ Swinging Light Test
- ♣ Accommodation Reflex
- ♥ Ciliospinal Reflex

Size

Note the size of the pupils at rest

Shape

Note the shape of the pupils at rest

Pupillary Light Reflexes

Test the patient's pupillary light reflexes with a torch. Flash the light twice into each eye in turn and note the direct and consensual light reflexes.

Swinging Light Test

Using a torch swing the light from one eye to the other. In the presence of an unilateral afferent pupillary defect, when the light shines in the normal eye both pupils will constrict due to the effect of the direct and consensual light reflexes. When the light shines in the affected eye no light reflex occurs and the pupils will dilate.

In a relative apparent pupillary defect (RAPD) when the light is initially shone in the affected eye both pupils will constrict due to the direct and consensual reflexes. When the light is shone in the unaffected eye again both pupils will constrict. When the light now swings back from the unaffected to the affected eye, the affected pupil will dilate instead of remaining constricted due to the effect of the contralateral consensual reflex being more powerful than the direct reflex in the affected eye. It indicates residual damage in the optic nerve following previous optic neuritis with apparent full recovery of vision.

Accommodation Reflex

The normal pupil constricts when the eyes focus on a near object.

Ciliospinal Reflex

The ciliospinal reflex refers to dilatation of the pupil when the skin of the ipsilateral side of the neck is pinched. It would be absent in Horner's syndrome.

Face

Note any abnormality of structure of the scalp, the forehead, the eyelids, the malar region, the chin.

Seventh Nerve

Examine the seventh nerve. Note the following:

♥ Position

♠ Size

♦ Movements at rest

♣ Power

♥ Reflexes

♠ Buccofacial Apraxia

♦ Taste Sensation

Position

Note the presence of the naso-labial fold and the position of the angle of the mouth. Observe whether the furrows on the skin of the forehead are equal on the two sides.

Size

Note the size of the facial muscles.

Movements at Rest

Observe the patient's facial expressions. One should note whether facial expressions are present or whether the face remains expres-sionless or whether there are any abnormal movements.

Power

Ask the patient to raise the eyebrows and wrinkle the forehead. Ask the patient to shut the eyes tightly. Attempt to open the patient's eyes whilst the patient offers resistance. Ask the patient to puff the cheeks out, tap the puffed out cheeks. Air will be pushed out more easily if one side is weak. Ask the patient to say "eee" and note movement of the lips and the lower part of the face. (Do not say, " Show me your teeth," as this may prompt the patient to remove his or her dentures and display them or point to a denture pot.)

Look for contraction of the facial muscles in the forehead, around the eyes and around the mouth. Look for contraction of the platysma.

Reflexes

The reflexes that may be elicited in relation to the facial nerve are the following:

♥ **Corneal Reflex**

The efferent arc of the corneal reflex is the facial nerve. This reflex will be discussed later.

♠ **Glabella Tap**

Place the fingers of one's left hand on the patient's forehead with the pulp of the middle finger on the glabella. One's hand should be brought in from above the patient's forehead with the palm facing the patient's forehead. Repeatedly tap the glabella with the finger. Unless there is an

404

abnormality, after a few initial blinks, the patient should stop blinking. In Parkinsonism the patient would go on blinking without cessation.

♦ **Snout Reflex**

In the snout reflex, gentle pressure against the patient's lips would, cause puckering of the lips.

♣ **Sucking Reflex**

In the sucking reflex, light contact near the corners of the mouth would result in opening of the mouth.

Buccofacial Apraxia (orofacial apraxia)

One may test for buccofacial apraxia if required. The method is to ask the patient to perform functions such as lick his or her lips or blow out matches.

Taste Sensation

Test taste sensation if required.

Ask the patient to rinse his or her mouth out with water. Then ask the patient to protrude his or her tongue and place the solutions provided on the tongue and ask the patient to indicate whether the taste is sensed before withdrawing the tongue. The solutions used are sugar, salt, citric acid and quinine to test sweet, salt, sour and bitter taste sensations. Test each solution separately and ask the patient to rinse out the mouth with water between tests. Test the bitter taste last.

Face and Jaws

Examine the structure of the jaws and then examine the functions of the trigeminal nerve.

Fifth Nerve (The Trigeminal)

The trigeminal nerve has two components:

♥ Motor Component

♠ Sensory Component

Motor Component (The Muscles of Mastication)

Examination of the motor component of the trigeminal nerve involves examination of the following:

♦ Size

♣ Power

♥ Reflexes

Size

Look for wasting of the temporalis and masseter muscles.

Power

Ask the patient to clench the teeth. Feel for contraction of the masseters and the temporalis muscles. Ask the patient to open the mouth whilst offering resistance by placing one's hand under the patient's chin. This will test the pterygoids. In unilateral weakness of the pterygoids, the jaw deviates to the side of the lesion.

Reflexes

The reflex that may be elicited in relation to the motor component of the trigeminal nerve is the:

♦ **Jaw Jerk**

Ask the patient to keep the mouth partially open. Place the middle finger of one's left hand over the patient's chin. The long axis of the finger should be parallel to the patient's lips. Gently strike the finger with a tendon hammer, which should be held lightly with one's right hand.

Sensory Component

Sensory examination is best left until examination of the lower limbs is concluded. But if required in a professional examination one should follow the system that will be described later.

♣ **Corneal reflex**

Test the corneal reflex if required. Remember that the afferent arc of the corneal reflex is the fifth nerve and the efferent is the seventh.

Hold a finger above the patient's head and ask the patient to look at it. With a wisp of cotton held in one's other hand, touch the exposed inferior aspect of the cornea. This should provoke blinking of the eyelids. For the contralateral eye remember to use a separate wisp of cotton to prevent the possibility of transmission of infection from one eye to the other.

Mouth

Examine the structure of the mouth. After this examine the functions of the 9th, 10th and 12th nerves.

Cranial Nerves Nine, Ten and Twelve (Glossopharyngeal, Vagus and Hypoglossal)

These nerves have a:

♥ Motor component

♠ Sensory component

Motor Component

Examination of the motor component of these nerves consists of examination of the soft palate and the tongue.

Soft Palate

Ask the patient to open his or her mouth. Note the following features of the soft palate.

♦ Position

♣ Movement

♥ Reflexes

Position

Note the position of the median raphe of the soft palate and the position of the uvula.

Movement

Ask the patient to say "Ah". Watch the movement of the soft palate. In unilateral lesions the soft palate would move to the normal side.

Reflexes

The reflex that is tested is the:

♠ **Gag Reflex**

Touch the soft palate with a spatula. Reflex contraction of the soft palate should be observed and the patient should be able to feel the touch of the spatula.

(In a professional examination this test should not be performed)

Tongue

Ask the patient to open the mouth. Note the following:

♦ Size

♣ Involuntary movements

♥ Tone

♠ Power

Size

Note the size of the tongue whilst the tongue rests on the floor of the mouth.

Involuntary Movements

Look for involuntary movements of the tongue whilst the tongue lies at rest on the floor of the mouth.

Tone

Note the tone as the tongue rests on the floor of the mouth.

Power

Ask the patient to put his or her tongue out and then move it first to one side and then to the other side.

In unilateral lesions the tongue would deviate to the affected side.

Sensory Component

Examination of the sensory component of the 9th nerve consists of the following:

♦ Touch sensation will be tested when performing the gag reflex.

♣ Test taste sensation in the posterior third of the tongue if required. This is rarely done in practice.

Neck and Shoulders

Look for any abnormality of structure of the neck and shoulders.

Eleventh Cranial Nerve (Accessory)

Note the following:

♥ Position

♠ Size

♦ Power

Position

Observe the position of the neck

Size

Note any wasting of the neck muscles and the trapezius.

Power

Place a hand on the patient's chin, ask the patient to turn the chin to one side and then to the other whilst offering resistance. Place one's hands on the patient's shoulders. Ask the patient to shrug the shoulders whilst offering resistance.

Ears

Examine the structure of the ears.

Eighth Cranial Nerve (Vestibulocochlear)

The eighth cranial nerve has two components the:

♥ Cochlear Component

♠ Vestibular Component

Cochlear Component (Hearing)

Test hearing by whispering in the patient's ears or by rubbing one's thumb, index and middle fingers together at the side of the patient's ears. Remember to close the patient's other ear by compressing the tragus with the thumb or fingers of one's other hand. Formal evaluation with a tuning fork may be required in which case one should perform Rinne's and Weber's test.

♦ **Weber's test**

Strike a 512 MHz tuning fork and hold it on the superior aspect of the frontal bone or on the vertex of the skull. Ask the patient in which ear he or she hears the sound better.

♣ **Rinne's test**

Strike a 512 MHz tuning fork and hold it near the patient' s ear. Then place it over the patient's mastoid process. Ask the patient where the sound is heard better.

Another way to do this is to ask the patient to say when the sound becomes indistinct and then hold the tuning fork in the alternative position and ask whether the sound is now heard more clearly.

Vestibular Component (Balance)

The tests done in relation to the vestibular component of the eighth nerve consist of looking for nystagmus and performing the Hallpike manoeuvre.

Hallpike Manoeuvre

Ask the patient to sit on the couch and look at the examiner's forehead. Rapidly lower the patient's head to a position below the horizontal. This will bring one ear into a dependent position. Repeat the manoeuvre on the other side. In a positive test the patient would develop vertigo and have nystagmus towards the dependent ear. Repetition of the test causes attenuation of the response.

This concludes examination of the cranial nerves. For ease of examination the order of examination has been rearranged. The order in which examination is performed is 1, 2, (3,4,6), 7, 5, (9,10,12), 11,8 or nose, eyes, face, mouth, neck, ears.

It would be best to pause at this point and make sure no structural abnormalities of the skull have been missed. Perform further evaluation of any structural abnormality by palpation. Perform auscultation over the orbits and the skull for bruits if required.

Summary of Examination of the Cranial Nerves

Although a complete system of examination of the cranial nerves has been described, in practice it would be difficult to perform such a comprehensive examination. Tests such as sensory examination of the face would usually be performed in conjunction with examination of the sensory system of the entire body, as this is more practical. In addition, in practice, taste sensation and olfactory sense are hardly ever formally examined. Hence, in practice examination of the cranial nerves would be as follows:

Nose

♥ Ask about sense of smell

Eyes

♠ Optic nerve

♦ 3rd, 4th and 6th nerves

Face

♣ Facial nerve

Mouth

♥ Test the motor component of the trigeminal then examine the 9th, 10th and 12th nerves

Neck and shoulders

♠ Test the accessory nerve

Ears

♦ Test hearing

Examination of the Cranial Nerves

♥ **Nose**	1st
♠ **Eyes**	2nd
	3rd, 4th, 6th
♦ **Face**	7th
	5th
♣ **Mouth**	
	Jaw 5th
	Palate 9th, 10th
	Tongue 12th
♥ **Neck**	11th
♠ **Ears**	8th

Examination of the Upper Limbs

One should examine:

♦ Structure

♣ Function

Examination of Structure

Look at the upper limbs. Note the following:

♥ Dimensions

♠ Integument (cover)

♦ Muscle mass (contents)

Dimensions

When examining the dimensions, note the following:

♠ Size

♦ Shape

409

Size

Note any change in the overall size of the limbs.

Shape

Note any deformity especially deformities of the hand

Integument

Note any trophic changes in the skin.

Muscle Mass

Note whether the muscle mass is normal, wasted or hypertrophied

Function

After examining the structure of the limbs one should proceed to examine function. The functions that are examined are:

♥ Motor Function

♠ Sensory Function

Motor Function

When examining motor function one should examine:

♠ Position

♦ Involuntary Movements

♣ Tone

♥ Power

♠ Reflexes

♦ Coordination

Position

Note the position of the limbs at rest.

Please remember that initially a functional change would result in a change in position. However, if the lesion were to be long standing structural changes occur and this would result in an alteration in shape (deformity).

Involuntary Movements

Observe whether there are any involuntary movements. If any involuntary movements are seen define them. The characteristics of involuntary movements that should be defined are:

♠ **Position**

Observe the position at which the involuntary movements occur.

They may be within muscle, involving a few muscle fascicles.

They may involve part of a limb or the whole limb.

♥ **Character**

Note the character of the movement. It may occur in a single plane or in multiple planes.

♠ **Quantity**

Note the degree of movement. It may be a slight movement or a large movement.

♦ **Rate**

Observe the rate at which the movements occur

♣ **Rhythm**

Note the rhythm displayed

♥ **Associated Features**

Note any associated features.

♠ **Modifying Factors**

Note whether movements occur at rest, whether they are postural or influenced by action.

Tone

First, test the tone of the muscles at the elbow and at the wrist. Support the patient's elbow with one hand and hold the patient's hand with the other. Note the tone whilst performing flexion and extension at the elbow, pronation and supination of the forearm and rotation at the wrist joint.

Next, raise the patient's arm up over the patient's head and let go allowing the arm to fall. Remember one should position one's other hand below the patient's arm to prevent the patient being hurt by the falling arm.

Myotonia

Shake hands with the patient. In myotonia the patient has difficulty letting go. This may have been noticed at the outset when one introduced oneself.

Percussion Myotonia

Percuss the thenar eminence. In percussion myotonia, a depression appears that fills up very slowly.

Power

Now test muscle power. Begin with an overall assessment and then test muscle groups.

Overall Assessment

Ask the patient to raise both upper limbs and hold them out in front of him or herself with the palms downwards. Look for a wrist drop. Next, ask the patient to turn the palms upwards. Now ask the patient to close his or her eyes. Observe any drift. There may be a drift upward, parietal drift, or a drift downwards with pronation, pronator drift.

Tap the patient's hands quite firmly. See whether they bounce back to their original position or whether they continue to drift down. Dysmetria may be assessed by this manoeuvre. In dysmetria the arm will overshoot its original position.

Muscle Groups

Next, examine muscle groups. Either begin at the shoulder and move distally or start at the hands and move proximally.

In this book we will start distally.

Hands

Before examining the power of the small muscles of the hands it would be wise to re-examine the structure of the hands in detail. Note:

♦ **Shape**

   Note any deformity

♣ **Size**

   Note any wasting of the small muscles of the hand and the distribution of the wasting

Then re-examine:

♦ **Position**

   Note the position of the hands and wrists at rest

Small Muscles of the Hand (T_1)

Ask the patient to turn the hands over with palms upwards. Test the power of thumb movements. One may test extension, flexion, abduction, adduction and opposition of thumb to fifth finger.

In practice one usually tests abduction and opposition. Ask the patient to push the thumb up towards the ceiling whilst offering resistance. Next, ask the patient to oppose the thumb and little finger and maintain opposition whilst one attempts to separate the thumb and little finger.

Now ask the patient to place the hands on a firm surface palms downwards. Test abduction and adduction of the fingers. Ask the patient to spread the fingers wide apart whilst one makes an attempt to bring them together. Next, ask the patient to grasp a sheet of paper between the fingers whilst one attempts to pull the paper away. Remember if the palms are not on a firm surface, contraction of the lumbricals could mimic function of the interossei and in radial nerve palsy a false impression of weakness of abduction and adduction may occur.

Long Flexors (C_8)

Next, test the long flexors of the fingers. This could be done by assessing grip strength or by an attempt to straighten the patient's partially flexed fingers.

Ask the patient to squeeze one's first and second fingers and assess grip strength. Remember to place the tips of one's fingers as far up the patient's palm as possible, preferably between the thenar and hypothenar eminences as this will prevent the patient attempting to crush one's fingers.

Alternatively, one may ask the patient to partially curl the fingers and ask the patient to prevent them being straightened whilst one attempts to straighten them. Remember to steady the patient's wrist with one's other hand whilst performing this test. This is probably the better test as it helps to differentiate weakness of flexion of the lateral and medial fingers.

Finger Extension ($C_{7,8}$)

Ask the patient to straighten the fingers. Fix the patient's hand with one hand and try to press the patient's fingers down with the other whilst the patient offers resistance.

Wrist (Flexion $C_{6,7}$ Extension $C_{7,6}$)

Now test flexion and extension at the wrist. Ask the patient to make a fist and then attempt to push the wrists first into a flexed and then into an extended position whilst the patient offers resistance.

Elbow (Flexion C_6, Extension C_7)

Test flexion and extension at the elbow. Ask the patient to flex the elbow and then push out whilst one offers resistance. Next, ask the patient to flex the elbow whilst one offers resistance.

Shoulder (Abduction C_5, Adduction C_6)

Test abduction and adduction at the shoulder. Ask the patient to flex the elbows and hold the flexed arms up so that the arms are in a horizontal position. One should then attempt to push the arms down. This tests the power of abduction. Next, from this position, ask the patient to bring his or her arms down to his or her side whilst resistance is offered to this movement. This tests adduction

Scapula

These tests would be performed only if indicated and are not usually done as a routine.

Serratus anterior (Long Thoracic Nerve $C_{5,6,7}$)

Ask the patient to push against resistance with outstretched arms. This would demonstrate winging of the scapulae in lesions affecting the long thoracic nerve.

Supraspinatus (Suprascapular Nerve C_5)

Ask the patient to initiate abduction with the arm against the patient's side whilst resistance is offered. Observe contraction of the muscle.

Infraspinatus (Suprascapular Nerve $C_{5,6}$)

Ask the patient to flex the elbow and keep the elbow by the side of the patient. Now ask the patient to externally rotate the arm whilst resistance is offered.

Summary of Examina Muscle Power of the Limbs

- ♥ **Raise Arms**
  Palms downwards
  Palms upwards
  Close eyes
  Tap palms
- ♠ **Thumbs**
  Abduction (T_1)
  Opposition (T_1)
- ♦ **Fingers**
  Abduction (T_1)
  Adduction (T_1)
  Flexion (C_8)
  Extension (C_7)
- ♣ **Wrist**
  Flexion (C_6)
  Extension (C_7)
- ♥ **Elbow**
  Flexion (C_6)
  Extension (C_7)
- ♠ **Shoulder**
  Abduction (C_5)
  Adduction (C_6)
- ♦ **Scapula**
  Serratus anterior
  Supraspinatus
  Infraspinatus

Grading of Muscle Power

Muscle power may be graded as:

- ♣ Grade 0: No movement
- ♥ Grade 1: A flicker of movement

- ♠ Grade 2: Movement with gravity eliminated
- ♦ Grade 3: Movement against gravity but not against resistance
- ♣ Grade 4: Movement against gravity and mild resistance
- ♥ Grade 5: Normal power

Reflexes

Examine the reflexes of the upper limb. They are as follows:

- ♠ Tendon reflexes
- ♦ Hoffman reflex
- ♣ Grasp reflex
- ♥ Palmomental reflex

Tendon Reflexes (Biceps, Triceps, Supinator)

Place the patient's partially flexed upper limbs across his or her torso. Hold the tendon hammer close to its pointed end and tap the tendon concerned. Allow the hammer to drop against the tendon rather than hitting the patient with it. Tap each tendon twice. Examine the:

- ♥ Biceps jerk
- ♠ Triceps jerk
- ♦ Supinator jerk.

Biceps Jerk

One's thumb or index finger should be placed over the biceps tendon. The tendon hammer should strike the examiner's thumb or index finger rather than the tendon directly.

Triceps Jerk

Raise the elbow slightly by holding the patient's hand or wrist so that movement at the elbow is not hindered by the examination bed or couch. Strike the tendon just above the elbow with the tendon hammer.

Supinator Jerk

Strike the distal end of the radius with the tendon hammer.

Reinforcement

If no reflexes are elicited, repeat with reinforcement. Ask the patient to clench his or her teeth.

Grading of Reflexes

The tendon reflexes may be graded as:

0: No reflex

1+: Slight response

2+: Brisk response

3+: Very brisk response

4+: Clonus

Hoffman Reflex

Hold the middle phalanx of the middle finger of one of the patient's hands with the thumb and index or middle fingers of one's left hand. Place the index or middle finger of one's right hand under the terminal interphalangeal joint of the patient's middle finger with the long axis of one's finger lying at right angles to the long axis of the patient's finger. Flick the tip of the patient's middle finger with one's thumb. That is, flex the distal phalanx and suddenly release. A positive response is flexion and adduction of the patient's fingers and thumb.

Repeat the test on the other side.

Grasp Reflex

Stroke the patient's palm in the area between the thumb and the index finger. In a positive response the patient will grasp the examiner's fingers and will not release the grip even when an attempt is made to distract the patient.

Palmomental Reflex

Scratch the skin near the thenar eminence with a key or pin. If the test is positive, brief contraction of the ipsilateral mentalis muscle occurs causing puckering of the chin.

Coordination

The tests performed are the:

- ♥ Finger nose test
- ♠ Dysdiadochokinesis
- ♦ Dysmetria

Finger Nose Test

Ask the patient to touch the tip of his or her nose with the tip of his or her extended index finger. Next, ask the patient to touch the tip of one's extended right index finger with the tip of his or her extended index finger. Repeat the process moving one's finger every time the patient touches the nose. Test both upper limbs.

Dysdiadochokinesis

Ask the patient to open one hand with the palm upwards. Then ask him or her to tap the open palm alternately with the palm of the other hand and the back of the other hand. Request the patient to do this as fast as he or she possibly can. Repeat the test on the other side.

Another method is to ask the patient to clap his or her hands together rapidly.

Dysmetria

Test for dysmetria by asking the patient to flex his or her elbows whilst one offers resistance initially and then suddenly lets go. Resistance is offered by holding the patient's forearm just proximal to the wrist. Remember to place one's other hand between the limb being tested and the patient's face to prevent the patient inadvertently hurting him or herself.

Dysmetria may have already been demonstrated when examining the outstretched arms.

Sensory System of the Upper Limbs

In practice, examination of the sensory system of the upper limbs would be best left until examination of the lower limbs is completed. However, in a professional examination if the instruction is to examine the upper limbs, one should perform sensory examination at this juncture. The method will be discussed later.

Tinel's Sign

Percuss over the flexor retinaculum. In the carpal tunnel syndrome this causes paraesthesiae (tingling) over the distribution of the median nerve. It is not only applicable to the median nerve and may be performed over any peripheral nerve.

Phalen's Sign

Flex the wrists for one minute. In the carpal tunnel syndrome, this causes tingling over the distribution of the median nerve.

Neck

Function of the neck muscles has already been examined when the accessory nerves were tested but remember to look for any structural lesion.

Chest

This is not an area that gives a lot of information in neurological assessment.

Motor Function

It is important to assess tidal volume in conditions where ascending paralysis could result in ventilatory failure.

Sensory Function

The main emphasis during examination of the chest will be the examination of the sensory system, which will be discussed later.

Abdomen

In the abdomen one may examine:

- ♥ Motor function
- ♠ Reflexes
- ♦ Sensory function

Motor Function

Look for any wasting and involuntary movements. Watch the respiratory movements of the abdomen. Paradoxical movement could occur in diaphragmatic palsy. Test power by asking the patient to lift up the head whilst lying on the bed or couch. Watch the umbilicus, as displacement of the umbilicus would demonstrate segmental weakness of the underlying abdominal musculature. One may also ask the patient to sit up from the supine position without using the hands.

Reflexes

Test the superficial reflexes by using the pointed end of the tendon hammer or an orange stick. Divide the abdomen into four quadrants and stroke each quadrant in turn. Use a radial movement from the periphery towards the umbilicus. Look for contraction of the underlying musculature. Movement of the umbilicus may be observed as evidence of a positive response.

Sensory Function

Testing of sensation may be left to be performed towards the end of the neurological examination.

Inguinal Region

In the inguinal region one would elicit the cremasteric reflex.

Cremasteric Reflex

Test the cremasteric reflex if required. Stroke the upper, inner part of the thigh. This causes contraction of the muscle and results in an upward movement of the testes.

Lower Limbs

Examine structure and function of the lower limbs.

Structure

Note the following:

- ♠ Dimensions
- ♦ Integument (cover)
- ♣ Muscle mass (contents)

Dimensions

When examining the dimensions note the following:

- ♥ Size
- ♠ Shape

Size

Note the overall size of the lower limbs.

Shape

Note any deformity

Integument

Note any trophic changes in the skin.

Muscle Mass

Note whether the muscle mass is normal, wasted or hypertrophied

Function

After examining the structure of the lower limbs one should proceed to examine function. The functions that are examined are:

- ♣ Motor Function
- ♥ Sensory Function

Motor Function

When examining motor function one should examine:

- ♥ Position
- ♠ Involuntary Movements
- ♦ Tone
- ♣ Power
- ♥ Reflexes
- ♠ Coordination

Position

Note the position of the limbs at rest.

Involuntary Movements

Look for any involuntary movements. Define them as discussed earlier.

Tone

Note the tone of the muscles at the:

- ♦ Hips
- ♣ Knees
- ♥ Ankles

Hips

With the patient lying with his or her lower limbs straight, roll the limb from side to side and note the tone.

417

Knees

Place one's right palm under the patient's knee and with a rapid movement raise the knee off the bed. Watch the foot and note its movement. This will give a very good assessment of muscle tone.

Ankle

Dorsiflex and plantarflex the foot and note the tone at the ankle.

Power

Begin assessment of power at the hips and work towards the foot.

Hips (Flexion $L_{1, 2}$, Extension L_5, S_1)

Test flexion of the hips. Place the palm of one's right hand just above the patient's knee and offer resistance whilst the patient is asked to lift the limb off the bed or couch.

Test extension of the hips. Lift the limb off the bed with one's hand under the patient's heel. Ask the patient to press the limb down to the bed and offer resistance.

Alternatively one may place the palm of one's right hand under the patient's thigh just above the knee. Raise the thigh off the bed and offer resistance whilst the patient is asked to press the thigh against the bed.

Hips (Abduction $L_{4, 5}$, Adduction $L_{2, 3}$)

Test abduction and adduction at the hip whilst offering resistance with one's palms just above the patient's knees.

Ask the patient to spread his or her limbs apart and offer resistance to abduction. Next, ask the patient to bring his or her limbs together and offer resistance to adduction.

Knee (Extension $L_{3, 4}$, Flexion L_5, S_1)

Place the patient's knee in a semi-flexed position. Hold the patient's leg with one's right hand just above the ankle and one's left hand on the patella steadying the knee. Ask the patient to flex the knee and offer resistance. Next, ask the patient to extend the knee and offer resistance.

Ankle (Dorsiflexion $L_{4, 5}$, Plantarflexion $S_{1, 2}$)

Test dorsiflexion and plantar flexion. Ask the patient to raise the foot up towards the head. Next, ask the patient to push the foot downwards. Offer resistance by placing one's right hand on the dorsum of the foot for dorsiflexion and on the sole of the foot for plantar flexion.

Eversion (L_5, S_1) and inversion (L_5, S_1) may be tested if required. Ask the patient to evert the foot against resistance and then ask the patient to invert the foot whilst offering resistance.

Toes (Big Toe Extension L_5, Flexion $S_{1, 2}$)

Test flexion and extension of the big toes. Offer resistance using one's thumb or fingers on the plantar and dorsal aspects of the toe.

Summary of Examination of Muscle Power in the Lower Limbs

♥ **Hips**

Flexion ($L_{1,2}$)

Extension (L_5)

Abduction (L_4)

Adduction (L_3)

♠ **Knees**

Flexion (L_5)

Extension (L_3)

♦ **Ankles**

Dorsiflexion (L_4)

Plantarflexion (S_2)

♣ **Big Toes**

Extension (L_5)

Flexion (S_1)

Reflexes

The reflexes that are tested are the:

♠ Tendon reflexes

♦ Superficial reflexes

Tendon Reflexes

The tendon reflexes tested in the lower limbs are the:

♣ Knee Jerk

♥ Ankle Jerk

Knee Jerk

Test the knee jerk by holding the semi-flexed knee up with one's left hand whilst the tendon hammer is used to strike the patellar tendon.

Ankle Jerk

Flex the patient's knee, externally rotate the hip and dorsiflex the ankle. Maintain this position with one's left hand holding the patient's forefoot and toes. Strike the Achilles tendon with the tendon hammer. Alternatively, one may place the ankle being tested over the contralateral lower leg and thus raise the ankle off the bedclothes.

Demonstrating the left ankle jerk is extremely difficult and should be practised a great deal. It is a good test of skill and one should take pride in being able to do this with ease.

Reinforcement

Remember, if it is not possible to elicit a reflex one should ask the patient to clench the teeth, make a fist or clasp the hands together and pull and thereby reinforce the reflex and retest before grading the reflex as absent.

Superficial Reflexes

The superficial reflex that is tested is the plantar response.

Plantar Response

Test the plantar response. Use the pointed end of the tendon hammer or an orange stick to perform this test. Draw the implement over the plantar aspect of the foot. First, move it along the lateral border of the foot beginning posteriorly and moving to the anterior aspect. When the anterior aspect is reached, draw the implement medially across the heads of the metatarsals. A positive response is fanning of the toes, dorsiflexion of the big toe, dorsiflexion at the ankle, flexion at the knee, flexion and external rotation at the hip.

In large corticospinal lesions, the receptive field or the area from which the response may be elicited increases. This allows other methods to be used to elicit this response. A number of eponymous reflexes have been described. They may be used if the standard test cannot be performed for any reason such as amputation of the toes or foot or dermatitis.

♣ **Chaddock**

Stroke the side of the foot from the external malleolus to the small toe.

♥ **Gordon**

Firmly squeeze the calf

♠ **Schaffer**

Pinch the Achilles tendon

♦ **Oppenheim**

Firmly press on the shin with one's knuckles and thumb and then run the knuckles and thumb down along the anterior tibia towards the foot.

♣ **Brissaud**

Elicit the plantar response in the usual fashion and note whether contraction of the tensor fascia latae muscle occurs.

Clonus

Clonus refers to a rhythmical contraction and relaxation of muscle in response to a suddenly applied and sustained stretch. Sustained clonus is abnormal and indicates an upper motor neurone lesion. Non-sustained clonus may occur in healthy people especially if they are tense or anxious. If exaggerated reflexes are observed, look for clonus at the:

♥ Knee

♠ Ankle

Knee

Place one's clenched right fist under the patient's knee and thus raise the knee off the bed. Grasp the patient's patella with the thumb and fingers of one's left hand (the thumb and fingers should be placed on either side of the patella). With a sudden movement push the patella inferiorly. Maintain this push and look for clonus.

Ankle

Place the ankle in the same position used to test the ankle jerk. Grasp the forefoot firmly with one's right hand and dorsiflex the foot with a sudden movement, which should be maintained. Observe if there is any clonus.

Coordination

Test coordination using the heel-shin test.

Heel-Shin Test

Place one of the patient's heels just below the contralateral knee and move this heel down the shin to the ankle. After this demonstration, ask the patient to perform the manoeuvre unaided. Test both sides.

Usually, this is the only test performed to test coordination in the lower limb. The other tests that may be performed are:

♥ Ask the patient to make circles with the foot by rotation around the ankle joint. (If proximal weakness precludes performance of the heel shin test)

♠ Ask the patient to rapidly tap the examiner's hand with the foot. (Dysdiadochokinesis)

Sensory System

Having completed examination of the motor system of the lower limb, this would be the best time to perform examination of the sensory system. Begin at the head and work down testing each dermatome in turn. Test all sensory modalities:

♦ Touch

♣ Light touch

♥ Pain

♠ Temperature

♦ Vibration sense

♣ Proprioception

Touch

For touch first demonstrate the test. Use the tip of the index finger to test touch. Tell the patient that they will be touched. Touch the patient and ask whether they can feel it. Then ask the patient to close his or her eyes and indicate verbally or by nodding the head whether an area is touched.

Light Touch

Use a wisp of cotton wool. Proceed in the same manner as for touch.

Pain and Temperature

When testing temperature and pain ask the patient whether they feel the change in temperature or the pain rather than touch. Use a disposable pin to test pain. Use bottles containing warm or cold water to test temperature sensation.

Vibration

For vibration sense use a 128 MHz tuning fork. Test by placing the tuning fork over a bony prominence. Ask specifically whether vibration is felt rather than touch.

Joint Position Sense

One may test joint position sense in the:

♦ Upper Limb

♣ Lower Limb

Upper Limbs

In the upper limbs test flexion and extension at the interphalangeal joint of the thumb. Hold the proximal phalanx of the patient's thumb with the thumb and forefinger of one hand and the distal phalanx of the patient's thumb with the thumb and forefinger of one's other hand. Hold the patient's thumb on either side and not anteriorly and posteriorly so that touch sensation does not come into play. Demonstrate the movement to the patient and explain what is expected and then ask the patient to shut his or her eyes and test. Flex and extend the joint and ask the patient to identify whether the joint is flexed or extended. It would be best not to alternate movements and thus create a pattern.

Lower Limbs

For the lower limbs test flexion and extension at the interphalangeal joint of the big toe. Hold the proximal phalanx of the big toe with the thumb and forefinger of one hand and the distal phalanx with the thumb and forefinger of one's other hand. Hold the toe on either side as for the thumb. Make sure that the first and second toes do not touch each other, as this will allow touch sensation to come into play.

Higher Sensory Function

If the sensory system is intact one may test higher sensory function.

♥ **Stereognosis**

Ask the patient to shut his or her eyes and then place a common object such as a coin or a key in the patient's palm and ask him or her to identify it.

♠ **Agraphaesthesia**

Ask the patient to shut the eyes. Draw a number or letter on the patient's skin and ask the patient to identify what has been drawn.

♦ **Two Point Discrimination**

Use a pair of blunt dividers to test the ability of the patient to differentiate between two points being stimulated simultaneously. Over the fingertips normally 2 mm of separation may be recognised. Over the toes a slightly wider separation may be recognised.

♣ **Sensory Inattention**

Ask the patient to close his or her eyes and then simultaneously stimulate corresponding points on the two sides of the body. The patient is asked to indicate which side or sides are being stimulated. In sensory inattention the patient does not perceive stimulation on the abnormal side.

Following examination of the lower limbs one should proceed to examine the perianal region and perform per rectal examination. This would not be expected in professional examinations and indeed even in practice most clinicians would not perform these examinations routinely.

Perianal Region

In the perianal region one may examine the anal reflex.

Anal Reflex

Test the anal reflex if required. Stroke or scratch the skin near the anus. Contraction of the anal sphincter should be observed.

Per Rectal Examination

Perform a rectal examination if required.

Anal Tone, Anal Squeeze Pressure

Note anal tone and test anal squeeze pressure by asking the patient to tighten the sphincter whilst performing rectal examination.

Next, examine the spine.

Spine

Examination of the spine is performed in three stages:

♥ Examination with the patient lying down

♠ Examination with the patient seated

♦ Examination with the patient standing up

Examination with the Patient Lying Down

One may examine:

♦ Structure

♣ Function

Structure

Look for:

♦ Neck stiffness

♣ Kernig's sign

♥ Straight leg raising

♠ Femoral stretch

These tests should be performed only if indicated.

Neck Stiffness

The patient should lie flat. Place one's left hand behind the patient's head. Gently rotate the head and feel for stiffness. Gently lift the head off the bed. Note any movement of the hips and knees. Pain in the neck, stiffness of the neck, flexion of the hips and knees indicates meningeal irritation.

Kernig's Sign

The patient should lie flat. Flex the patient's right hip and knee. Try to extend the knee. Resistance to straightening of the knee with pain and spasm of the hamstrings would mean Kernig's sign is positive.

Straight Leg Raising

The patient should lie flat. With one's right hand under the heel of the patient's foot, lift the straight leg up as far as possible. A positive sign is limitation of movement with pain radiating down the back of the limb. When this point is reached, lower the limb slightly and dorsiflex the foot. The pain should be reproduced.

Femoral Stretch

Ask the patient to lie prone. Flex the knee as far as possible. Limitation of flexion with pain radiating down the front of the limb is a positive sign.

Function (of the Spine)

The functions that may be examined are:

♦ Power

♣ Coordination

Power

This is rarely tested. Test the erector spinae by asking the patient to lie in the prone position and raise the head and or the lower limbs off the bed or couch. Note contraction of the erector spinae.

Coordination

Look for truncal ataxia.

423

Examination with the Patient Seated

Truncal Ataxia

Before assessing gait, ask the patient to sit on the edge of the bed and watch whether the patient is able to maintain balance. Ask the patient to fold his or her arms across the chest, as this will exaggerate any inability to maintain balance.

Gait

Now ask the patient to stand and walk a short distance, then turn and walk back. Observe and analyse gait.

Heel Toe Walking (Tandem Walking)

Ask the patient to walk in a straight line placing the heel of one foot directly in front of the toes of the other foot.

Analysis of Gait

Analyse gait using the usual procedure for analysing function.

♦ **Position**

One should observe the posture of the patient and the position of the limbs

♣ **Character**

Note the character of gait.

♥ **Quantity**

Make a note of the length of the steps taken.

♠ **Rate**

Note the rate at which the steps are taken.

♦ **Rhythm**

Note the rhythm with which the steps are taken

♣ **Associated Features**

Note whether arm swing is normal.

♥ **Modifying Factors**

Note the effect of asking the patient to perform tandem walking.

Romberg's Sign

Ask the patient to stand with his or her feet close together. Now ask the patient to shut his or her eyes and note whether the patient becomes unsteady. This is Romberg's sign. Remember to stand close to the patient and be prepared to steady the patient lest he or she falls.

Trendelenburg Test

Observe the patient from behind and ask the patient to stand on one leg. In health the hip with the leg raised should tilt upwards. If there is disease in the weight-bearing hip, the contralateral hip dips downwards.

Standing From a Seated or Squatting Position

Ask the patient to rise from a seated position and assess function of the pelvic girdle. Asking the patient to squat and assessing the ability to rise from the squatting position is a better test but it is not always possible to get the patient to do this in practice and in professional examinations.

Spine (with the patient standing)

If required one may examine the spine with the patient standing. The method of examination is described in the chapter on the locomotor system.

Apraxia

If no gross abnormality of motor or sensory function has been identified one may assess the patient's ability to perform complex tasks. The inability to perform complex tasks in the absence of a motor or sensory deficit is termed apraxia. The types of apraxia that occur are the following:

- ♠ Dressing Apraxia
- ♦ Reading
- ♣ Writing
- ♥ Constructional Apraxia

Dressing Apraxia

The ability to dress may be assessed by asking the patient to put on an item of clothing that has been turned inside out.

Reading and Writing

Assess the patient's ability to read and write if this has not been done already.

Constructional Apraxia

Test for constructional apraxia by asking the patient to draw a five-pointed star (the pen should not leave the paper whilst the star is being drawn) or a clock face (not a digital clock!)

Autonomic Nervous System

The autonomic nervous system is rarely examined in practice and hardly ever is this required in professional examinations.

The functions that are tested are:

- ♥ Pupils:

   Response to light and accommodation

- ♠ Skin:

   Sweating

- ♦ Pulse:

   Resting pulse rate

   Response to six maximal deep breaths

- ♣ Blood pressure:

   Postural variation

Pupils

In autonomic dysfunction the response of the pupils to light and accommodation would be abnormal

Skin

In autonomic dysfunction there would be a lack of sweating and the skin would be dry. This leads to a lack of friction as the skin becomes dry and powdery. If the skin is stroked with the back of one's finger this would be more obvious.

In conditions where a line of demarcation exists between normal autonomic function and abnormal autonomic function (for example unilateral Horner's syndrome, spinal transection), when the finger moves from the abnormal dry powdery area to the normal area with sweating, a change in resistance is felt by the finger. This test can also serve as a quick means of determining the sensory level in a spinal cord lesion.

Pulse

In autonomic dysfunction there would be a resting tachycardia and a lack of slowing in response to deep breaths.

Blood Pressure

Postural hypotension would be feature of autonomic dysfunction

This concludes examination of the nervous system.

Aide Memoire

The neurological history and examination may be simplified by thinking of it in terms of the cortex, the cranium, the cranial nerves, the spinal cord, the connections of the cord (the peripheral nerves) and the canal through which the spinal cord runs (the spine). Thus history and examination may be thought of as follows:

CNS

Cortex *(cerebral hemispheres)*

Cranium

Cranials

Cord

Connections *(motor, sensory, autonomic)*

Canal *(of the spinal cord, the spine)*

This gives **7 C**'s

Nerve Supply

It is important to have an idea of the nerve supply of the skin, the muscles and the reflexes. As an aid to remembering a summary follows:

Dermatomes

The dermatomes may be remembered as:

- ♠ **Trigeminal nerve: Face**
- ♦ **C_2: Back of scalp**
- ♣ **C_3: Neck**
- ♥ **C_4: Shoulder tip**

  C_5: Upper arm lateral aspect

C_6: Forearm lateral aspect

C_7: The middle fingers and the middle of the hand

C_8: Forearm medial aspect

T_1: Upper arm medial aspect

♠ **T_2: Axilla**

T_1 to T_3: Upper chest

♦ **T_4: Nipples**

T_4 to T_{10}: Nipples to umbilicus

♣ **T_{10}: Umbilicus**

T_{10} to L_1: Umbilicus to inguinal region

♥ **L_1 :Inguinal region**

L_2: Thigh medial aspect

L_3: Thigh lateral aspect

L_4: Lower leg lateral aspect

L_5: Lower leg medial aspect to dorsum of foot

♠ **S_1: Stand (Sole of foot)**

S_2, S_3: Narrow band at the back of lower limb

♦ **S_3: Sit (Buttocks)**

S_4: Between buttocks and anus

♣ **S_5: Around anus**

Remember the areas supplied by the Trigeminal nerve, C_2, C_4, T_2, T_4, T_{10}, L_1, S_1, S_3 and S_5. The other areas can be easily filled in as the dermatomes are consecutive.

Reflexes

The reflexes may be remembered as:

♥ Plantar 1

♠ Ankle Jerk 2

♦ Knee Jerk 3,4

♣ Supinator 5

♥ Biceps 6

♠ Triceps 7

Start at the bottom and work up and this makes it easy to remember the nerve supply of the reflexes.

Motor Supply

The motor supply may be remembered as:

Upper Limb

Start at the shoulder and work down

♦ Shoulder abduction is C_5

♣ Flexion of the elbow is C_6

♥ Extension of the elbow is C_7

♠ The long flexors are C_8

♦ The small muscles of the hand are T_1

Lower Limb

Start at the hip, work downwards to the toes along the anterior aspect and then back up again to the hip along the posterior aspect.

The inguinal region is L_1

Hip

♣ Hip flexion is L_1, L_2

♥ Hip adduction is L_3 (L_2)

♠ Hip abduction is L_4 (L_5)

♦ Hip Extension is L_5 (S_1)

Rest of the Lower Limb

♣ Hip flexion is L_1, L_2

♥ Knee extension is L_3, (L_4) (*Knee Flexion is L_5 (S_1)*)

♠ Ankle dorsiflexion is L_4, (L_5)

♦ Big toe extension is L_5

427

♣ Big toe flexion is S_1

♥ Ankle Plantar flexion is S_2 (S_1)

♠ Knee Flexion is L_5 (S_1)

As an aid to memorising the nerve roots of the lower limb, remember that the roots begin with L_1 at the hip and then go down the roots as they go down the anterior compartment to L_5. The sole of the foot is S_1 and plantar flexion S_2. Then come up the roots as they come back up from S_1 along the posterior compartment.

Lesions of the CNS

When considering lesions of the nervous system one should study lesions that affect the following:

♦ Brain

♣ Spinal cord

♥ Nerve roots

♠ Plexus lesions

♦ Peripheral nerves

♣ Neuromuscular junction

♥ Muscles

♠ Sensory organs

♦ Autonomic nerves

Brain

When studying lesions of the brain it would be best to categorise them into lesions involving the following:

♣ Ventricles

♥ Brain tissue

♠ Meninges

♦ Dural venous sinuses

♣ Skull

Ventricles

The ventricles may be affected by:

♥ Hydrocephalus

♠ Intraventricular haemorrhage

♦ Choroid plexus papilloma

Brain Tissue

Brain tissue may be affected by:

♠ Vascular lesions

♥ Neoplasms

♠ Inflammation

♦ Trauma

♣ Degeneration

♥ Functional disorders

♠ Cerebral oedema

Vascular Lesions of the Brain

The major vascular lesions of the brain are:

♦ Ischaemia

♣ Haemorrhage

Ischaemia

Ischaemia of the brain may be due to:

♥ Arterial Obstruction

♠ Venous Obstruction

Arterial Obstruction

Arterial obstruction may be caused by:

♦ **Luminal Factors**

Thrombosis, embolism, hypoperfusion (cardiovascular collapse), red cell disorders such as sickle cell disease, falciparum malaria

♣ **Mural Factors**

Atheroma, hypertension (damage to the vessel wall), vasculitis

Venous Obstruction

Venous obstruction may be due to:

♥ **Luminal Factors**

Thrombosis

♠ **Mural Factors**

Phlebitis

Haemorrhage

Haemorrhage may be due to:

♦ **Luminal Factors**

Bleeding diathesis, clotting disorders, hypertension

♣ **Mural Factors**

Aneurysm, hypertensive changes

♥ **External Factors**

Trauma

Distribution of Vascular Lesions of the Brain

Vascular lesions of the brain may be:

♠ Focal Lesions

♦ Diffuse Lesions

Cerebral Ischaemia

The distribution of cerebral ischaemia may be:

♣ **Focal Cerebral Ischaemia**

Focal cerebral ischaemia presents as an infarction

♥ **Global Cerebral Ischaemia (diffuse hypoxic/ischaemic encephalopathy)**

Global cerebral ischaemia results from a severe hypotensive episode

Cerebral Haemorrhage

The distribution of cerebral haemorrhage may be:

♠ **Focal**

This results in a localised intra-parenchymal haemorrhage.

♦ **Diffuse**

Hypertensive Encephalopathy

Hypertensive encephalopathy causes diffuse cerebral oedema and petechial haemorrhages

Neoplasms of Brain Tissue

Neoplasms affecting the nervous system may be:

♣ **Secondary Deposits**

Secondary deposits are the common lesions

♥ **Lymphoma**

Lymphoma occurs in the immunocompromised

♠ **Primary Lesions**

Primary lesions do not affect the neurones but affect the connective tissue cells

Primary Neoplasms of the Nervous System

Primary neoplasms of the nervous system may be:

♦ Neurofibroma

♣ Meningioma

♥ Glioma either Astrocytoma or Oligodendroglioma

Other lesions that may occur are:

♠ Ependymoma from the ependymal lining of the ventricles usually the fourth

- ◆ Choroid plexus papilloma
- ♣ Chordoma of the skull base
- ♥ Cerebellar tumours such as medulloblastoma, which usually occurs in childhood, cerebellar haemangioblastoma
- ♠ Glomus tumour; a vascular tumour of the jugular bulb

The intracranial glands may give rise to:

- ◆ Pinealoma
- ♣ Pituitary tumours, craniopharyngioma

Inflammation of Brain Tissue

Inflammation of brain tissue may be acute or chronic. Depending on the component involved the result may be:

- ♥ **Encephalitis**: inflammation involving nerve cells
- ♠ **Demyelination**: inflammation involving the myelin sheath
- ◆ **Vasculitis**: inflammation involving blood vessels
- ♣ **Cerebral Abscess**: acute inflammation and suppuration involving the parenchyma
- ♥ **Granuloma**: chronic inflammation involving the parenchyma

Encephalitis

Encephalitis is caused by:

- ♠ **Viruses** Echo, Coxsackie, mumps, herpes simplex, Japanese B, rabies

Demyelination

Demyelination may be due to:

- ◆ **Multiple Sclerosis**

- ♣ **Acute Disseminated Encephalomyelitis**

Acute disseminated encephalomyelitis may be due to:

Viral Infections: measles, chicken pox, rubella

Immunisation. It occurs following immunisation for small pox, rabies, pertussis

- ♥ **Acute Necrotising Haemorrhagic Encephalomyelitis**

Acute necrotising haemorrhagic encephalomyelitis is a syndrome that may occur after a respiratory infection.

- ♠ **Central Pontine Myelinolysis**

Central pontine myelinolysis occurs following rapid correction of hyponatraemia

Vasculitis

Vasculitis may be associated with conditions involving the:

- ◆ **LMS** systemic lupus erythematosus, rheumatoid arthritis, scleroderma, relapsing polychondritis, temporal arteritis, Lyme disease
- ♣ **GIT** coeliac disease, ulcerative colitis
- ♥ **RS** Wegener's granulomatosis, sarcoidosis
- ♠ **HS** lymphoma, hairy cell leukaemia, serum sickness, cryoglobulinaemia, Henoch-Schonlein purpura
- ◆ **RAG** syphilis, AIDS
- ♣ **Toxins** cocaine

Brain Abscess

A brain abscess may be due to:

- ♥ Pyogenic bacteria
- ♠ Fungi
- ♦ Amoebae

Primary Focus of Infection

The primary focus of infection, from which a cerebral abscess arises, may be:

- ♣ **Undefined**
- ♥ **Local External**

  Nose, paranasal sinus, middle ear, skull fracture

- ♠ **Systemic**

  Heart, lungs, abdomen

Granuloma

Granulomata of the brain may be due to:

- ♦ Tuberculosis
- ♣ Sarcoidosis
- ♥ Syphilis

Trauma

Trauma to the brain may result in:

- ♠ Contusion
- ♦ Laceration
- ♣ Diffuse Axonal Injury
- ♥ Cerebral Oedema (as a secondary phenomenon)

Degeneration

Degeneration of brain tissue may be due to:

- ♣ **Internal Factors**

Inherited diseases: Huntington's disease

Acquired conditions: viral infections, prion disease, Alzheimer's disease, Pick's disease, Parkinson's disease

- ♦ **External Factors**

External factors that cause degeneration of brain tissue are:

Compression: hydrocephalus, chronic subdural haematoma

Trauma: repetitive trauma as in professional boxers

- ♣ **Systemic Factors**

Systemic factors that result in degeneration of brain cells are conditions affecting the:

E&M Vitamin deficiencies like thiamine, vitamin B_{12}, niacin (pellagra), chronic hypoglycaemia, magnesium toxicity, manganese toxicity, hypothyroidism

RS non-metastatic manifestations of bronchial neoplasm

RAG AIDS, syphilis

KUS dialysis dementia

Toxins alcohol, lead

Functional Disorders

Under functional disorders one may include diseases where no definite pathological process has been demonstrated. This may be due to:

- ♥ **Internal Factors**

  Epilepsy

- ♠ **Systemic Factors**

  Failure of other systems (respiratory failure, liver failure, nutritional failure, renal failure, cardiac failure). This initially results in a functional disorder but if it is persistent it progresses to cell degeneration and death.

Cerebral Oedema

Cerebral oedema occurs:

- ♦ As a consequence of a primary pathological process in the brain
- ♣ Secondary to major organ failure

Meninges

Conditions that involve the meninges are:

- ♥ Benign intracranial hypertension
- ♠ Meningitis both acute and chronic
- ♦ Meningeal infiltration
- ♣ Subarachnoid haemorrhage
- ♥ Subdural haemorrhage
- ♠ Extradural Haemorrhage
- ♦ Meningioma

Dural Venous Sinuses

The dural venous sinuses may be affected by:

- ♦ Thrombosis
- ♣ Phlebitis

Skull

Conditions that affect the skull are:

- ♥ Fractures
- ♣ Tumours
- ♦ Inflammatory lesions
- ♠ Platybasia refers to flattening of the base of the skull. This may be congenital or occur in Paget's disease
- ♦ Basilar invagination refers to invagination of the base of the skull with upward movement of the odontoid peg.

Lesions of the Spinal Cord

When studying lesions of the spinal cord one should consider lesions affecting the:

- ♣ Central canal
- ♥ Cord
- ♠ Meninges
- ♦ Vertebral column
- ♣ External Factors

Central Canal

The central canal of the spinal cord may be affected by lesions such as:

- ♥ Syringomyelia

Cord

The cord may be affected by:

- ♠ Neoplasms
- ♦ Vascular lesions
- ♣ Degeneration
- ♥ Inflammatory lesions

Neoplasms

Neoplasms that occur in the spinal cord are similar to those that occur in the brain. The commonest secondary deposits are those from the lung, breast, kidney and prostate.

Vascular Lesions

Vascular lesions are similar to those that occur in the brain. They may be ischaemic or haemorrhagic.

Degeneration

Degeneration of the spinal cord may be due to:

- ♣ Motor neurone disease
- ♥ HTLV-1 infection
- ♠ Vitamin B_{12} deficiency
- ♦ Tabes dorsalis

Inflammatory Lesions

The inflammatory lesions that affect the brain may also affect the spinal cord. Important lesions in relation to the spinal cord are:

- ♣ Multiple sclerosis
- ♥ Transverse myelitis

Meninges

Lesions that occur in the meninges overlying the spinal cord are:

- ♠ Meningioma
- ♦ Meningitis
- ♣ Subarachnoid haemorrhage
- ♥ Meningeal infiltration

Vertebral Column

The vertebral column may be affected by:

- ♣ Fractures
- ♥ Osteoporotic collapse
- ♠ Prolapsed intervertebral disc
- ♦ Spondylosis

- ♣ Tumours usually secondaries
- ♥ Myeloma
- ♠ Inflammatory lesions such as rheumatoid arthritis, ankylosing spondylitis
- ♦ Abscess
- ♣ Tuberculosis

External Factors

External factors that cause lesions of the spinal cord are:

- ♥ Radiation myelopathy
- ♠ Trauma

Lesions of the Nerve Roots (Radiculopathy)

The nerve roots may be affected by:

- ♦ **Inflammatory Disorders**

  Inflammation of the nerve roots occurs in:

  Acute Inflammatory Demyelinating Polyradiculoneuropathy (Guillain-Barre syndrome)

  Chronic Inflammatory Demyelinating Polyradiculoneuropathy

- ♣ **Compression**

  Compression of the nerve roots occurs in:

  Spondylosis, slipped disc

Plexus Lesions

Plexus lesions are usually due to:

- ♥ Trauma
- ♠ Malignant infiltration

433

- Thoracic outlet syndrome

Peripheral Nerves

Lesions of the peripheral nerves may be classified as:

- ♣ Mononeuropathy
- ♥ Mononeuritis Multiplex
- ♠ Distal Symmetrical Polyneuropathy

Mononeuropathy

Mononeuropathy refers to a disease process involving a single nerve. It may be due to:

- **Internal Factors**

    Neuralgic amyotrophy, neurofibroma

- ♣ **External Factors**

    Entrapment neuropathy like carpal tunnel syndrome, meralgia paraesthetica

    Malignant infiltration or compression by tumours. This may give rise to cranial nerve palsies, obturator palsy from pelvic malignancies

    Trauma

- ♥ **Systemic Factors**

    Conditions affecting the:

    E&M diabetic amyotrophy

Remember a mononeuropathy may be part of mononeuritis multiplex.

Mononeuritis Multiplex

Mononeuritis multiplex refers to a disease process involving several nerves. It may occur in conditions affecting the:

- ♠ **E&M** diabetes mellitus
- ♦ **LMS** rheumatoid arthritis, systemic lupus erythematosus, polyarteritis nodosa, Sjogren's syndrome, Lyme disease
- ♣ **RS** Churg-Strauss syndrome, sarcoidosis
- ♥ **IS** leprosy
- ♠ **HS** amyloidosis

It may also occur in carcinoma

Distal Symmetrical Polyneuropathy

Distal symmetrical polyneuropathy refers to a diffuse, bilateral, symmetrical disease process involving the peripheral nerves. This usually begins distally and progresses proximally. It may be due to:

- **Internal Factors**

    Hereditary Diseases

    Hereditary Motor Sensory Neuropathy Type I (autosomal dominant inheritance, early onset, skeletal deformity common)

    Hereditary Motor Sensory Neuropathy Type II (autosomal dominant commonly, less severe course, tends to be confined to the lower limbs, skeletal deformity less common)

    Hereditary Motor Sensory Neuropathy Type III (Dejerine-Sottas disease a severe, slowly progressive disease with onset in childhood)

    X-linked Hereditary Motor Sensory Neuropathy (similar to HMSN I)

Hereditary Sensory and Autonomic Neuropathy (HSAN) several types have been described

Familial Amyloid Polyneuropathies (sensory neuropathy with autonomic involvement, cardiomyopathy, renal failure)

Hereditary Neuropathy with liability to Pressure Palsies (HNPP diffuse distal neuropathy with isolated mononeuropathy)

Refsum's disease

♣ **Systemic Factors**

Systemic factors that cause distal symmetrical polyneuropathy are conditions affecting the:

E&M diabetes mellitus, vitamin deficiencies B_1, B_6, B_{12}, porphyria (acute intermittent porphyria, variegate porphyria, hereditary coproporphyria)

Toxins alcohol, heavy metals

Drugs isoniazid, nitrofurantoin, metronidazole, ethambutol amiodarone, cyclosporin, gold, vincristine, thalidomide

KUS uraemia

Paraneoplastic effect of tumours

Critical illness polyneuropathy occurs in patients who are in intensive care units and have sepsis and multiple organ failure

Neuromuscular Junction

The neuromuscular junction may be affected by:

♥ Myasthenia gravis

♠ Eaton-Lambert syndrome

♦ Botulism

♣ Snake venom

Muscle

Disorders of muscle may be due to:

♥ **Internal Factors**

Internal factors that cause disorders of muscle are:

Genetic Disorders: muscular dystrophies, channelopathies, abnormalities of lipid metabolism, mitochondrial myopathies, glycogen storage diseases

Inflammatory Disorders: myositis

Necrosis: rhabdomyolysis

♠ **Systemic Disorders**

Systemic disorders that result in lesions of the muscles are conditions affecting the:

E&M thyrotoxicosis, Cushing's syndrome, acromegaly, hypocalcaemia

Paraneoplastic syndrome

Muscular Dystrophies

Muscular dystrophies are primary diseases of muscle caused by a genetic defect. They cause muscular weakness and are usually progressive. The types are:

♦ Facioscapulohumeral (autosomal dominant, onset late childhood or adolescence with weakness in the face progressing to involve the shoulder girdle)

♣ Limb Girdle Muscular Dystrophies

435

This refers to a group of disorders that present with weakness of the proximal musculature. Genetic defects have been identified for many of them and several distinct syndromes are defined.

♥ Emery-Dreifuss (X-linked recessive, autosomal dominant and autosomal recessive forms may occur. It causes wasting and weakness of the scapulohumeral and peroneal muscles)

♠ Oculopharyngeal (autosomal dominant, late presentation, causes ptosis and dysphagia)

♦ Pseudohypertrophic Muscular Dystrophy (Dystrophin Deficiency)

This refers to two X-linked conditions that result from deletions of the dystrophin gene.

Duchenne (more severe, occurs in childhood)

Becker (much milder, presents later)

♣ Myotonic Dystrophy

This refers to muscular dystrophy with myotonia. Two types are known:

Dystrophia myotonica (autosomal dominant affects eyes, face, jaw, larynx, hand and foot)

Proximal myotonic dystrophy (onset in adult life with stiffness, muscle pain, proximal weakness)

♥ Congenital Muscular Dystrophies. These disorders have very early childhood onset. A number of disorders have been described.

Channelopathies (Ion Channel Myopathies)

This refers to inherited disorders of ion channels. They usually present with abnormalities of muscle tone. The abnormalities may be:

♠ **Hypotonia**

Periodic paralysis, which may be normokalaemic, hypokalaemic or hyperkalaemic

♦ **Myotonia**

Myotonia congenita, which may be of two types:

Thomsen's disease (autosomal dominant, muscle hypertrophy and myotonia)

Becker type (autosomal recessive, later onset, myotonia may be more severe)

Paramyotonia congenita (autosomal dominant, myotonia on exercise or exposure to cold)

♣ **Malignant Hyperthermia**

Malignant hyperthermia causes muscular rigidity and a hypermetabolic state on exposure to anaesthetic agents

Abnormalities of Lipid Metabolism

Abnormalities of lipid metabolism may present with muscular weakness. They are:

♥ Carnitine palmitoyl transferase deficiency (autosomal recessive, presents in adolescence or early adulthood with muscle pain, rhabdomyolysis, myoglobinuria precipitated by fasting, exercise, infection)

♠ Carnitine deficiency

♦ Defects of beta-oxidation

♣ Myoadenylate   deaminase deficiency

Mitochondrial Myopathies

In these disorders there is an abnormality of the mitochondrial respiratory chain. The mitochondrial myopathies are:

♥ Chronic progressive external ophthalmoplegia (presents in childhood or early adult life with ptosis and ophthalmoplegia)

♠ Kearns-Sayre syndrome (chronic progressive external ophthalmoplegia with retinitis)

♦ Myopathy, Encephalopathy, Lactic Acidosis and Stroke-Like Episodes (MELAS); presents in childhood with short stature and any of the above

♣ Myoclonic Epilepsy with Ragged Red Fibres (presents in adolescence or early adulthood with proximal muscle weakness, ataxia, deafness, seizures)

♥ Leber's hereditary optic atrophy

♠ Leigh syndrome (relapsing encephalopathy with cerebellar and brainstem signs)

Glycogen Storage Diseases

Several of the glycogen storage diseases present with skeletal muscle involvement. They are:

♦ Acid maltase deficiency (may present as an adult form with proximal limb girdle myopathy

and symptoms of respiratory failure)

♣ Myophosphorylase deficiency (McCardle's disease); an adult form may occur with muscle cramps, exercise intolerance, wasting, weakness and myoglobinuria.

♥ Other disorders are:

Phosphofructokinase deficiency, debrancher enzyme deficiency, defects of distal glycolysis

♠ Adult Onset Nemaline Myopathy (cardiomyopathy associated with proximal and distal weakness presenting in the fourth and fifth decades)

Inflammatory Myopathies (Myositis)

Inflammation of the muscles may occur in:

♦ Polymyositis

♣ Dermatomyositis

♥ Infections: coxsackie virus infection, gas gangrene, leptospirosis, pyogenic infection following trauma, *Trichinella spiralis*

Rhabdomyolysis

Rhabdomyolysis or necrosis of muscle may be due to:

♠ **Internal Factors**

Internal factors that result in rhabdomyolysis are the following:

Genetic Disorders: glycolytic enzyme deficiencies, fatty acid oxidation disorders (carnitine palmitoyl transferase II

deficiency), mitochondrial myopathies

Infections: viral or bacterial

♦ **Mural Factors**

Ischaemia

♣ **External Factors**

Rhabdomyolysis may be due to compression as in:

Compartment syndromes, pressure necrosis in unconscious patients

♥ **Systemic Factors**

Systemic factors that result in rhabdomyolysis are conditions affecting the:

LMS unaccustomed exertion

Drugs alcohol, opiates, statins

CNS prolonged seizures, neuroleptic malignant syndrome

Sensory Organs

Specific problems that would be encountered are those related to the special senses. These disorders will be dealt with later under the relevant sections.

Autonomic Nerves

Abnormalities of autonomic function may be caused by lesions of the autonomic nervous system that result from conditions affecting the following:

♠ **CNS**

Hereditary Conditions: hereditary sensory and autonomic neuropathy, familial amyloid polyneuropathy

Degenerative Conditions: multi-system atrophy, pure autonomic failure (young to middle aged patients with orthostatic hypotension, nocturia, constipation)

Inflammatory Conditions: Guillain-Barre syndrome, transverse myelitis

Toxins tetanus

♦ **E&M** diabetes mellitus, porphyria, vitamin B_{12} deficiency

♣ **Toxins** alcohol, heavy metals, Botulinum toxin

♥ **Drugs** vincristine, cisplatin

♠ **LMS** rheumatoid arthritis, systemic lupus erythematosus, Raynaud's phenomenon, erythromelalgia

♦ **GIT** liver failure

♣ **KUS** uraemia

♥ **HS** amyloidosis

♠ **RAG** HIV infection

♦ **IS** leprosy

♣ **Paraneoplastic syndrome**

Degenerative Disorders of Motor Function

Degenerative disorders of motor function are not common but they are long lasting and are often seen in professional examinations. It would be wise to study these conditions when preparing for exams.

Anatomical Regions Affected

The anatomical regions that are affected in these conditions are the:

- ♥ Motor Neurones
- ♠ Basal ganglia
- ♦ Cerebellum
- ♣ Peripheral nerves
- ♥ Muscles

Motor Neurones

Degenerative disorders that affect the motor neurones may involve the:

- ♠ Upper Motor Neurones
- ♦ Lower Motor Neurones
- ♣ Combination of Upper and Lower Motor Neurones

Upper Motor Neurones

Degenerative disorders that affect the upper motor neurones are:

- ♥ **Primary Lateral Sclerosis**

  Primary lateral sclerosis is a rare, sporadic form of motor neurone disease. Average age of onset fifty years.

- ♠ **Pure Hereditary Spastic Paraplegia**

  Pure hereditary spastic paraplegia is an inherited, slowly-progressive, spastic paraparesis. Onset fourth to sixth decade.

- ♦ **Complex Hereditary Spastic Paraparesis**

  In complex hereditary spastic paraparesis, in addition to spastic paraparesis patients have other features such as mental retardation, optic atrophy, retinopathy,

deafness, ataxia, extrapyramidal features, muscle wasting, peripheral neuropathy and skin changes. Several syndromes have been described.

Lower Motor Neurones

Degenerative disorders that affect the lower motor neurones are:

- ♣ **Proximal Hereditary Motor Neuronopathy**

  This may present as:

  Acute Infantile form (Werdnig-Hoffman a fatal autosomal recessive disorder of childhood)

  Childhood form (Kugelberg-Welander autosomal recessive, onset infancy to early teens)

  Adult Onset Form (autosomal recessive, starts from fifteen to sixty years)

- ♥ **Focal Spinal Muscular Atrophy**

  Focal spinal muscular atrophy presents in young adult males with distal wasting and weakness of one forearm or hand. This progresses for about two years after which it stabilises or the rate of progression slows.

- ♠ **X-liked Recessive Bulbospinal Neuronopathy**

  X-linked recessive bulbospinal neuronopathy affects the face and bulbar muscles. Mild proximal weakness may have been present for years, gynaecomastia, testicular atrophy and diabetes mellitus may also feature

- ♦ **Hereditary Bulbar Palsy of Infancy and Childhood**

Hereditary bulbar palsy of infancy and childhood usually presents in the teens with bilateral sensorineural deafness followed by bulbar, facial, limb and respiratory weakness (sometimes)

Combination of Upper and Lower Motor Neurones

Degenerative disorders that affect the upper and lower motor neurones are:

♣ **Amyotrophic Lateral Sclerosis**

Amyotrophic lateral sclerosis starts off as bulbar or spinal disease although both become evident as the disease progresses.

Basal Ganglia

Degenerative disorders that affect the basal ganglia are:

♥ Parkinsonism

♠ Parkinsonism-plus syndromes

♦ Huntington's disease

♣ Wilson's disease

Cerebellum

Degenerative disorders that affect the cerebellum result in cerebellar ataxia.

Cerebellar Ataxia

Cerebellar degeneration resulting in cerebellar ataxia may be:

♥ Inherited

♠ Acquired

The acquired forms will be discussed later.

Inherited Ataxic Disorders

Inherited ataxic disorders are:

♦ Congenital ataxias (several types described, they are not dealt with here)

♣ Autosomal recessive cerebellar ataxia

♥ Autosomal dominant cerebellar ataxia

Autosomal Recessive Ataxias

Autosomal recessive ataxias are usually of early onset (before twenty years of age). They are:

♠ Friedrich's ataxia

♦ Early onset cerebellar ataxia with other associated features:

Pigmentary retinopathy, cataract, deafness, optic atrophy, hypogonadism, myoclonus, retained tendon reflexes

♣ Autosomal recessive late onset ataxia

Autosomal Dominant Ataxias

Autosomal dominant ataxias are usually of later onset, after twenty years of age. They are:

♥ Autosomal Dominant Cerebellar Ataxia type I. This is a progressive cerebellar ataxia with associated extracerebellar features such as optic atrophy, ophthalmoplegia, peripheral neuropathy, pyramidal and extrapyramidal signs

♠ Autosomal Dominant Cerebellar Ataxia type II. This is a cerebellar syndrome with pigmentary macular dystrophy

- Autosomal Dominant Cerebellar Ataxia type III. This is a pure cerebellar syndrome

Peripheral Nerves

Disorders of the peripheral nerves have been discussed earlier

Muscles

Degenerative disorders of the muscles are:

Muscular Dystrophies

Muscular dystrophies have been discussed earlier

Parkinsonism-plus Syndromes

Parkinsonism-plus syndromes refer to conditions in which there are features of Parkinsonism together with additional features. The conditions are:

- ♣ Multisystem Atrophy
- ♥ Progressive Supranuclear Palsy
- ♠ Cortico Basal Ganglion Degeneration
- ♦ Dementia with Lewy Bodies

Multisystem Atrophy

Conditions included in this category are:

- ♣ **Olivopontocerebellar Degeneration**

   The distinguishing feature is ataxia
- ♥ **Striato Nigral Degeneration**

   The distinguishing feature is rigidity, no tremor

- ♠ **Shy-Drager Syndrome**

   The distinguishing feature is autonomic dysfunction

Progressive Supranuclear Palsy

The features of progressive supranuclear palsy are:

- ♦ It affects eye movements; inability to move the eyes up and down.

It also results in:

- ♣ Neck dystonia
- ♥ Dysarthria
- ♠ Tendency to suddenly lose balance

Cortico Basal Ganglion Degeneration

The features of cortico basal ganglion degeneration are:

- ♦ Asymmetry of features
- ♣ Apraxia
- ♥ Action myoclonus; jerky abnormal movements superimposed on normal movements
- ♠ Stimulus sensitive myoclonus

Lewy Body Dementia

The features of Lewy body dementia are:

- ♦ Progressive dementia
- ♣ Fluctuations in cognitive impairment
- ♥ Visual hallucinations (sometimes auditory)
- ♠ Paranoid delusions
- ♦ Mild extrapyramidal features or sensitivity to neuroleptics

♣ Falls

♥ Variations in consciousness

Blood Supply of the Brain

It is important to have a sound knowledge of the blood supply of the brain in order to understand cerebrovascular disease. The blood vessels that supply the brain are the following:

♠ **Anterior Cerebral Artery**

The anterior cerebral artery supplies the orbital surface of the frontal lobe and the whole of the medial surface of the cerebral hemisphere above the corpus callosum to the parieto-occipital sulcus. It supplies the motor and sensory areas of the opposite lower limb and the perineum and also supplies the micturition and defecation centres.

♦ **Middle Cerebral Artery**

The middle cerebral artery supplies the motor and sensory areas of the opposite half of the body except the lower limb and perineum. It also supplies the speech and auditory areas.

♣ **Posterior Cerebral Artery**

The posterior cerebral artery supplies the inferomedial aspect of the temporal lobe, the occipital lobes and the upper brain stem. The macular area is supplied by the middle cerebral artery.

♥ **Anterior Choroidal Artery**

The anterior choroidal artery supplies the optic tract and radiation, the lateral geniculate body, the posterior part of the internal capsule, basal nuclei and limbic system.

♠ **Midbrain**

The midbrain is supplied by the posterior cerebral and the superior cerebellar arteries

♦ **Pons**

The pons is supplied by the basilar artery

♣ **Medulla**

The blood supply of the medulla is:

Ventrally: the vertebral and basilar arteries

Laterally and dorsally: the posterior inferior cerebellar arteries

Internal Capsule

The internal capsule carries afferent fibres to the cortex and efferent fibres from the cortex. It has an:

♥ Anterior Limb

♠ Genu

♦ Posterior Limb

Anterior Limb

The anterior limb lies between the head of the caudate nucleus medially and the lentiform nucleus laterally. It carries frontopontine fibres

Genu

The genu lies at the apex of the globus pallidus. It caries corticonuclear fibres from the cortex to the cranial nerve nuclei.

Posterior Limb

The posterior limb lies between the thalamus medially and the lentiform nucleus laterally. The anterior two thirds of the posterior limb carry corticospinal fibres; (from anterior to posterior) arm, hand, trunk, leg, perineum. Posterior to these fibres lie the sensory, visual and auditory fibres.

Anterior Perforated Substance

The anterior perforated substance receives branches from the middle cerebral artery. They supply the internal capsule, the thalamus and the basal nuclei.

Posterior Perforated Substance

The posterior perforated substance receives branches from the posterior cerebral artery. They supply the thalamus and the basal ganglia.

Spinal Cord

The blood supply of the spinal cord is from the:

♣ **Anterior Spinal Artery**

The anterior spinal artery supplies the whole of the cord anterior to the posterior grey columns.

♥ **Posterior Spinal Artery**

The posterior spinal artery supplies the white and grey posterior columns of its own side.

Lesions of Motor Function

Evaluation of motor function follows a well-defined routine. It is assessment of:

♠ Muscle Mass
♦ Involuntary Movements
♣ Muscle Tone
♥ Muscle Power
♠ Reflexes
♦ Coordination

It is easy to classify lesions of the motor system on this basis.

Muscle Mass

On examination one may note that the muscle mass is:

♣ Normal
♥ Wasted
♠ Hypertrophied

Wasting

Wasting may be due to:

♦ Lower motor neurone disease
♣ Myopathy
♥ Disuse

Hypertrophy

Hypertrophy may be:

♠ Physiological

Or it may be due to:

♦ Myopathy

Generalised hypertrophy is seen in myotonia congenita

Localised hypertrophy (calf muscles) occurs in Duchenne and Becker muscular dystrophy

Involuntary Movements

Involuntary movements may be caused by lesions at various levels of the motor system. These lesions may be at the level of:

- ♣ Muscle
- ♥ Neuro-Muscular Junction
- ♠ Lower Motor Neurone
- ♦ Upper Motor Neurone
- ♣ Basal Ganglia
- ♥ Cerebellum
- ♠ Higher Centres
- ♦ Systemic Factors

Muscle

Involuntary movements caused by lesions at muscle level are:

- ♣ Tetany due to hypocalcaemia

Neuro-Muscular Junction

Denervation causes:

- ♥ Fibrillation of the muscles however this is not detectable clinically

Lower Motor Neurone

Lesions at the level of the lower motor neurone cause:

- ♠ Fasciculation

Upper Motor Neurone

Lesions at the level of the upper motor neurone cause:

- ♦ Myoclonus

Basal Ganglia

Lesions at the level of the basal ganglia commonly result in involuntary movements. These involuntary movements may be:

- ♣ Chorea
- ♥ Ballism
- ♠ Parkinsonism
- ♦ Dyskinesia
- ♣ Dystonia
- ♥ Torticollis
- ♠ Gilles de la Tourette syndrome. This is an inherited disorder; autosomal dominant with variable penetrance. It presents with tics, involuntary noises, coprolalia (obscene language), echolalia (repetition of words spoken to the patient)

Cerebellum

Involuntary movements caused by lesions at the level of the cerebellum are:

- ♦ **Benign Essential Tremor**

  Benign essential tremor is characterised by postural tremor of the arms and head. A positive family history is obtained in the majority of patients. The pathophysiology is not definite, abnormalities of the cerebellum, the red nucleus and the thalamus have been observed

Higher Centres

Involuntary movements caused by lesions at the level of the higher centres are:

♣ Tics, habits and ritualistic movements. These usually begin in childhood. They are compulsive movements that are under voluntary control.

Systemic Factors

Systemic factors that result in involuntary movements are:

♥ **Physiological Tremor (Fine Tremor)**

This refers to the fine, rapid physiological tremor that is inherent in all muscles. It may be exaggerated in:

Nervousness, thyrotoxicosis, alcoholism

♠ **Flapping Tremor (Asterixis)**

Flapping tremor or metabolic tremor occurs in organ failure such as liver, cardiac, respiratory, renal failure and Wernicke's encephalopathy. It is a jerky, irregular flexion-extension movement usually seen at the wrist and metacarpophalangeal joints. It can also be demonstrated at the hip joint. (Ask the patient to lie supine with the knees bent and the feet flat on the bed or couch. Get the patient to relax the legs and as they fall to the sides flapping of the limbs would be noted as a result of movements at the hip joint.)

Description of Involuntary Movements

Involuntary movements:

♦ May occur within muscles

♣ They may affect groups of muscles

♥ They may affect the limbs, torso, head

Muscle

Involuntary movements that occur within muscles are:

♠ **Fasciculation**

Fasiculation refers to contractions of groups of muscle fibres. It occurs in:

Lower Motor Neurone Lesions

Fasciculation is seen in lower motor neurone damage, which may be caused by:

Syringomyelia, motor neurone disease, poliomyelitis, syphilitic amyotrophy, prolapsed disc, cervical spondylosis, neuralgic amyotrophy, Hereditary Motor Sensory Neuropathy

Groups of Muscles

Involuntary movements may occur within groups of muscles. They could be:

♦ Sustained contractions or tetany

♣ Spasmodic contractions or myoclonus

♥ Oscillations or tremor

♠ Drug induced involuntary movements or dyskinesia

♦ Repetitive, habitual normal movements or tics

Tetany

Tetany causes spasm of muscles. The spasm may be brought on by stimuli such as tapping on the muscles or by tests such as Trousseau's sign. Tetany is usually due to hypocalcaemia but may also occur in alkalosis, potassium deficiency, magnesium deficiency.

Myoclonus

Myoclonus refers to rapid, irregular, jerk like movements. Myoclonus may occur in epilepsy, encephalitis, degenerative disorders of the cerebellum

Tremor

Tremor refers to involuntary movements caused by rhythmical, alternating contractions of opposing groups of muscles. These could be:

♣ Simple tremors

♥ Compound tremors

Simple Tremor

Movement may be in a single plane (simple tremor). This may be:

♠ Physiological tremor

♦ Flapping tremor

Physiological Tremor

Exaggerated physiological tremor may occur in:

♣ **Anxiety States**

♥ **Systemic Disorders**

Systemic disorders could result in an exaggerated physiological tremor. These would be conditions such as:

Thyrotoxicosis, alcoholism, treatment with beta agonists

Flapping Tremor (Asterixis, Metabolic Tremor)

Flapping tremor may be due to:

♠ Hepatic failure

♦ Uraemia

♣ Hypercapnoea

♥ Congestive cardiac failure

♠ Wernicke's encephalopathy

Compound Tremor

Compound tremor refers to a tremor in which movements occur in more than one plane.

♦ **Parkinsonian Tremor**

Parkinsonian tremor is a compound tremor involving more than one plane of movement.

Dyskinesia

Dyskinesia refers to drug-induced involuntary movements, which usually affect the facial and peri-oral musculature.

Tics

Tics refer to simple normal movements, which have become a habit. They may be associated with verbal manifestations in the Gilles de la Tourette syndrome.

Limbs, Torso, Head

Involuntary movements may affect one or more of the following parts of the body:

♥ Limbs

♠ Torso

♦ Head

These involuntary movements may be:

♣ Chorea

♥ Ballism

♠ Athetosis

- ♦ Dystonia
- ♣ Choreoathetosis
- ♥ Benign Essential Tremor

Chorea

Chorea refers to a dance like movement. The word chorea means dance.

Chorea occurs in conditions affecting the:

- ♠ **CNS**

  Rheumatic fever (Sydenhams chorea), Huntington's disease, drug induced, senile chorea, post-encephalitis, idiopathic

- ♦ **Systemic Factors**

  Systemic factors that cause chorea are:

  Hypocalcaemia, thyrotoxicosis, systemic lupus erythematosus

Ballism

Ballism refers to violent movements where the limb is flung about. Ballism is usually caused by:

- ♣ Vascular lesions that affect the ipsilateral subthalamic nucleus. It is usually unilateral; Hemiballism

Athetosis

Athetosis refers to slow, writhing movements. They are seen in:

- ♥ Cerebral palsy caused by kernicterus or perinatal asphyxia

Dystonia

Dystonia refers to a sustained increase in tone with the result that an abnormally maintained posture is demonstrated. Dystonia may be:

- ♠ **Generalised Dystonia**

  Generalised dystonia affects the whole body

- ♦ **Segmental Dystonia**

  Segmental dystonia affects adjacent parts of the body. Segmental dystonia could be:

  Cranial affecting the eyes, mouth, jaw, bulbar muscles

  Torticollis and a dystonic arm

- ♣ **Focal Dystonia**

  Focal dystonia affects one part of the body. It occurs in conditions such as:

  Spasmodic torticollis, writer's cramp, blepharospasm, oromandibular dystonia, spasmodic dysphonia, axial dystonia

Choreoathetosis

Choreoathetosis refers to a combination of chorea and athetosis. It occurs in:

- ♥ Cerebral palsy, Wilson's disease

Benign Essential Tremor

Benign essential tremor usually presents with a slowly progressive tremor of the arms and the head. A positive family history may be obtained in more than half of the patients and small or moderate doses of alcohol suppress the tremor.

Analysis of Involuntary Movements

In analysis of involuntary movements one should use the system for analysis of function.

447

Position

Note the position at which the involuntary movements occur. Involuntary movements may occur in the following regions:

♠ **Head**

In the head one may observe:

Oro-facial dyskinesia, tics, dystonia such as occulo-gyric crisis, titubation or tremor of the head occurs in benign essential tremor. Paucity of movement would be seen in Parkinsonism.

♦ **Hands**

In the hands one may observe physiological tremor, flapping tremor, Parkinsonian pill-rolling tremor.

♣ **Limbs**

In the limbs one may note chorea, ballism, athetosis

♥ **Neck**

In the neck the abnormality observed would be dystonia causing torticollis (turtle-neck)

♠ **Torso**

In the torso one would note dystonia causing lordosis or scoliosis

Rate

Variations in the rate of the involuntary movements may be:

♦ Slow movements are seen in athetosis.

♣ Rapid movements occur in ballism and physiological tremor.

♥ Intermediate rate is seen in flapping tremors, chorea and Parkinsonism

Rhythm

Variations in the rhythm of the involuntary movements are:

♠ Parkinsonism, flapping tremor and physiological tremor are rhythmical.

♦ Chorea and ballism do not show a rhythm

Quantity

Variations in the length of the excursion made by the involuntary movements are:

♣ Physiological tremor, flapping tremor, Parkinsonism the excursion is small.

♥ In chorea, ballism the excursion is greater

Character

Note whether the involuntary movement is simple that is in a single plane of movement or compound involving more than one plane.

♠ Physiological tremor, flapping tremor movements are in one plane

♦ Chorea, ballism, Parkinsonism the movements are compound. They are in more than one plane

Modifying Factors

Factors that may modify the involuntary movements are:

♣ **Resting**

In Parkinsonism movements are greater at rest.

♥ **Postural**

Flapping tremor and physiological tremor are dependent upon the position of the limbs.

Benign essential tremor is a postural tremor.

♠ **Quasi-Purposive**

In chorea the patient tries to hide involuntary movements by pretending that they have a purpose.

♦ **Intention Tremor**

Intention tremor, or tremor brought on by the patient attempting to perform an action, occurs in cerebellar disease.

Muscle Tone

Muscle tone may be affected by lesions in:

♣ Muscles

♥ Lower motor neurones

♠ Upper motor neurones

♦ Basal ganglia

♣ Cerebellum

♥ Afferent side of the reflex arc

Types of abnormality

Muscle tone may be:

♣ Decreased

♥ Increased

Decreased Tone (Flaccidity)

Flaccidity would be seen in:

♠ Lesions of the sensory side of the reflex arc such as tabes dorsalis

♦ Myopathies

♣ Lower motor neurone lesions

♥ Ipsilateral cerebellar lesions

♠ In the early stage of upper motor neurone lesions, the stage of spinal shock

Increased Tone

Increased tone may be:

♦ Spasticity

♣ Rigidity

♥ Stiffness

♠ Myotonia

♦ Paratonia

Spasticity

Spasticity occurs in upper motor neurone lesions. It results in a clasp-knife type of increased tone. Clasp-knife type of increased tone refers to initial resistance to movement followed by a sudden loss of resistance similar to opening a clasp-knife (pen-knife)

Rigidity

Rigidity occurs in lesions of the basal ganglia. The result may be either cogwheel or lead pipe type of rigidity and this occurs in Parkinsonism. Lead pipe rigidity refers to uniform stiffness of the limbs when they are moved. Cogwheel rigidity refers to rigidity with a series of interruptions or "gives" when the limbs are moved.

Stiffness

Stiffness of muscles may be due to:

♣ Central Causes

♥ Peripheral Causes

449

Central Causes of Stiffness

Central causes of stiffness are:

♠ Stiff Man Syndrome

♦ Tetanus

Stiff Man Syndrome

Stiff man syndrome is a condition caused by antibodies directed against a subpopulation of spinal neurones. It causes slowly progressive, aching and stiffness of muscles with painful cramps and spasms, which may lead to tendon and muscle rupture. On examination the features are normal power, tendon reflexes, coordination and sensation. Axial and abdominal wall rigidity would be noted and proximal limb muscle stiffness would be detected with opposing muscles acting simultaneously.

Tetanus

Tetanus is a condition where tetanus toxin binds to and inhibits the action of inhibitory interneurones in the spinal cord.

Peripheral Causes of Stiffness

Peripheral stiffness may be caused by:

♣ **Neuromyotonia**

   Neuromyotonia is a condition, which is associated with antibodies against voltage-gated potassium channels. Neuromyotonia may be paraneoplastic and occur in association with thymoma and small cell lung cancer. It causes muscle spasms and rigidity, which may be brought on by activity.

Myotonia

Myotonia refers to slow relaxation of muscle following contraction. It occurs in myotonia dystrophica and myotonia congenita.

Paratonia

In paratonia the patient resists attempts to move his or her limbs. It occurs in bilateral frontal lobe damage.

Muscle Power

Muscular weakness may be caused by lesions at various levels. They are at the level of:

♣ Muscle

♥ Neuromuscular junction

♠ Lower motor neurone

♦ Upper motor neurone

Muscles

Lesions of the muscles that result in weakness are:

♣ Myositis

♥ Myopathy (caused by genetic disorders or systemic disease)

Neuromuscular Junction

Lesions that occur at the neuromuscular junction and result in weakness are:

♠ Myasthenia gravis

♦ Eaton-Lambert syndrome

♣ Botulinum toxin

♥ Snake venom

Lower Motor Neurone

Lesions of the lower motor neurone that result in weakness are:

- ♠ Peripheral neuropathy
- ♦ Plexus lesions
- ♣ Radiculopathy
- ♥ Anterior horn cell lesions

Upper Motor Neurone

Lesions of the upper motor neurone that result in weakness are lesions at:

- ♠ Spinal level
- ♦ Brain stem level
- ♣ Internal capsule level
- ♥ Cortical level

Distribution of Weakness

The distribution of muscular weakness is characteristic of the site of the lesion. The distribution may be:

- ♠ Generalised Weakness
- ♦ Head
- ♣ Hemiplegia
- ♥ Monoplegia
- ♠ Quadriparesis
- ♦ Paraparesis
- ♣ Spinal Segment
- ♥ Proximal Large Muscle
- ♠ Part of Limb
- ♦ Localised Weakness
- ♣ Distal Symmetrical Weakness

Generalised Weakness

Generalised muscular weakness may be due to:

- ♥ Neuromuscular junction lesions
- ♠ Radiculopathy

Head

Lesions of the muscles of the head may be due to:

- ♦ Myopathy
- ♣ Myasthenia gravis
- ♥ Cranial nerve lesions
- ♠ Upper motor neurone lesions

Hemiplegia

Hemiplegia refers to weakness of one side of the body it may be due to lesions at:

- ♦ Cortical level
- ♣ Internal capsule level
- ♥ Brain stem level
- ♠ Spinal level

Monoplegia

Monoplegia refers to weakness of a limb.

- ♦ **Brachial Monoplegia**

  Atrophic brachial monoplegia is an uncommon presentation. It may be the result of poliomyelitis, syringomyelia, motor neurone disease, brachial plexus lesions.

- ♣ **Crural Monoplegia**

  Crural monoplegia is caused by lesions in the thoracic or lumbar cord such as trauma, tumour, myelitis, multiple sclerosis, progressive muscular atrophy

  Atrophy is uncommon.

451

Quadriparesis

Quadriparesis refers to weakness of all four limbs. It may be due to lesions at:

♥ Brain stem level

♠ Spinal cord level

♦ Radiculopathy

Paraparesis

Paraparesis refers to weakness of both lower limbs. It may be due to:

♣ Parasagittal lesions

♥ Spinal cord lesions

♠ Cauda equina lesions

♦ Radiculopathy

Spinal Segment

Muscular weakness in the distribution of a spinal segment may be due to:

♣ Anterior horn cell lesions

♥ Radiculopathy such as prolapsed disc

Proximal Large Muscle Weakness

Weakness of the proximal large muscles, the limb girdle muscles, may be due to lesions at the level of:

♠ Muscle (myopathy)

♦ Neuromuscular junction (Eaton-Lambert syndrome)

♣ Nerve lesions like neuralgic amyotrophy, diabetic amyotrophy

♥ Systemic Factors

Proximal Myopathy

Proximal myopathy may be due to:

♥ **Internal Factors**

Degenerative Hereditary Myopathies: Becker muscular dystrophy, facio-scapulo-humeral, limb girdle dystrophy mitochondrial myopathy

Inflammatory Disorders: dermatomyositis, polymyositis

♠ **Systemic Factors**

E&M Cushing's syndrome, thyrotoxicosis, osteomalacia, hypocalcaemia, hypokalaemia

Toxins alcohol

Drugs amiodarone, chloroquine, beta-blockers, lithium, isoniazid

Malignancy (carcinomatosis)

KUS renal failure

Weakness of Part of a Limb

Muscular weakness of part of a limb would occur as a result of:

♠ Plexus lesions

Localised Weakness

Localised muscular weakness may be caused by:

♦ Nerve lesions

♣ Radiculopathy

Distal Symmetrical Weakness

Distal symmetrical muscular weakness may be caused by:

♥ Peripheral neuropathy

♠ Syringomyelia

Reflexes

The reflexes tested are:

♦ Tendon reflexes

♣ Superficial reflexes

Tendon Reflexes

Abnormalities that may be identified when examining tendon reflexes are the following:

♥ Loss of reflexes

♠ Exaggerated reflexes

♦ Pendular reflexes

♣ Delayed relaxation time

Loss of Reflexes

Loss of reflexes may be due to an:

♥ Afferent defect

♠ Spinal segment lesion

♦ Efferent defect

♣ Muscular lesion

Exaggerated reflexes

Exaggerated reflexes are due to :

♥ Upper motor neurone lesions

Pendular Reflexes

Pendular reflexes occur in:

♠ Cerebellar lesions

Delayed Relaxation Time

Delayed relaxation time occurs in:

♦ Hypothyroidism

Superficial Reflexes

Superficial reflexes change when:

♣ Cortical inhibition is lost

Coordination

The functions of the cerebellum are the maintenance of coordination, tone and balance. The central part of the cerebellum (the vermal zone) subserves balance, the most primitive function, the surrounding area (the paravermal zone) subserves tone and the periphery (lateral zones) subserves coordination. Hence, lesions of the cerebellum may result in disorders affecting one or more of these functions depending on the region of the cerebellum that is affected.

Ataxia

Ataxia or incoordination of movement may be of several types. They are:

♥ Truncal or positional

♠ Gait

♦ Appendicular

Truncal Ataxia (Positional)

In truncal ataxia, when the patient sits on the edge of the bed or couch he or she tends to drift backwards into a supine position. This is exaggerated by asking the patient to fold his or her arms across the chest.

Gait Ataxia

Gait ataxia refers to incoordination whilst walking. It may be seen during a normal attempt at walking or it

453

may be evident only when the patient attempts to perform tandem walking in which case it signifies a midline or vermis lesion.

Appendicular Ataxia (Limb Ataxia)

Appendicular ataxia refers to ataxia of the limbs.

Cerebellar Lesions

Cerebellar lesions may be:

- ♣ Unilateral lesions
- ♥ Bilateral lesions
- ♠ Midline (vermis) lesions

Unilateral Cerebellar Lesions

Unilateral lesions may be due to:

- ♦ Demyelination
- ♣ Vascular lesions
- ♥ Trauma
- ♠ Tumour
- ♦ Abscess

Bilateral Cerebellar Lesions

Bilateral lesions may be due to conditions affecting the:

- ♣ **CNS** demyelination, extrapontine myelinolysis due to hyponatraemia, vascular disease, hereditary cerebellar degenerations (autosomal recessive, autosomal dominant), idiopathic late onset cerebellar degeneration (refers to isolated cases of cerebellar degeneration presenting after the age of twenty), posterior fossa tumours
- ♥ **Systemic Factors**

  Drugs anticonvulsants

Toxins alcohol

Paraneoplastic disease

E&M hypothyroidism, zinc deficiency, vitamin E deficiency

Inherited metabolic disorders such as sphingomyelin lipidoses, metachromatic leucodystrophy, hexosaminidase deficiency, galactosylceramide lipidosis, adrenoleucomyeloneuropathy, cholestanolosis

RS pneumonia such as mycoplasma, legionella

HS *Plasmodium falciparum* malaria, ataxia telangiectasia

GIT typhoid fever

Viral Infections echo, herpes simplex. Epstein Barr, varicella

Vermis Lesions

The causes of vermis lesions are similar to the causes of bilateral cerebellar disease

Sensory System

Sensory loss may be due to lesions at various levels. The lesions may be at the level of:

- ♠ Sense Organs
- ♦ Distal Symmetrical Polyneuropathy
- ♣ Mononeuropathy
- ♥ Plexus lesions
- ♠ Nerve Roots (Radiculopathy)
- ♦ Cauda Equina
- ♣ Spinal Cord
- ♥ Pons and Medulla
- ♠ Mid Brain

- ♦ Thalamus
- ♣ Internal Capsule
- ♥ Cortical Level

Distribution of Sensory Loss

The distribution of the sensory loss would be a good guide to the level of the lesion.

♥ Special Senses

The special senses may be affected by lesions of the components of these complex structures. The special senses will be analysed when dealing with the relevant cranial nerves.

♠ Distal Symmetrical Polyneuropathy

Distal symmetrical polyneuropathy would result in a glove and stocking sensory loss. The sensory loss usually affects all modalities but in some instances proprioception and vibration sense may be affected earlier and to a greater degree than pain, temperature and touch.

♦ Mononeuropathy

Nerve lesions would result in a localised sensory loss

♦ Plexus Lesions

Plexus lesions result in a sensory loss in the distribution of the specific nerve trunks that are damaged.

♣ Radiculopathy

Radiculopathy would result in a sensory loss restricted to the relevant dermatomes

♥ Cauda Equina Lesion

A cauda equina lesion would result in a loss of sensation in the saddle area

♠ Spinal Cord Lesions

Spinal cord lesions could be:

Transection

Complete sensory loss below the level of the lesion would occur in transection of the cord. All modalities would be lost.

Hemisection

Brown-Sequard Syndrome. In hemisection of the cord, ipsilateral joint position sense and vibration sense would be lost together with contralateral loss of pain and temperature sensation

Central Cord Lesion

A central cord lesion would cause dissociate loss. There would be loss of pain and temperature sensation with preserved touch, vibration and proprioception. This is caused by intramedullary lesions like syringomyelia

Posterior Column Lesion

Posterior column lesions would result in loss of joint position sense and loss of vibration sense.

Anterior Spinal Syndrome

The anterior spinal syndrome would result in bilateral loss of pain and temperature sensation with preserved joint position sense and vibration sense. This is caused by lesions affecting the anterior spinal artery.

◆ Pons and Medulla

Unilateral lesions of the pons and medulla would result in ipsilateral numbness and loss of sensation in the face with contralateral hemianaesthesia.

In the lateral medullary syndrome the lateral leminiscus is damaged and this results in contralateral loss of pain and temperature sensation. The fifth nerve nucleus may also be affected giving rise to ipsilateral loss of pain and temperature sensation in the face.

In the medial medullary syndrome the medial leminiscus is damaged and this results in loss of postural sense in the limbs of the opposite side of the body.

♣ Mid-Brain

Unilateral lesions at the level of the mid-brain would result in contralateral hemianaesthesia

♥ Thalamus

Unilateral lesions at the level of the thalamus would result in deep pain felt on the contralateral side of body. There would be impaired pain, temperature and touch sensation (contralateral). It may be associated with a homonymous hemianopia and choreoathetosis.

◆ Internal Capsule

In unilateral lesions at the level of the internal capsule the patient would have a contralateral hemisensory loss and may have an associated hemiplegia and homonymous hemianopia

◆ Cortical lesion

Cortical lesions that affect the higher functions of tactile sensation would result in loss of two-point discrimination, astereognosis and agraphaesthesia.

Findings on History

The findings that one may obtain on history taking are as follows:

Loss of Consciousness

Loss of consciousness may be due to:

♣ Internal Factors

Internal factors may be:

- Ventricular lesions
- Localised lesions affecting the brain
- Generalised lesions affecting the brain

Ventricular Lesions

Lesions that affect the ventricles and result in loss of consciousness are:

Ventricular haemorrhage

Obstructive hydrocephalus

Localised Lesions affecting the Brain

Localised lesions could be:

Infarct, haemorrhage, abscess, granuloma, tumour

Generalised Lesions affecting the Brain

Generalised lesions could be:

Cerebral oedema, encephalitis, epilepsy

♥ **Mural Factors**

Mural factors or factors that affect the coverings of the brain and result in loss of consciousness are:

Meningitis, sub-arachnoid haemorrhage, sub-dural haematoma, dural venous thrombosis, extradural haemorrhage

♠ **External Factors**

External factors that may result in loss of consciousness are:

Trauma

♦ **Systemic Factors**

Systemic factors that result in loss of consciousness are those that affect the:

GIT liver failure

KUS renal failure

RS respiratory failure

CVS cardiac failure or cardiac arrhythmia

E&M hypothermia, hyperthermia, hypoglycaemia, hypothyroidism, fever

Seizures

Seizures may be due to:

♣ **Epilepsy**

Epilepsy can result in generalised or partial seizures:

Epilepsy

Epilepsy may cause:

♥ Partial seizures

♠ Generalised seizures

Partial Seizures

Partial seizures may be

♦ Simple Partial Seizures (consciousness not impaired)

These seizures may be

- Motor
- Sensory
- Autonomic
- Psychic

♣ Complex Partial Seizures (consciousness impaired)

♥ Partial Seizures Evolving to Secondary Generalised Seizures

- Simple partial to generalised
- Complex partial to generalised
- Simple partial to complex partial to generalised

Generalised Seizures

♥ Generalised seizures may be

♠ Absence seizures

♦ Atypical absence seizures

♣ Myoclonic

♥ Clonic

♠ Tonic

♦ Tonic-clonic

♣ Atonic

Other causes of seizures are:

♣ **Internal Factors**

Internal factors that may result in seizures are:

Localised Lesions: vascular lesions of the brain, tumours, cerebral abscess, granuloma

Generalised Lesions: encephalitis, degenerative disorders

♥ **Mural Factors**

Meningitis, cortical venous thrombosis

♠ **External Factors**

Trauma

♦ **Systemic Factors**

E&M hypoglycaemia, hypocalcaemia, hyponatraemia, porphyria

RS hypoxia

GIT liver failure

KUS uraemia

Drugs phenothiazines, tricyclic antidepressants

Toxins alcohol (either during periods of drinking or abstinence)

Headaches

Headaches may be due to:

♣ **Internal Factors**

Internal factors that may cause headaches are space-occupying lesions of the brain such as:

Haemorrhage, tumour, abscess, granuloma

These headaches increase in the morning or after a nap because hypoventilation increases the intracranial pressure.

♥ **Mural Factors**

Meningitis, sub-arachnoid haemorrhage, dural venous sinus thrombosis, Benign Intracranial Hypertension

♠ **Local (External) Factors**

Conditions affecting the:

CNS trigeminal neuralgia, postherpetic neuralgia, glaucoma

CVS migraine, cluster headaches

LMS tension headache, temperomandibular joint lesions, temporal arteritis

RS sinusitis

♦ **Systemic Factors**

Systemic disturbances that result in headache are

E&M fever, hypoglycaemia

KUS uraemia

Toxins alcohol

Vertigo

Vertigo is defined as a sensation of movement of the affected individual or his or her surroundings. It may be due to conditions affecting the:

♣ **Sense Organ (Vestibule)**

Meniere's disease, benign positional vertigo

♥ **Nerve**

Vestibular neuronitis

♠ **Cerebello-Pontine Angle**

Acoustic neuroma, meningioma, secondary deposits

♦ **Medulla**

Lateral medullary syndrome

♣ **Blood Supply**

Vertebro-basilar insufficiency

♥ **Systemic Factors**

Systemic factors that may cause vertigo are:

Drugs amionoglycosides, anticonvulsants

Toxins alcohol

Bladder and Bowel Function

Control of Micturition

The muscles involved in the control of micturition are the detrusor muscle and the external sphincter of the urinary bladder. The parasympathetic nerve supply to these structures is from the pelvic splanchnic nerves $S_{2, 3, 4}$ and the sympathetic supply is from $L_{1, 2.}$ Problems with micturition arise from damage at various levels. They are as follows:

♣ **Frontal Lobe**

Frontal lobe damage causes detrusor hyperreflexia. This results in urge incontinence.

♦ **Basal Ganglia**

Damage to the basal ganglia causes detrusor hyperreflexia.

♣ **Pons**

Damage at the level of the pons results in difficulty in voiding due to detrusor-sphincter dyssynergia. This is especially so if the lesion is close to the median longitudinal fasiculus.

♥ **Spinal Cord**

Damage at the level of the spinal cord causes detrusor hyperreflexia and an automatic bladder.

♣ **Conus Medullaris and Cauda Equina**

In conus medullaris and cauda equina lesions, the bladder is decentralised. It usually results in detrusor hyporeflexia.

♦ **Peripheral Innervation**

Damage to the peripheral innervation of the bladder results in decreased bladder contractility; detrusor areflexia.

♣ **Sensory Neuropathy**

Sensory neuropathy results in detrusor areflexia

♥ **Muscle**

Muscle damage may affect the:

• Detrusor

• Sphincter

Detrusor

The detrusor muscle may be affected in myotonic dystrophy and this results in bladder symptoms and megacolon.

Sphincter

The sphincter is usually affected in surgical trauma or birth trauma and this results in incontinence.

Functional Abnormalities of the Bladder

Several types of abnormality may be identified with respect to the function of the urinary bladder. They are the following:

- ♠ Frontal Bladder
- ♦ Spinal Bladder
- ♣ Peripheral Neurogenic Bladder (Autonomous Bladder)
- ♥ Sensory Bladder

Frontal Bladder

In the frontal bladder there is loss of the voluntary control of micturition. The patient has uncontrolled voiding of large quantities of urine. There is no residual urine. Normal anal tone. This occurs in:

- ♠ Frontal lobe lesions
- ♦ Dementia
- ♣ Normal pressure hydrocephalus

Spinal Bladder

The spinal bladder occurs in:

- ♥ Spinal Cord Lesions

  Initially there is retention with overflow, later the patient voids small quantities of urine automatically. The bladder is distended. The patient is constipated. The anal tone is normal.

Peripheral Neurogenic Bladder (Autonomous Bladder)

The peripheral neurogenic bladder causes painless distension of the bladder with overflow incontinence. There is associated faecal incontinence. Anal tone is reduced. It is seen in:

- ♠ Cauda equina lesions
- ♦ Peripheral nerve lesions

Cauda Equina Lesions

Cauda equina lesions may be caused by:

- ♣ Lumbar disc prolapse
- ♥ Spina bifida
- ♠ Neurofibroma
- ♦ Ependymoma
- ♣ Chordoma
- ♥ Metastases

Peripheral Nerve Lesions

Peripheral nerve lesions may be caused by:

- ♠ Diabetes mellitus
- ♦ Pelvic surgery
- ♣ Malignancy

Sensory Bladder

The sensory bladder is similar to the autonomous bladder. It may be caused by:

- ♥ Tabes dorsalis
- ♠ Subacute combined degeneration of the cord
- ♦ Multiple sclerosis

Urinary Incontinence

Incontinence may be classified as:

- ♣ Continuous Incontinence (Total)
- ♥ Stress Incontinence
- ♠ Urge Incontinence
- ♦ Overflow Incontinence

Continuous Incontinence (Total)

Continuous incontinence refers to continuous leakage of urine due to urinary tract fistulae such as:

♣ Vesico-vaginal fistula

♥ Ectopic ureter

Stress Incontinence

Stress incontinence refers to urinary leakage with increased intra-abdominal pressure. The causes of stress incontinence are the following:

♠ **Females**

In females, stress incontinence is caused by weakening of the pelvic floor muscles

♦ **Males**

In males, stress incontinence is caused by damage to the external urethral sphincter following prostatectomy

Urge Incontinence

Urge incontinence is the inability to control voiding when the patient has an urge to pass urine. It may be caused by:

♣ Cystitis

♥ Frontal bladder, which is caused by detrusor hyperreflexia

♠ Advanced bladder outflow obstruction

Overflow Incontinence

Overflow incontinence refers to urinary retention with overflow. It may be caused by chronic urinary outflow obstruction, autonomous bladder and sensory bladder.

Enuresis

Enuresis refers to incontinence that occurs during sleep

Findings On Examination

The abnormalities that may be detected on physical examination of the patient are as follows:

General Examination

The abnormalities that may be detected on general examination of the patient are abnormalities in relation to the following:

♣ Dress

♥ Posture

♠ Integument

Dress

The patient may be improperly dressed and this could indicate:

♦ Dementia

♣ Depression

Posture

Variations that one may note in the patient's posture are:

♥ A hemiplegic posture with flexion and pronation in the upper limb and extension in the lower limb would indicate a contralateral upper motor neurone lesion

Integument

On examination of the integument, the lesions that may be detected are:

- Phakomatoses
- Icthyosis

Phakomatoses

The phakomatoses or neurocutaneous syndromes involve nerve and cutaneous tissue. Many syndromes have been described. The important syndromes are neurofibromatosis, tuberose sclerosis and Sturge-Weber syndrome.

- Neurofibromatosis. The features are multiple neurofibromata and café au lait spots, axillary freckling, Lisch nodules (hamartoma) in the iris
- Tuberose sclerosis. The features are angiofibromatous papules on the face, nail fold fibromas, ash leaf patches (hypopigmented macules), shagreen patches (flesh coloured plaques) over the lower back, lesions in the retina, pulmonary lesions, tumours of the heart, brain and kidney.
- Sturge-Weber syndrome. The features are cutaneous haemangioma with associated intracranial lesions.

Icthyosis

Icthyosis occurs in:

- Refsum's disease (phytanic acid storage disease). This is an autosomal recessive inherited disease where the abnormalities are anosmia, retinitis pigmentosa, pupillary abnormalities, nerve deafness, motor and sensory polyneuropathy, cerebellar ataxia, cardiomyopathy, epiphyseal dysplasia (short fourth metatarsal, syndactyly, hammer toe, pes cavus, osteochondritis dessicans)

Regional Examination

The abnormalities that may be detected on regional examination of the patient are as follows:

Cortex

Abnormalities that may be detected are those that affect the following:

Higher Functions

Abnormalities of the higher functions that may be detected are as follows:

Level of Consciousness

The causes of a decreased level of consciousness have already been documented.

Speech

The abnormalities that may be detected in relation to speech are:

- Aphonia
- Dysphonia
- Dysarthria
- Dysphasia

Aphonia

Aphonia may be caused by lesions in the:

- **Vocal Cords**

  Laryngitis, carcinoma

- **Neuromuscular junction**

  Myasthenia gravis

462

♦ **Vagus Nerve**

Involvement of the vagus nerve and its branches may result in aphonia

♣ **Pons**

Basal Pontine Syndrome

The basal pontine syndrome or locked in syndrome is caused by lesions of the basis pontis. It results in the loss of the ability to speak together with quadriplegia. Consciousness is preserved, as the ascending reticular activating system is not affected. Voluntary vertical eye movements are preserved.

The causes of the locked in syndrome are:

Infarction (basilar artery occlusion, vertebrobasilar dissection, hypotension), haemorrhage, hypoxia, trauma (brain stem contusion), tumours (primary or secondary infiltration), demyelination (multiple sclerosis, central pontine myelinolysis), inflammation (abscess, encephalitis)

Dysphonia

Dysphonia may be due to:

♣ Palatal palsy resulting in nasal speech

♥ Hypothyroidism resulting in a hoarse voice

Dysarthria

Dysarthria may be caused by lesions at various levels. They are the following:

♠ Local Causes in the Mouth

♦ Muscle Lesions

♣ Neuromuscular Junction Lesions

♥ Lower Motor Neurone Lesions

♠ Upper Motor Neurone Lesions

♦ Basal Ganglia Lesions

♣ Cerebellar Lesions

Local Causes in the Mouth

Local causes in the mouth that result in dysarthria are:

♥ Amyloidosis causing a large tongue

♠ Mouth ulcers

♦ Parotitis

♣ Temperomandibular joint disease

Muscle

Lesions in the muscles that may result in dysarthria are:

♥ Dystrophia myotonica

Neuromuscular Junction

Lesions at the neuromuscular junction that may cause dysarthria are:

♠ Myasthenia gravis

Lower Motor Neurone Lesions

Lower motor neurone lesions that result in dysarthria are those that involve the following cranial nerves:

♦ 5th

♣ 7th

♥ 10th

♠ 12th

Upper Motor Neurone Lesions

Upper motor neurone lesions that result in dysarthria occur at the level of the:

463

♥ **Internal Capsule**

Lesions of the internal capsule may be:

Unilateral Lesions. These cause a mild dysarthria

Bilateral Lesions. Pseudobulbar palsy, which may occur as a result of bilateral internal capsule lesions, causes more severe dysarthria

♠ **Cortical lesions**

General Paralysis of the Insane (tertiary syphilis) results in dysarthria

Basal Ganglia Lesions

Basal ganglia lesions that result in dysarthria include:

♦ Parkinsonism (slow, monotonous, slurred speech)

♣ Huntington's chorea

Cerebellar Lesions

Cerebellar lesions result in staccato speech. Cerebellar lesions cause dysarthria if they affect the vermis, the whole cerebellum or its connections. If one lateral hemisphere alone is affected dysarthria may not occur.

Aphasia

When analysing aphasia one should consider lesions involving the:

♥ Sensory component

♠ Motor component

♦ Communication between the two components

♣ Combinations of the two components

Sensory Component

The sensory component or the area involved in the ability to understand speech is located in Wernicke's area. This area, which is in the midst of the sensory cortices, is ideally located to receive multiple sensory inputs from all modalities and relate them to one another and thus enable understanding of speech. Lesions in this area will thus produce a failure to understand speech.

Motor Component

The motor component is situated in Broca's area, which is in the pre-motor cortex and is thus ideally positioned to communicate with the multiple motor areas involved in the production of speech. Lesions in this area will thus cause an inability to produce speech.

Communication

If the communicating fibres between these two areas are damaged the result is a failure to repeat words and phrases.

Combination

Damage to the motor and sensory areas will cause an inability to understand speech as well as an inability to produce speech.

Types of Aphasia

Aphasia may be classified as:

♥ Sensory or Wernicke's Aphasia

♠ Motor or Broca's Aphasia

♦ Conduction Aphasia

♣ Global Aphasia

♥ Nominal Aphasia

Sensory or Wernicke's Aphasia

Sensory aphasia refers to an inability to understand speech. It may be associated with right homonymous hemianopia in right-handed individuals; the converse will apply in left-handed individuals.

Motor or Broca's Aphasia

Motor aphasia refers to an inability to produce speech. It may be associated with a right hemiparesis in right-handed individuals; the converse will apply in left-handed individuals.

Conduction Aphasia

Conduction aphasia causes a failure of repetition. When asked to do so, the patient is unable to repeat words or phrases that are spoken to him or her.

Global Aphasia

Global aphasia refers to an inability to understand speech and produce speech. This results from extensive damage to the dominant hemisphere due to infarction. The patient may also have a hemiplegia and hemianopia.

Nominal Aphasia

Nominal aphasia refers to an inability to name common objects. It occurs in lesions of the posterior superior temporal region and adjacent inferior parietal lobe.

Frontal Lobe

In relation to the higher cerebral functions, lesions of the frontal lobe result in:

♠ Delirium

♦ Dementia

The frontal lobe is also involved in motor function and in inhibition of primitive reflexes. These will be discussed later.

Delirium

Delirium refers to a state of disorientation and confusion. Thoughts and speech are incoherent. Delusions occur and there may be hallucinations, which are usually visual. The causes of delirium are:

♣ **Internal Factors (Brain)**

Tumours, abscess, encephalitis, epilepsy, cerebrovascular accident, hypertensive encephalopathy

♥ **Mural Factors**

Subarachnoid haemorrhage, meningitis

♠ **External Factors**

Trauma

♦ **Systemic Factors**

Conditions affecting the:

E&M fever, hypoglycaemia, vitamin deficiencies such as thiamine, nicotinic acid, vitamin B_{12}

RS hypoxia, pneumonia

KUS renal failure, urinary tract infections

GIT hepatic failure

LMS systemic lupus erythematosus

Drugs anticonvulsants, anticholinergics, opiates

Toxins alcohol withdrawal

Septicaemia

Dementia

In dementia there is chronic impairment of multiple higher cortical functions including orientation, thoughts, memory, calculation, comprehension, language.

The causes of dementia are:

♣ **Internal Factors (Brain)**

Normal pressure hydrocephalus, Alzheimer's disease, frontotemporal dementia, Lewy body dementia, Huntington's chorea, Parkinson's disease, prion disease, encephalitis, multiple cerebral infarctions, multiple sclerosis, tumour

♥ **Mural Factors**

Chronic subdural haematoma, meningioma

♠ **External Factors**

Chronic traumatic encephalopathy

♦ **Systemic Factors**

Conditions affecting the:

E&M hypothyroidism, hypoparathyroidism, pellagra, thiamine deficiency, vitamin B_{12} deficiency, Wilson's disease, prolonged hypoglycaemia

RS prolonged anoxia

GIT chronic hepatic encephalopathy, Wilson's disease, Whipple's disease

KUS uraemia, dialysis

LMS systemic lupus erythematosus

RAG General Paralysis of the Insane, AIDS

Drugs and Toxins barbiturates, alcohol, heavy metals

Paraneoplastic effects of tumours

Temporal Lobe

The temporal lobe serves the functions of:

♣ Memory

♥ Mood

Memory

Memory loss occurs in damage to the medial aspect of the temporal lobe and its connections. The causes of memory loss are:

♠ **Internal Factors (Brain)**

Encephalitis (herpes simplex), bilateral tumours, dementia, infarction, neurosarcoidosis

♦ **Mural Factors**

Chronic meningitis (tuberculosis)

♣ **External Factors**

Head injury

♥ **Systemic Factors**

Conditions affecting the:

RS anoxia

Toxins alcohol, solvent abuse, arsenic

E&M hypoglycaemia, thiamine deficiency

Mood

Mood abnormalities may be categorised as:

♥ Mania

♠ Depression

♦ Emotional lability

Mania

Mania refers to an elevation of mood. It is a feature of manic-depressive psychosis but may also occur in conditions caused by:

♣ **Internal Factors (Brain)**

Acute schizophrenia, dementia

♥ **Systemic Factors**

Conditions affecting the:

E&M hyperthyroidism

Drugs and Toxins amphetamines, steroids, cannabis

Depression

This refers to depression of mood and may be primary depression in manic-depressive psychosis. Depression may be secondary to:

♠ **Internal Factors (Brain)**

Schizophrenia, anxiety neurosis, dementia

♦ **Systemic Factors**

Any chronic debilitating illness may be compounded by depression. In addition depression may be due to:

Drugs and Toxins corticosteroids, oestrogens and progesterone, antihypertensives that act centrally, alcohol, drug abuse

Emotional Lability

Emotional lability is a feature of:

♣ Pseudobulbar palsy

Parietal Lobe

Lesions that affect the higher functions of the parietal lobe result in:

♥ Agnosia

♠ Apraxia

Agnosia

Agnosia refers to the failure of recognition despite intact sensory modalities

Apraxia

Apraxia refers to the failure of performance of tasks despite intact motor function

Dominant Parietal Lobe

Lesions of the dominant parietal lobe result in abnormalities of:

♦ Writing

♣ Numeracy

Writing

An inability to write would indicate a lesion in the dominant parietal lobe.

Numeracy

An inability to calculate would indicate a lesion in the dominant parietal lobe.

Non-Dominant Parietal Lobe

Lesions of the non-dominant parietal lobe result in:

♥ Sensory Inattention

♠ Anosognosia

♦ Astereognosis

♣ Constructional Apraxia

♥ Dressing Apraxia

Sensory Inattention

Sensory inattention refers to an inability to perceive stimulation of one side of the body when homologous points on opposite sides of the body are stimulated. It indicates a lesion in the non-dominant parietal lobe.

Anosognosia

Anosognosia refers to the failure of realisation that a limb is paralysed. This indicates a non-dominant parietal lobe lesion.

Astereognosis

Astereognosis refers to the failure of recognition of familiar objects by touch alone; despite intact sensory function. It indicates a lesion in the non-dominant parietal lobe.

Constructional Apraxia

Constructional apraxia refers to an inability to draw complex figures despite intact motor and sensory function. It indicates a lesion in the non-dominant parietal lobe but may also occur in hepatic encephalopathy.

Dressing Apraxia

Dressing apraxia refers to the patient's inability to put on his or her clothes despite intact motor and sensory function. It indicates a lesion in the non-dominant parietal lobe

Lesions of the Parietal Lobe

Lesion of the parietal lobe may be due to:

♠ **Internal Factors** (Brain)

   Tumours, stroke

♦ **Systemic Factors**

   Conditions affecting the:

   GIT hepatic encephalopathy

Occipital Lobe

The higher function of the occipital lobe is higher visual function.

Higher Visual Function

Lesions that affect the occipital regions, which lie in proximity to the primary visual cortex, result in a failure of recognition visually despite intact visual pathways. This may result in:

♣ Visual Agnosia

♥ Prosopagnosia

Visual Agnosia

Visual agnosia refers to the failure of recognition of objects despite intact visual pathways. It indicates posterior left hemisphere pathology

Prosopagnosia

Prosopagnosia refers to the inability to recognise familiar faces despite intact visual pathways. This is usually due to lesions in the right occipitotemporal region.

Head

When examining the head one may detect abnormalities of the following:

♠ Dimensions

♦ Movement

Dimensions

Abnormalities that one may note with respect to the dimensions of the head are:

♠ Enlargement of the skull may be seen in Paget's disease of bone where there may be associated deafness caused by cranial nerve entrapment or involvement of the ossicles by the disease. Paget's disease may be associated with platybasia and basilar invagination.

Movement

The abnormal movement of the head that may be noted would be:

♦ Titubation

Titubation

Titubation or tremor of the head would occur in:

♣ Cerebellar disease

♥ Benign essential tremor

Examination of the Cranial Nerves

Abnormalities that may be detected on examination of the cranial nerves are as follows:

Nose

Olfactory Nerve

Anosmia

Anosmia or loss of the sense of smell may result from lesions at various levels. They are:

♠ **Sensory Organ**

   Local lesions such as the common cold, chronic sinusitis

♦ **Nerve Lesions**

   Nerve lesions may be caused by:

   Skull fractures, meningioma

♣ **Central Connections**

Lesions that involve the central connections include frontal lobe tumours and Kallman's syndrome.

Eyes

Abnormalities of structure and function may be noted. Functions would be in relation to the functions of the optic nerve and the 3rd, 4th and 6th cranial nerves.

Structure

Abnormalities that one may note in the structure of the eyes are:

♥ Chemosis would occur in cavernous sinus thrombosis, retro-orbital tumour

♠ A bruit would be heard over the eye in carotico-cavernous fistula

Functions of the Eyes

One may detect abnormalities of the:

♦ Optic nerve

♣ 3rd, 4th and 6th nerves

Optic Nerve

Abnormalities that may be detected are those concerning:

♥ Visual acuity

♠ Higher visual function

♦ Visual fields

Visual Acuity

Abnormalities that may be detected are:

♣ Refractory errors

469

♥ Diminished vision

Refractory Errors

The common cause of a problem with visual acuity is an error of refraction. This could be:

- ◆ Short sight
- ♣ Long sight
- ♥ Astigmatism

Diminished Vision

The causes of diminished vision may be classified as lesions in the:

- ♠ Cornea
- ◆ Anterior Chamber
- ♣ Iris
- ♥ Lens
- ♠ Vitreous
- ◆ Retina
- ♣ Blood Vessels
- ♥ Choroid
- ♠ Optic Nerve
- ◆ Visual Cortex

Cornea

Lesions of the cornea that result in diminished vision are:

- ♣ Keratomalacia
- ♥ Keratitis

Anterior Chamber

Lesions of the anterior chamber of the eye that result in diminished vision are:

- ♠ Glaucoma

Iris

Diminished vision may occur if the iris is affected by:

◆ Anterior uveitis

Lens

Diminished vision would occur if a cataract forms in the lens.

Cataract

Cataract refers to the lens becoming opaque due to a change in its protein structure. The causes of cataract are the following conditions:

- ♣ **Degenerative**: senile cataract
- ♥ **Genetic**: Down's syndrome, dystrophia myotonica, retinitis pigmentosa
- ♠ **Metabolic**: diabetes mellitus, hypoparathyroidism, Wilson's disease
- ◆ **Drugs**: chlorpromazine, steroids, chloroquine
- ♣ **Inflammatory**: syphilis, rubella, chronic anterior uveitis
- ♥ **Trauma**
- ♠ **Radiation**

Vitreous

Lesions of the vitreous that result in diminished vision are:

- ◆ Vitreous haemorrhage,
- ♣ Subhyaloid haemorrhage

Retina

Lesions of the retina that result in diminished vision are:

- ♥ Retinopathies:

    Retinitis pigmentosa

    Diabetic retinopathy
- ♠ Retinal detachment
- ◆ Age related macular degeneration

♣ Cancer Associated Retinopathy. This refers to retinal degeneration occurring in the presence of systemic tumour growth, most commonly small cell carcinoma of the lung but breast and gynaecological malignancies may also be involved.

♥ Melanoma Associated Retinopathy. This refers to night-blindness associated with metastatic cutaneous melanoma

Blood Vessels

Diminished vision may be due to conditions affecting the blood vessels of the eye:

♣ Retinal artery embolism

♥ Retinal vein thrombosis

Choroid

Lesions of the choroid that result in diminished vision are:

♠ Posterior uveitis

Optic Nerve

Diminished vision may be the result of:

♦ Optic neuritis commonly due to multiple sclerosis

♣ Toxic neuropathy due to drugs, tobacco

♥ Ischaemic neuropathy in giant cell arteritis, central retinal artery thrombosis or embolism

♠ Compression by tumours

♦ Increased intracranial pressure may cause infarction of the optic nerve in benign intracranial hypertension

♣ Primary optic atrophy. Any condition that causes primary optic atrophy will result in diminished vision. The causes of primary optic atrophy are discussed later.

Visual Cortex

Diminished vision may be the result of:

♦ **Bilateral Vascular Lesions**. This results in cortical blindness. The entire visual field may be lost but more commonly a small area of central vision is retained. This macular sparing is due to the alternative blood supply of the posterior pole of the occipital lobe.

♠ **Anton's syndrome**. This is caused by extensive damage to both the primary visual cortex and the association areas. The patient is unable to see but denies any visual disorder (anosagnosia)

Higher Visual Function

Visual agnosia and prosopagnosia have already been discussed.

Visual Fields

Visual field defects are caused by lesions affecting the:

♠ Visual cortex

♦ Optic radiation

♣ Internal capsule

♥ Optic tract

♠ Optic chiasma

♦ Optic nerve

♣ Optic disc

♥ Retina

471

Types of Field Defect

The types of field defect that arise as a consequence of lesions of the above are as follows:

- ♠ Homonymous Hemianopia
- ♥ Homonymous Hemianopia with Macular Sparing
- ♣ Upper Quadrantopia
- ♦ Lower Quadrantopia
- ♠ Bitemporal Hemianopia
- ♦ Binasal Hemianopia
- ♣ Altitudinal Field Defects
- ♥ Tunnel Vision
- ♠ Central Scotoma
- ♦ Homonymous Central (Macular) Hemiscotoma
- ♣ Enlarged Blind Spot

Homonymous Hemianopia

Homonymous hemianopia refers to the loss of vision in the same (congruent) halves of the visual fields in both eyes. It is caused by lesions in the:

- ♥ Optic tract
- ♠ Internal capsule
- ♦ Optic radiation

Homonymous hemianopia may be due to:

- ♣ Cerebrovascular disease
- ♥ Tumour

Homonymous Hemianopia with Macular Sparing

Homonymous hemianopia with macular sparing occurs in:

- ♠ Unilateral posterior cerebral artery occlusion.

Upper Quadrantopia

A defect affecting one quadrant of the visual field is referred to as a quadrantopia. Upper quadrantopia is caused by a:

- ♦ Temporal lobe lesion

Lower Quadrantopia

Lower quadrantopia is caused by a:

- ♠ Parietal lobe lesion

Bitemporal Hemianopia

Bitemporal hemianopia refers to a visual field loss affecting the temporal or outer halves of both visual fields. It is due to lesions of the optic chiasma caused by:

- ♥ Pituitary tumour
- ♠ Craniopharyngioma
- ♦ Suprasellar aneurysm
- ♣ Granuloma
- ♥ Suprasellar meningioma
- ♠ Glioma
- ♦ Metastases

Binasal Hemianopia

Binasal hemianopia refers to the loss of the nasal halves of the visual fields in both eyes. It is uncommon. It may occur in:

- ♣ Bilateral lesions affecting the uncrossed fibres on either side of the optic chiasma
- ♥ Open angle glaucoma

Altitudinal Field Defects

Altitudinal field defects refer to the loss of the upper or lower halves of the field of vision. They are uncommon.

Unilateral Altitudinal Field Defects

Unilateral altitudinal field defects may be caused by:

♠ Optic nerve damage due to ischaemia or trauma

Bilateral Altitudinal Field Defects

Bilateral altitudinal field defects may be caused by:

♦ Occipital lesions

Tunnel Vision

Tunnel vision refers to concentric constriction of the visual field. It is caused by:

♣ Glaucoma

♥ Retinitis pigmentosa

♠ Choroidoretinitis

♦ Long-standing papilloedema

♣ Bilateral lesions of the visual cortex

Central Scotoma

Central scotoma refers to a zone of loss of vision confined to the centre of the visual field. It is caused by lesions affecting the optic nerve or the macula. They are:

♥ Retrobulbar neuritis, pressure on the optic nerve

♠ Local disease of the choroid or retina in the vicinity of the macula

♦ Vitamin B$_{12}$ deficiency

♣ Alcoholism

The scotoma may affect only one eye; toxic causes usually affect both eyes

Homonymous Central (Macular) Hemiscotoma

Homonymous central (macular) hemiscotoma is caused by a lesion of:

♥ One occipital pole

Enlarged Blind Spot

An enlarged blind spot occurs in:

♠ Papilloedema

Optic Fundus

It is convenient to classify lesions of the optic fundus according to the structure that is primarily affected by the condition. Lesions of the fundus may affect the:

♦ Red Reflex (a combination of structures)

♣ Optic Disc

♥ Blood Vessels

♠ Choroid and Retina

♦ Vitreous

Red Reflex

The abnormality that may be detected is an absent red reflex.

Absent Red Reflex

If the red reflex cannot be seen when the fundus is examined the conditions to be considered are:

♣ Opacities in the lens

♥ Vitreous haemorrhage

♠ Retinal detachment

473

Optic Disc

When inspecting the optic disc the lesions that may be identified are the following:

♦ **Deep Cup**

A deep cup could be due to:

Glaucoma

♣ **Swollen Disc**

A swollen disc could be due to:

Papilloedema, papillitis, central retinal vein thrombosis

♥ **Pale Disc**

A pale disc may be due to:

Optic atrophy, central retinal artery occlusion

♠ **Myelinated nerve fibres**

Myelinated nerve fibres are a:

Normal variant

Blood Vessels

The blood vessels may be affected by:

♦ Diabetic retinopathy

♣ Hypertensive retinopathy

♥ Branch retinal artery occlusion

♠ Branch retinal vein thrombosis

♦ Angioid streaks (although not strictly speaking a lesion of the blood vessels this is best considered here)

Choroid and Retina

The choroid and retina may be affected by:

♣ Choroiditis; acute and chronic

♥ Retinitis pigmentosa

♠ Drusen

♦ Retinal detachment

♣ Age related macular degeneration

♥ Scarring

Vitreous

The vitreous may be affected by:

♣ Haemorrhage

♥ Asteroid Hyalosis

♠ Synchysis scintillans

♦ Subhyaloid haemorrhage

Descriptions and Causes of Lesions in the Fundus

A description of lesions that may occur in the fundus and their causes follows:

Papilloedema

In papilloedema, the optic cup is filled. The disc becomes pinker and approaches the colour of the surrounding retina and the margins of the disc cannot be defined. The veins are engorged and become non-pulsatile. The blood vessels disappear as they traverse the swollen edge of the disc.

The causes of papilloedema are:

♣ **Internal Factors (Brain)**

Space occupying lesions of the brain, cerebral oedema

♥ **Mural Factors**

Meningitis, subarachnoid haemorrhage, benign intracranial hypertension

♠ **External Factors**

Sagittal sinus thrombosis, cavernous sinus thrombosis, Guillain-Barre syndrome

♦ **Systemic Factors**

Conditions affecting the:

RS hypercapnoea

E&M Grave's disease, hypoparathyroidism, vitamin A toxicity

HS severe anaemia

CVS hypertension (grade 4 retinopathy), superior vena cava obstruction

LMS Paget's disease, Hurler's syndrome, systemic lupus erythematosus

Drugs and Toxins poisoning by vitamin A, lead, tetracycline, nalidixic acid

Foster-Kennedy Syndrome

The Foster-Kennedy syndrome refers to papilloedema in one eye with optic atrophy in the other. It is caused by a tumour in the posterior inferior frontal region compressing the optic nerve and raising intracranial pressure.

Papillitis

In papillitis the disc is swollen, it is red and appears cloudy with exudates on the disc and in the overlying vitreous humour. The veins are not distended.

Papillitis may be due to:

♣ Multiple sclerosis

Optic Atrophy

In optic atrophy the optic disc would be pale, even white. The number of blood vessels crossing the disc is reduced from the usual 7-10.

Optic atrophy may be classified as:

♥ Primary

♠ Secondary

♦ Consecutive

Primary Optic Atrophy

In primary optic atrophy the margins of the disc are distinct.

Secondary Optic Atrophy

Secondary optic atrophy is a consequence of papilloedema. In secondary optic atrophy, the margins of the disc are indistinct.

Consecutive Optic atrophy

Consecutive optic atrophy is where optic atrophy is secondary to primary retinal disease

Causes of Optic atrophy

The causes of Optic atrophy are:

♣ **Primary Optic Atrophy**

  Primary optic atrophy may be due to:

  - **Inflammation**: multiple sclerosis, tabes dorsalis
  - **Degeneration**: compression by a tumour or an aneurysm, Paget's disease of bone
  - **Vascular lesions**: retinal artery occlusion
  - **Metabolic and Toxic Causes**

    Vitamin B_{12} deficiency

    Toxins: alcohol, methyl alcohol, quinine
  - **Genetic Causes**: Leber's hereditary optic atrophy, DIDMOAD syndrome (diabetes insipidus,

475

diabetes mellitus, optic atrophy, deafness), Friedrich's ataxia

♥ **Consecutive Optic Atrophy**

Consecutive optic atrophy may occur following:

Choroidoretinitis, retinitis pigmentosa

Glaucoma

In glaucoma the optic cup would be deepened. The blood vessels appear to climb out of the cup, which looks like a well.

Myelinated Nerve Fibres

Myelinated nerve fibres appear as bright white streaks at the edge of the disc. They are a normal variant.

Central Retinal Artery Occlusion

In central retinal artery occlusion, the fundus would be pale with very few vessels, which are thin. A cherry red spot would be seen at the macula. The causes of central retinal artery occlusion are conditions affecting the:

♠ **CVS** embolism

♦ **LMS** temporal arteritis, connective tissue disorders

♣ **HS** sickle cell disease

♥ **RAG** syphilis

♠ **Drugs** cocaine abuse

Branch Retinal Artery Occlusion

In branch retinal artery occlusion, the territory supplied by the occluded branch would appear white. The embolus may be seen and give a characteristic appearance.

♦ **Cholesterol**

Glistening white or yellow pieces of cholesterol

♣ **Calcified Heart Valve**

Debris from a calcified valve appear as:

Large, solid, rounded, white emboli

♥ **Fibrin or Platelet**

Emboli from a thrombosed plaque or cardiac thrombus appear:

Dark or grey

Angioid Streaks

Angioid streaks are linear, dark-red or grey streaks that lie beneath the retinal vessels. They are seen in conditions affecting the:

♠ **IS** pseudoxanthoma elasticum, Ehlers-Danlos syndrome

♦ **LMS** Paget's disease of bone

♣ **HS** sickle cell anaemia

Central Retinal Vein Occlusion

In central retinal vein occlusion (thrombosis), the veins are tortuous and engorged. Multiple haemorrhages and soft exudates would be seen. Papilloedema would be observed. The causes of central retinal vein occlusion are:

♥ Hypertension

♠ Hyperlipidaemia

♦ Diabetes mellitus

♣ Hyperviscosity syndromes (Waldenstrom's macroglobulinaemia, myeloma)

Branch Retinal Vein Occlusion

In branch retinal vein thrombosis, the appearance would be a wedge shaped sector of haemorrhage with the apex pointing towards the disc. The occlusion is usually at an arteriovenous crossing.

Choroidoretinitis

In choroidoretinitis there would be yellowish-white, patchy, exudates with haemorrhages in the acute phase. In the chronic phase there would be white scars with pigmented edges.

The causes of choroidoretinitis are:

♥ Cytomegalovirus infection in AIDS

♠ Syphilis

♦ Sarcoidosis

♣ Tuberculosis

♥ Toxoplasmosis

♠ Toxaemia

♦ Trauma

Retinitis Pigmentosa

In retinitis pigmentosa, black pigment would be seen scattered throughout the retina. The appearance of the pigmentation is similar to bone corpuscles. Optic atrophy may occur.

Conditions that are associated with retinitis pigmentosa are the following:

♣ Laurence-Moon-Biedl syndrome

♥ Refsum's disease

♠ Hereditary ataxias

♦ Neuronal lipidoses

♣ Familial neuropathies

♥ Abetalipoproteinaemia

Phakomata

Yellow hamartoma are seen in the fundus in tuberose sclerosis

Drusen

Drusen appear as multiple, discrete, yellow-white spots around the macula and the posterior aspect of the retina

Age-Related Macular Degeneration

The features of age-related macular degeneration are drusen, areas of hypopigmentation and hyperpigmentation, choroidal neovascularistion. It is the commonest cause of blindness in the elderly.

Retinal Detachment

In retinal detachment, the area detached would lose its pink colour and appear grey and opaque. If a large subretinal fluid collection occurs the area would appear ballooned out and have numerous folds.

Retinal detachment may be:

♠ Rhegmatogenous Retinal Detachment

♦ Traction Retinal Detachment

♣ Secondary Retinal Detachment

Rhegmatogenous Retinal Detachment

Rhegmatogenous retinal detachment is where a hole or break occurs in the retina and this allows fluid from the vitreous to track into the subretinal space.

The causes are:

♥ Trauma

♠ Following surgery

Traction Retinal Detachment

Traction retinal detachment is caused by traction on the retina. The causes are:

♦ Diabetic retinopathy

♣ Intraoccular foreign body

♥ Eye injuries (perforating)

♠ Cataract surgery causing loss of vitreous

Secondary Retinal Detachment

Secondary retinal detachment refers to detachment secondary to diseases such as:

♦ Hypertension

♣ Chronic glomerulonephritis

♥ Retinal vasculitis

♠ Retinal vein occlusion

♦ Toxaemia of pregnancy

Subhyaloid Haemorrhage

Subhyaloid haemorrhage refers to haemorrhage into the pre-retinal space. It obscures the retinal vessels and tends to settle inferiorly. The causes of subhyaloid haemorrhage are:

♣ Subarachnoid haemorrhage

♥ Diabetic retinopathy.

Vitreous Haemorrhage

Vitreous haemorrhage presents as loss of vision in one eye or as a floating shadow in the field of vision. A large bleed causes loss of the red reflex. It has the fundoscopic appearance of a featureless, grey haze. It may be due to:

♠ Trauma

♦ Hypertension

♣ Diabetes mellitus

♥ Bleeding disorders

Asteroid Hyalosis

In asteroid hyalosis a large number of tiny, white opacities would be seen in the vitreous. This is commonly unilateral. Visual function is not affected.

Synchysis Scintillans

Synchysis scintillans refers to golden, cholesterol crystals in the vitreous. It is commonly bilateral.

3ʳᵈ, 4ᵗʰ and 6ᵗʰ nerves

The nerve supply to individual muscles may be remembered as **LR₆ (SO₄)₃.** *That is, lateral rectus 6, superior oblique 4 and all the rest 3*

The 3ʳᵈ, 4ᵗʰ and 6ᵗʰ nerves are related functionally as they act in concert to control movements of the eyes. In addition, in certain parts of their anatomical course they are closely related.

Lesions of these nerves may occur at various levels. They are at the level of the:

♦ Brain Stem (3rd, 4th)

♦ Lower part of the pons (6th)

♣ Sub-Arachnoid Space

♥ Cavernous Sinus

♠ Superior Orbital Fissure

♦ Orbit

Brain Stem

In the brain stem the third and fourth nerves may be damaged. Associated features caused by involvement of the neighbouring structures would be observed.

Lower Part of the Pons

Here the sixth nerve would be involved. Neighbouring structures may be involved as well.

Sub-Arachnoid Space

In the subarachnoid space isolated lesions of the nerves occur

Cavernous Sinus

In the cavernous sinus, features due to involvement of the neighbouring structures would be noted.

Superior Orbital Fissure

In the superior orbital fissure, features of involvement of the neighbouring structures would be noted.

Orbit

Lesions in the orbit are rare.

Examination of cranial nerves 3, 4 and 6

On examination of cranial nerves 3, 4 and 6, abnormalities may be detected in relation to the:

♥ Eyelids

♠ Eyeball

♦ Eye movements

♣ Pupils

Eyelids

On examination of the eyelids, abnormalities may be noted of their position.

Position of the Eyelids

The abnormality that may be noted in neurological examination is ptosis.

Ptosis

Ptosis refers to drooping of the upper eyelid. It occurs due to weakness of elevation of the upper eyelid. The elevators of the upper eyelid are the levator palpebrae superioris, which is supplied by the third nerve and the superior tarsal muscle, which is a smooth muscle that is supplied by the cervical sympathetic nerves.

Types of Ptosis

Ptosis may be:

♦ Complete

♣ Partial

Ptosis may also be:

♥ Unilateral

♠ Bilateral

Complete Ptosis

Complete ptosis with closure of the eyelid occurs in:

♦ Third nerve lesions

Partial Ptosis

Partial ptosis occurs in:

♣ Horner's syndrome

♥ Neuromuscular junction lesions

♠ Muscular weakness

Unilateral Ptosis

Unilateral ptosis may be:

♦ **Congenital**

Or it may occur due to lesions of the:

♣ **Muscle**

Dystrophia myotonica

♦ **Neuromuscular Junction**

Myasthenia gravis

♣ **Third Cranial Nerve**

Lesions of the third cranial nerve cause complete ptosis

♥ **Cervical Sympathetic**

In Horner's syndrome partial ptosis occurs

Bilateral Ptosis

Bilateral ptosis may be:

♠ **Congenital**

Or it may be due to lesions in the:

♦ **Muscle**

Ocular myopathy, oculopharyngeal muscular dystrophy, dystrophia myotonica

♣ **Neuromuscular Junction**

Myasthenia gravis

♥ **Sympathetic Nerve Lesions**

Bilateral Horner's syndrome in syringomyelia

♠ **Central Lesions**

Tabes dorsalis

Eyeballs

On examination of the eyeballs one may note abnormalities of:

♦ Size

♣ Position.

Size

The eyes may be larger or smaller than normal.

Large

Buphthalmos or ox-eye may occur in the:

♥ Sturge-Weber syndrome

Small

Microphthalmia may occur in:

♠ Ocular toxoplasmosis

Position

The position of the eyeball may deviate from normal. This deviation may be:

♦ Proptosis

♣ Enophthalmos

♥ Squint

Proptosis

Proptosis refers to forward protrusion of the eyeballs. Proptosis may be:

♦ Bilateral

♣ Unilateral

Bilateral Proptosis

Bilateral proptosis could be due to lesions in the:

♥ Cavernous Sinus

Cavernous sinus thrombosis, carotico-cavernous fistula

♠ Orbit

Grave's ophthalmopathy

Unilateral Proptosis

Unilateral proptosis could be due to lesions in the:

♦ Orbit

Grave's ophthalmopathy, orbital tumour, orbital cellulitis, granuloma

Enophthalmos

Apparent enophthalmos (the eye looks retracted and smaller than normal) occurs in:

♠ Horner's syndrome.

Strabismus or Squint

Strabismus or squint refers to a condition where the visual axes of the two eyes do not meet at the point of fixation. Strabismus may be divided into:

♣ Non-paralytic (concomitant squint)

♦ Paralytic squint

Non-Paralytic Squint

Non-paralytic squint begins in early childhood. The deviating eye has defective vision. There is no diplopia. When each eye is tested separately movements are full.

Paralytic Squint

Paralytic squint is the result of weakness of the extraocular muscles. The patient has diplopia but visual acuity is not affected. The image from the unaffected eye is projected on the macula and is clear. The image from the affected eye is not projected on the macula and is thus blurred and indistinct. This is called the false image. Covering the affected eye will make the false image disappear.

Eye Movements

On testing eye movements one may observe:

♥ Spontaneous ocular movements

♠ Abnormalities of the range of eye movements

♦ Nystagmus

Spontaneous Ocular Movements

In unconscious patients one may observe spontaneous ocular movements. They may indicate:

♥ A posterior fossa lesion

♠ Tricyclic overdosage

Range of Eye Movements

Abnormalities of the range of eye movements may be due to:

♦ Nerve palsies

♣ External Ophthalmoplegia

♥ Abnormalities of conjugate gaze

♠ Lesions of the medial longitudinal fasiculus

♦ Gaze apraxia

Nerve Palsies

The nerve palsies that result in abnormalities of the range of eye movements are those involving the:

- ♣ 3rd nerve
- ♥ 4th nerve
- ♠ 6th nerve

Third Nerve

In third nerve palsy there is complete ptosis and the eye is deviated outwards and downwards. The pupillary fibres run outside the nerve and the pupil is affected early in compressive lesions. In pathology affecting the vasa nervorum, the pupil is spared.

The third nerve may be affected in the:

- ♦ Midbrain
- ♣ Subarachnoid Space
- ♥ Cavernous Sinus and Superior Orbital Fissure
- ♠ Orbit

Midbrain

In third nerve lesions that occur in the midbrain, other structures in the midbrain may be affected thus aiding localisation. The resulting syndromes are:

- ♦ **Weber's syndrome**

  Weber's syndrome refers to a lesion of the third nerve associated with contralateral hemiplegia.

- ♣ **Benedikt's syndrome**

  Benedikt's syndrome refers to a lesion of the third nerve with involuntary movements of the opposite limbs due to involvement of the red nucleus as well

- ♥ **Claude's syndrome**

  Claude's syndrome refers to a palsy of the third nerve with contralateral ataxia and tremor due to involvement of the red nucleus and cerebellar pathways.

- ♠ **Nothnagel's syndrome**

  Nothnagel's syndrome refers to a lesion of the third nerve with ipsilateral cerebellar ataxia

The above lesions may be caused by:

- ♦ Syringobulbia
- ♣ Cerebrovascular disease
- ♥ Demyelination
- ♠ Tumours such as brain stem glioma or metastases
- ♦ Trauma

Subarachnoid Space

In its path from the midbrain to the cavernous sinus the third nerve may be subject to:

- ♣ Compressive lesions
- ♥ Involvement of the vasa nervorum
- ♠ Cranial polyradiculitis

Compression

Compression of the 3rd nerve may be due to:

- ♦ Aneurysm of the posterior communicating artery
- ♣ Herniation of the uncus of the temporal lobe in supratentorial lesions
- ♥ Subacute meningitis

♠ Meningeal infiltration due to leukaemia or neoplasia

Vascular Lesions

Vascular lesions of the 3rd nerve are due to involvement of the vasa nervorum and may occur in:

♦ Ophthalmoplegic migraine

♣ Mononeuritis multiplex

Cranial Polyradiculitis

Cranial polyradiculitis affecting the 3rd nerve may occur as part of:

♥ Guillain-Barre syndrome

Or it could be:

♠ Isolated polyradiculitis

Cavernous Sinus and Superior Orbital Fissure

In these locations, lesions of other cranial nerves also occur. Lesions that may occur are:

♦ Cavernous sinus thrombosis

♣ Carotico-cavernous fistula

♥ Parasellar neoplasm

♠ Sphenoidal wing meningioma

♦ Tolosa-Hunt syndrome

Orbit

Lesions in the orbit are rare. They may be due to:

♣ Trauma

♥ Grave's disease

♠ Tumours

♦ Granuloma

Fourth Nerve

Lesions of the fourth nerve cause impairment of the ability to move the eye downwards. On attempting to look downwards in the mid-position of gaze, the eyeball would be rotated outwards. Isolated lesions of the fourth nerve are rare. The causes of 4th nerve lesions are:

♣ Head injury

♥ Lesions affecting the cerebral peduncles

♠ Vascular disease

♦ Neoplasms of the brain stem

Sixth Nerve

Lesions of the sixth nerve impair outward movement of the affected eye. Convergent squint may occur.

Isolated sixth nerve lesion may be due to:

♣ Central lesions

♥ Subarachnoid space lesions

Central Lesions

Central lesions that involve the 6th nerve are:

♠ Multiple sclerosis

♦ Thiamine deficiency (Wernicke-Korsakoff syndrome)

Subarachnoid Space

In the subarachnoid space the 6th nerve may be affected by:

♣ Mononeuritis multiplex

♥ Increased intracranial pressure (as a false localising sign)

♠ Aneurysm of an ectatic basilar artery

♦ Subacute meningitis or meningeal infiltration: carcino-matous, lympomatous, fungal

(AIDS), tuberculosis, meningo-vascular syphilis

External Ophthalmoplegia

External ophthalmoplegia or weakness of the extraocular muscles may be due to:

- ♣ Multiple Ocular Nerve Palsies
- ♥ Neuromuscular Junction Lesions
- ♠ Myopathy

Multiple Ocular Nerve Palsies

Multiple ocular nerve palsies occur in:

- ♦ Cavernous sinus lesions
- ♣ Lesions of the superior orbital fissure like the Tolosa-Hunt syndrome (a painful external ophthalmoplegia due to a granulomatous angiitis)

Neuromuscular Junction Lesions

Involvement of the neuromuscular junction occurs in:

- ♥ Myasthenia gravis

Myopathy

Disease of the muscles occurs in:

- ♠ Ocular myopathy
- ♦ Oculopharyngeal myopathy
- ♣ Grave's ophthalmopathy

Conjugate Gaze

Horizontal gaze is controlled by centres in the frontal lobe and pons. Vertical gaze is controlled by centres in the midbrain at the level of the superior and inferior colliculus. The medial longitudinal fasiculus is the other system that is involved in the control of conjugate gaze.

Lesions that may result are:

- ♥ Horizontal Gaze Palsies
- ♠ Vertical Gaze Palsies

Horizontal Gaze Palsies

Horizontal gaze palsies could be due to lesions in the:

- ♦ Frontal lobe
- ♣ Pons

Frontal Lobe

Frontal lobe lesions result in conjugate deviation with the eyes deviated toward the lesion

Aide Memoire

Frontal **L**ooks at the **L**esion

Pontine Lesions

Pontine lesions cause conjugate deviation towards the paralysed side

Aide Memoire

Pontine **P**eers (**Peeps**) at **P**aralysis

Vertical Gaze Palsies

Vertical gaze palsies may be due to lesions in the:

- ♥ Superior Colliculus
- ♠ Inferior Colliculus

Superior Colliculus

Lesions in the superior colliculus cause paralysis of upward gaze.

Parinaud's syndrome consists of paralysis of upward gaze and convergence. Lesions in this area are uncommon. They could be due to:

- ♦ Compression from a supratentorial mass

♣ Brain stem tumour

Inferior Colliculus

Lesions in the inferior colliculus cause paralysis of downward gaze.

Progressive Supranuclear Palsy

Progressive supranuclear palsy affects voluntary eye movements. Initially vertical gaze is affected, particularly downward, but progression occurs and later horizontal gaze is affected as well.

Median Longitudinal Fasiculus

Lesions in the medial longitudinal fasiculus cause:

♥ Internuclear Ophthalmoplegia

♠ Divergent Squint

♦ Convergent Squint

Internuclear Ophthalmoplegia

Internuclear ophthalmoplegia results in weakness of adduction and nystagmus of the abducting eye on attempted lateral gaze. The lesions may be:

♣ **Unilateral Lesions** are usually due to ischaemia. Unilateral lesions are caused by pathology in the ipsilateral medial longitudinal fasiculus. The side of the lesion is the side of impaired adduction not the side of nystagmus.

♥ **Bilateral Lesions** are caused by multiple sclerosis

Divergent Squint

Divergent squint is caused by paralysis of the medial recti. It occurs in:

♠ Multiple sclerosis

♦ Vascular lesions

Convergent Squint

Convergent squint is due to weakness of abduction of both eyes. It may be differentiated from bilateral sixth nerve palsy as each eye moves normally when tested independently.

Gaze Apraxia

Gaze apraxia refers to an inability to direct the eyes towards an object and maintain fixation in the setting of an intact visual field and the absence of an oculomotor palsy and where random eye movements and oculo-cephalic reflexes are normal. It is associated with:

♣ Biparietal damage

Nystagmus

Nystagmus may be defined as a disturbance of ocular movements where there are involuntary, rhythmical oscillations of the eyes. Nystagmus may be:

♥ Pendular

♠ Horizontal

♦ Vertical

♣ Rotary

♥ Positional

485

Pendular Nystagmus

Pendular nystagmus refers to pendular, side-to-side movements with no distinct slow and fast component. The amplitude is equal in all directions. Pendular nystagmus may be:

- ♠ Familial
- ♦ It may occur when visual defects have been present from the early years of life. These could be lesions such as macular abnormalities, albinism, choroidoretinitis, high infantile myopia.

Horizontal Nystagmus

The direction of nystagmus is defined as the direction of the fast component.

- ♣ **Peripheral (labyrinth) Lesions**: The direction is away from the side of the lesion
- ♥ **Cerebellar Lesions**: The direction is towards the side of the lesion
- ♠ **Cerebello-Pontine Angle Lesions**: There are both peripheral and central effects but the amplitude of the movement is greater towards the side of the lesion (more central).

Ataxic Nystagmus (Dissociate Nystagmus)

In ataxic nystagmus, on attempted lateral gaze there is defective adduction of one eye with nystagmus of the abducting eye. It occurs in lesions of the medial longitudinal fasiculus commonly in:

- ♦ Multiple sclerosis
- ♣ Ischaemia

Convergence Nystagmus

In convergence nystagmus, on attempted upgaze, nystagmus is observed with the fast phase inwards, in a convergent manner. It indicates:

- ♥ Lesions of the upper midbrain close to the pineal gland

Vertical Nystagmus

Vertical nystagmus may be:

- ♠ Upbeat
- ♦ Downbeat

Upbeat Nystagmus

In upbeat nystagmus, the fast phase is upwards. It occurs in lesions of the:

- ♣ Floor of the fourth ventricle
- ♥ Pontine tegmentum
- ♠ Anterior cerebellum

Downbeat Nystagmus

In downbeat nystagmus, the fast phase is downwards. It occurs in lesions at the level of the foramen magnum such as:

- ♦ Herniation of the cerebellar tonsil

Rotary Nystagmus

Rotary nystagmus occurs in:

- ♣ Central lesions involving the medial vestibular nucleus

Positional Nystagmus

Positional nystagmus is demonstrated by moving the patient from an upright, seated position to a horizontal position with the head lowered below the horizontal. This is done rapidly. Positional nystagmus may be:

♥ Benign Positional Nystagmus

♠ Central Positional Nystagmus

Benign Positional Nystagmus

In benign positional nystagmus, the direction of nystagmus is towards the dependent ear. Nystagmus occurs after a short latent period, it is transient and is accompanied by vertigo. Benign positional nystagmus indicates:

♦ Utricular damage

Central Positional Nystagmus

In central positional nystagmus, the direction is not towards the dependent ear, it is persistent and there is no vertigo. It indicates:

♣ Central Damage (tumour or multiple sclerosis)

Pupils

When examining the pupils one may note abnormalities of:

♥ Size

♠ Shape

♦ Mobility

Size

On examination of the size of the pupils one may note that they are:

♣ Normal

♥ Dilated

♠ Constricted

Dilated Pupils

Dilated pupils may be due to:

♦ **Afferent Lesions**

The pupils would be dilated in amblyopic eyes (both eyes should be affected)

♣ **Third Nerve Lesion**

In a 3rd nerve lesion, one would observe a dilated pupil not reacting to light.

♥ **Holmes-Adie Pupil**

In the Holmes-Adie pupil one would observe a dilated pupil with poor contraction to light and slow response to accommodation. Abnormal tendon reflexes may occur.

♠ **Systemic Factors**

Systemic factors that result in dilated pupils are:

Drugs anticholinergics, cocaine

Constricted Pupils

Constricted pupils are caused by lesions in the:

♦ **Iris**

Iritis

♣ **Cervical Sympathetic**

The cervical sympathetics may be affected in:

Horner's Syndrome. In Horner's syndrome there would be a small pupil, ptosis, enophthalmos, lack of sweating on that side of the face and an absent cilio-spinal reflex.

♥ **Mid Brain**

Small pupils may be caused by lesions in the midbrain such as:

Argyll-Robertson Pupil. In Argyll-Robertson pupils there would be small, irregular pupils. They do not react to light but react to accommodation. Argyll-Robertson pupils occur in tabes dorsalis and in diabetes mellitus

♠ **Pontine Lesions**

Pontine lesions cause bilateral constricted pupils

♦ **Systemic Factors**

Systemic factors that could cause constricted pupils are:

Drugs opiate use causes bilateral constricted pupils

Toxins organophosphate poisoning

Shape

The shape of the pupils may change and the pupils may be irregular.

Irregular Pupils

Irregular pupils could be due to:

♣ Coloboma of the iris

♥ Previous episodes of anterior uveitis

♠ Argyll-Robertson pupil

Mobility

The pupil constricts in response to light and accommodation. It dilates in response to stress. The abnormalities that may be elicited are:

♦ Absent Light Reflex

♣ Relative Apparent Pupillary Defect (RAPD)

♥ Holmes-Adie Pupil

♠ Argyll-Robertson Pupil

♦ Hippus

♣ Ciliospinal Reflex

Absent Light Reflex

An absent light reflex could be due to an:

♣ Afferent Defect

♥ Efferent Defect

Afferent Defect

An afferent defect would include:

♠ Most causes of blindness

Efferent Defect

An efferent defect would be due to:

♦ Third nerve palsy

Relative Apparent Pupillary Defect (RAPD)

This defect may be demonstrated using the swinging light test. When light is initially shone in the affected eye both the affected pupil and the unaffected pupil constrict. When the light is shone in the unaffected eye both direct and consensual reflexes occur and both pupils constrict. However, when light is now shone back into the affected eye the pupil dilates instead of constricting. This indicates that the consensual light reflex is more powerful than the direct. It occurs when there is incomplete damage to one optic nerve as in previous retrobulbar neuritis where there has been apparent full recovery of vision.

Holmes-Adie Pupil

In the Holmes-Adie pupil reaction to light and or accommodation is delayed or absent.

Argyll-Robertson Pupil

In Argyll-Robertson pupils reaction to light is absent. Both direct and consensual light reflexes cannot be elicited. The pupils react to accommodation. The causes are:

- ♥ **CNS** syringobulbia, brainstem encephalitis, pinealoma
- ♠ **RAG** syphilis
- ♦ **E&M** diabetes mellitus
- ♣ **LMS** Lyme disease
- ♥ **RS** sarcoidosis

Hippus

In hippus, there is rhythmical constriction and dilatation of the pupil either spontaneously or in response to light. It is usually of no significance but it may be seen in:

- ♠ Retrobulbar neuritis

Ciliospinal Reflex

The pupil dilates when the skin over the ipsilateral side of the neck is pinched. This is called the ciliospinal reflex.

Absent Ciliospinal Reflex

The ciliospinal reflex is absent in:

- ♦ Horner's syndrome

Horner's syndrome

Horner's syndrome consists of partial ptosis, constricted pupils, abolition of the ciliospinal reflex, absence of sweating on that side of the face, apparent enophthalmos.

Horner's syndrome could be due to:

- ♥ **Hemisphere Lesions**: massive cerebral infarction
- ♠ **Brainstem Lesions**: pontine glioma, lateral medullary syndrome
- ♦ **Cervical Cord Lesions**: syringomyelia, cord tumours
- ♣ **Chest Lesions**: Pancoast's syndrome, aortic aneurysm
- ♥ **Neck Lesions**: cervical rib, brachial plexus trauma, neck surgery or trauma, carotid aneurysm, cervical lymphadenopathy

Lack of Sweating in Horner's Syndrome

- ♠ **Central lesions**

  Central lesions affect sweating over the ipsilateral half of the head, arm and upper trunk

- ♦ **Neck lesions**

  Lesions in the neck proximal to the superior cervical ganglion cause reduced facial sweating

- ♣ **Lesions distal to the superior cervical ganglion**

  These lesions do not affect sweating at all

489

Colour of the Pupil

In congenital Horner's syndrome the ipsilateral iris is lighter in colour (heterochromia of the iris). The lesion is thought to be caused by birth trauma.

Face

Examination of the face involves examination of the structure of the face and examination of the functions of the seventh nerve and the sensory component of the fifth nerve.

Structure of the Face

On examination of the structure of the face one may note abnormalities of the following:

- ♥ Skin
- ♠ Circulation

Skin

The lesions that may be detected are:

- ♦ **Dystrophia myotonica**: Frontal balding
- ♣ **Sturge-Weber syndrome**: Port-wine stain or capillary haemangioma
- ♥ **Tuberose sclerosis**: Salmon-coloured papules

Circulation

The temporal artery would be tender and non-pulsatile in:

- ♠ Temporal arteritis

Facial Nerve

On examination of the facial nerve one may detect abnormalities of the following:

- ♦ Position
- ♣ Size
- ♥ Involuntary movements
- ♠ Power
- ♦ Reflexes
- ♣ Buccofacial apraxia
- ♥ Sensation

Position (at rest)

In relation to the facial nerve, when assessing the position of the facial muscles at rest, one may note:

- ♦ In facial nerve palsy, loss of the naso-labial fold and drooping of the angle of the mouth would occur.
- ♣ In lower motor neurone lesions there would be no wrinkling of the forehead on the affected side.

Size

On examination of the size of the facial muscles one may note:

- ♥ Wasting of the facial muscles occurs in dystrophia myotonica.

Involuntary Movements of the Face

When assessing involuntary movements of the face one may note:

- ♠ Lack of Facial Expression
- ♦ Orofacial Dyskinesis

490

Lack of Facial Expression

Lack of facial expression would occur in generalised loss of facial muscle function. This occurs in:

- ♣ Myopathies
- ♥ Bilateral facial nerve palsy
- ♠ Parkinsonism

Orofacial Dyskinesis

Orofacial dyskinesis refers to orofacial movement, lip smacking and tongue protrusion. It is a chronic tardive dyskinesia and occurs as a result of chronic treatment with neuroleptics.

Muscle Power

Weakness of the facial muscles may be due to a:

- ♣ **Lower Motor Neurone Lesion**

  Weakness of both the upper and lower parts of the face occur in lower motor neurone lesions

- ♥ **Upper Motor Neurone Lesion**

  The upper part of the face is spared in upper motor neurone lesions

Bell's Sign

This refers to upward movement of the eye on attempted eye closure in lower motor neurone facial palsy.

Causes of Facial Palsy

Facial nerve lesions may be:

- ♠ Unilateral
- ♦ Bilateral

Unilateral Lesions of the Facial Nerve

Unilateral lesions of the facial nerve may be:

- ♣ Unilateral Upper Motor Neurone Lesions
- ♥ Unilateral Lower Motor Neurone Lesions

Unilateral Upper Motor Neurone Lesions

Unilateral upper motor neurone lesions occur in:

- ♠ Cerebrovascular disease

Unilateral Lower Motor Neurone Lesions

Unilateral lower motor neurone lesions of the facial nerve may occur at the level of the:

- ♦ Pons
- ♣ Cerebello-Pontine Angle
- ♥ Nerve Pathway

Pons

The facial nerve may be affected at the level of the pons in:

- ♠ Cerebrovascular disease. This is associated with contralateral weakness of the limbs, the Millard-Gubler syndrome. The sixth nerve may be affected as well.
- ♦ Brain stem tumours
- ♣ Poliomyelitis

Cerebello-Pontine Angle

The facial nerve may be affected at the cerebello-pontine angle in:

- ♥ Acoustic neuroma

Nerve Pathway

The nerve may be affected along its path by:

- ♠ Mononeuritis multiplex
- ♦ Basal meningitis
- ♣ Meningeal carcinomatosis
- ♥ Middle ear disease
- ♠ Bell's palsy
- ♦ Ramsay-Hunt syndrome
- ♣ Trauma
- ♥ Parotid tumours

Bilateral Facial Weakness

Bilateral facial weakness may be due to:

- ♠ Bilateral Upper Motor Neurone Lesions
- ♦ Bilateral Lower Motor Neurone Lesions
- ♣ Neuromuscular Junction Lesions
- ♥ Myopathy

Bilateral Upper Motor Neurone Lesions

Bilateral upper motor neurone lesions of the facial nerve occur in:

- ♠ Pseudobulbar palsy

Bilateral Lower Motor Neurone Lesions

Bilateral lower motor neurone lesions of the facial nerve may be due to:

- ♦ Congenital facial diplegia (Mobius' syndrome). The features are congenital bilateral facial palsy with third and sixth nerve palsies
- ♣ Motor neurone disease
- ♥ Poliomyelitis
- ♠ Basal meningitis
- ♦ Carcinomatous infiltration of the meninges
- ♣ Guillain-Barre syndrome
- ♥ Bilateral Bell's palsy
- ♠ Lyme disease
- ♦ Sarcoidosis

Neuromuscular Junction Lesions

Neuromuscular junction lesions involving the facial muscles could be due to:

- ♣ Myasthenia gravis

Myopathy

Myopathy involving the facial muscles could be due to:

- ♥ Muscular dystrophy (facioscapulohumeral, dystrophia myotonica)

Dystrophia myotonica

The features are cataract, frontal balding, ptosis, wasted facial muscles, atrophic temporalis, transverse smile, sternomastoid wasting. Limb weakness is predominantly distal. Dysphagia, cardiomyopathy and gonadal atrophy also occur.

Reflexes

The reflexes that involve the facial nerve are the:

- ♠ Corneal Reflex
- ♦ Glabella Tap
- ♣ Snout Reflex

Corneal Reflex

The corneal reflex would be lost in:

♥ Lower motor neurone lesions of the facial nerve

Glabella Tap

Glabella tap would be positive in:

♠ Parkinsonism

Snout Reflex

The snout reflex refers to puckering or protrusion of the lips on stroking the upper lip. This occurs in:

♦ Frontal lobe lesions

♣ Bilateral upper motor neurone facial lesions

Buccofacial (orofacial) Apraxia

Buccofacial apraxia may be associated with motor aphasia.

Sensation

Sensory abnormalities that occur in relation to the facial nerve are abnormalities of:

♥ Taste sensation

♠ Hearing

Taste Sensation

Loss of taste sensation over the anterior two-thirds of the tongue would occur in facial nerve lesions proximal to the origin of the chorda tympani nerve.

Hyperacusis

Hyperacusis would occur if the nerve supply to the stapedius were affected.

Trigeminal Nerve

On examination of the trigeminal nerve one may note abnormalities of the:

♥ Motor component

♠ Sensory component

♦ Corneal reflex

Motor Component of the Trigeminal Nerve

On examination of the motor component of the trigeminal nerve one may note abnormalities of:

♦ Size

♣ Power

♥ Reflexes

Size of Muscles

Wasting of the masseter and temporalis may occur in:

♦ **Myopathies**: myotonia dystrophica, facioscapulohumeral dystrophy

♣ **Lower motor neurone involvement**: motor neurone disease

Power of Muscles

Weakness of the muscles of mastication occurs in:

♥ **Myopathies**: dystrophia myotonica, facioscapulohumeral dystrophy

♠ **Neuromuscular Junction Involvement**: myasthenia gravis

♦ **Lower Motor Neurone Involvement**: motor neurone disease

Reflexes

In relation to the trigeminal nerve one would test the jaw jerk.

Jaw Jerk

The jaw jerk would be brisk in pseudobulbar palsy

Causes of Pseudobulbar Palsy

Pseudobulbar palsy may be caused by:

- ♥ Cerebrovascular disease (bilateral)
- ♠ Multiple sclerosis
- ♦ Motor neurone disease
- ♣ High brain stem tumour
- ♥ Head injury

Sensory Component of the Trigeminal Nerve

On examination of the sensory component of the trigeminal nerve one may note:

- ♠ Sensory Loss
- ♦ Loss of the corneal reflex

Sensory Loss

Sensory loss over the distribution of the trigeminal nerve may be due to lesions at the following sites:

- ♣ Peripheral Sensory Loss
- ♥ Apex of Petrous Bone
- ♠ Cerebello-Pontine Angle Lesions
- ♦ Pontine Lesions

Peripheral Sensory Loss

Peripheral sensory loss may be over the:

- ♣ Ophthalmic Division
- ♥ Maxillary Division
- ♠ Mandibular Division
- ♦ Isolated Trigeminal Neuropathy

Ophthalmic Division of the Trigeminal Nerve

Lesions of the ophthalmic division may be due to:

- ♣ Trauma
- ♥ Herpes zoster

Or it may be due to lesions at the:

- ♠ **Superior Orbital Fissure**

  Tumour invading the superior orbital fissure. This would be associated with an ophthalmoplegia due to involvement of the 3rd, 4th and 6th nerves and proptosis due to compression of the ophthalmic vein.

  Tolosa-Hunt syndrome

- ♦ **Cavernous Sinus**

  Lesions in the cavernous sinus are associated with 3rd, 4th, 6th nerve lesions, proptosis, chemosis, engorgement of the retinal veins and papilloedema (sometimes). The maxillary division may also be involved. (Bilateral involvement is considered diagnostic of cavernous sinus thrombosis although in some instances features may be unilateral)

Maxillary Division of the Trigeminal Nerve

Lesions of the maxillary division are usually due to:

- ♣ Trauma
- ♥ Cavernous sinus lesions

Mandibular Division of the Trigeminal Nerve

Lesions of the mandibular division are not common. Causes include:

- ♠ Impacted molars
- ♦ Metastases

It may be associated with a motor lesion of the fifth.

Isolated Trigeminal Neuropathy

Isolated trigeminal neuropathy may occur in:

- ♣ Sjogren's syndrome
- ♥ Systemic Sclerosis
- ♠ Amyloidosis
- ♦ Idiopathic

Apex of Petrous Bone

Lesions at the apex of the petrous temporal bone may be associated with a 6th nerve lesion; Gradenigo's syndrome. It is due to:

- ♣ Osteomyelitis

Cerebello-Pontine Angle Lesions

Lesions at the cerebello-pontine angle are associated with 7th, 8th nerve lesions. The lesions that could occur are:

- ♥ Acoustic neuroma
- ♠ Meningioma
- ♦ Aneurysm of the basilar artery

Pontine Lesions

Pontine lesions cause checkerboard anaesthesia; sensory loss over the face and contralateral sensory loss over the limbs. Pontine lesions may be due to:

- ♣ Vascular lesions

- ♥ Syringobulbia

Corneal Reflex

The corneal reflex would be absent in fifth nerve lesions that affect the ophthalmic division.

Glossopharyngeal, Vagus, Hypoglossal and Accessory Nerves

These four cranial nerves are closely related at their sites of origin and their nerve pathways. When considering lesions of these nerves the anatomical localisation should be considered in terms of:

- ♦ Intramedullary Lesions
- ♣ Posterior Fossa Lesions
- ♥ Foramen Lesions:

  Jugular foramen lesions

  Hypoglossal canal lesions
- ♦ Cervical Lesions
- ♣ Thoracic Lesions (in the case of the vagus nerve)

Glossopharyngeal, Vagus, Hypoglossal Nerves (9th, 10 th, 12th)

When examining the 9th, 10th and 12th nerves one may note abnormalities of the:

- ♥ Mouth
- ♠ Palate
- ♦ Tongue

Mouth

On examination of the mouth one may note:

♣ Drooling of saliva. This would be a feature of Parkinsonism

Palate

When examining the palate one may note abnormalities of:

♥ Structure

♠ Involuntary movements

♦ Power

♣ Gag reflex

Structure

A high arched palate occurs in:

♥ Friedrich's ataxia

Involuntary Movement

One may observe:

♠ Palatal Myoclonus. This refers to persistent, rhythmical contraction of the soft palate. It may cause dysarthria. It is due to an infarct or demyelination in the brainstem resulting in damage to the dentato-rubro-olivary pathway.

Power (Palatal Movement)

Palatal movement would be abnormal in upper and lower motor neurone lesions.

♦ **Unilateral Lesions**

In unilateral lesions the uvula would move away from the paralysed side as it is pulled by the contracting muscle.

♣ **Bilateral Lesions**

In bilateral lesions there would be no palatal movement.

Gag Reflex

In relation to the 9th and 10th cranial nerves the reflex that would be tested is the gag reflex.

♥ The gag reflex would be absent in both upper and lower motor neurone lesions and in sensory loss. In sensory loss the patient would not perceive an unpleasant sensation.

Tongue

When examining the tongue one may note abnormalities of:

♠ Size

♦ Tone

♣ Power

♥ Sensation

Size

Variations in the size of the tongue would be seen in:

♣ **Lower Motor Neurone Lesions**

In lower motor neurone lesions wasting would be observed on the affected side of the tongue

♦ **Upper Motor Neurone Lesions**

In bilateral upper motor neurone lesions the tongue would be small and spastic.

Tone

Abnormalities of tone would be:

♣ The tongue would be spastic in bilateral upper motor neurone lesions

♥ Percussion myotonia may be observed in dystrophia myotonia; indentation made by the teeth fill out slowly

Involuntary Movements

Involuntary movements that may be seen in the tongue are:

♥ Fasciculations would be seen in motor neurone disease affecting the lower motor neurones

♠ Trombone tremor would be observed in Parkinsonism and in general paralysis of the insane. The tongue moves in and out like the movement of a trombone.

♦ Continuous rotatory movement would be observed in drug-induced dyskinesia. The drugs that are most likely to cause this are the phenothiazines.

♣ In patients with chorea, the tongue would dart in and out of the mouth if the patient were asked to keep his or her mouth open.

Power

On asking the patient to protrude his or her tongue it will deviate to the affected side in lower motor neurone lesions.

Sensory System

Taste in the posterior third of tongue would be lost in glossopharyngeal lesions. This would hardly ever be tested in practice.

Lesions of the 9th, 10th, 12th Nerves

Lesions of the 9th, 10th and 12th nerves could be:

♣ Upper Motor Neurone Lesions

♥ Lower Motor Neurone Lesions

Upper Motor Neurone Lesions

Upper motor neurone lesions of the 9th, 10th, 12th nerves could be:

♠ Bilateral lesions

♦ Unilateral lesions

Bilateral Lesions

Bilateral lesions of the 9th, 10th and 12th nerves occur in:

♣ Pseudobulbar palsy, which may result from bilateral stroke, multiple sclerosis, motor neurone disease

Unilateral Lesions

Unilateral lesions cause mild and short lasting clinical features.

Lower Motor Neurone Lesions

Lower motor neurone lesions of the 9th, 10th, 12th nerves occur in:

♠ Lateral Medullary Syndrome

♦ Medial Medullary Syndrome

♣ Bulbar Palsy

♥ Jugular Foramen Syndrome

♠ Hypoglossal Canal Syndrome

♦ Cervical Lesions

♣ Thoracic Lesions

497

Lateral Medullary Syndrome

In the lateral medullary syndrome there would be:

- ♥ Dysphagia and dysarthria due to involvement of the ninth and tenth nuclei
- ♠ Ipsilateral cerebellar signs
- ♦ Ipsilateral Horner's syndrome
- ♣ Vertigo, vomiting and hiccup
- ♥ Loss of pain and temperature sensation in the face
- ♠ Loss of pain and temperature sensation in the contralateral limbs

The lateral medullary syndrome involves the 9th and 10th nuclei, nucleus ambiguus, vestibular nuclei, inferior cerebellar peduncle, descending autonomic fibres, 5th nerve nucleus, lateral leminiscus. The lesion is usually due to involvement of the posterior inferior cerebellar artery.

Medial Medullary Syndrome

In the medial medullary syndrome there would be:

- ♦ Weakness and loss of position sense of the contralateral limbs
- ♣ Ipsilateral weakness of the tongue

The medial medullary syndrome involves the pyramidal tract, the medial leminiscus and the 12th nerve nucleus. The lesion is due to involvement of the vertebral artery or one of its branches or a branch of the lower basilar artery.

Bulbar Palsy

Bulbar palsy may be due to:

- ♥ Nuclear Damage
- ♠ Posterior Fossa Lesions

Nuclear Damage

Nuclear damage may be due to:

- ♦ Motor neurone disease (progressive bulbar palsy)
- ♣ Syringobulbia
- ♥ Poliomyelitis

Posterior Fossa Lesions

Posterior fossa lesions may be due to:

- ♠ Meningeal involvement caused by lymphoma, carcinoma, meningo-vascular syphilis
- ♦ Guillain-Barre syndrome

Jugular Foramen Syndrome

The jugular foramen syndrome affects the 9th, 10th and 11th nerves and is caused by:

- ♣ Middle ear infection
- ♥ Granulomatous meningitis
- ♠ Neurofibroma
- ♦ Epidermoid tumours
- ♣ Cerbellopontine angle lesions
- ♥ Glomus or carotid body tumours
- ♠ Metastases

Hypoglossal Canal Syndrome

The hypoglossal canal syndrome affects the hypoglossal nerve only and is caused by tumours in this region.

Cervical Lesions

Cervical lesions are caused by:

- ♣ Trauma
- ♥ Cancer

Thoracic Lesions

Thoracic lesions affect the recurrent laryngeal nerve. Lesions are caused by:

- ♠ Bronchial cancer
- ♦ Aortic aneurysm
- ♣ Surgery

Neck

Abnormalities may be noted of:

- ♥ Structure
- ♠ Function

Structure

One may note abnormalities of

- ♦ Size
- ♣ Circulation

Size

Abnormalities of the size of the neck are:

- ♥ A short neck would be seen in the Klippel-Feil syndrome (reduction in the number of cervical vertebrae with fusion of two or more), which is associated with syringomyelia. The other features are a low hairline (posteriorly), webbing of the neck. Rotation of the neck is limited.
- ♠ Wasted neck muscles occur in facioscapulohumeral dystrophy

Circulation

When examining the circulation one may note:

- ♥ A bruit over the carotids indicating stenosis

Function

When examining function one may detect abnormalities of:

- ♦ Position
- ♣ Power

Position

When observing the position of the neck one may note:

Torticollis

In torticollis the neck is held in a twisted position.

- ♦ Spasmodic torticollis is a type of adult onset focal dystonia.

Power

When examining power one may note weakness of the:

- ♣ Sternomastoid
- ♥ Trapezius

Sternomastoid Weakness

Sternomastoid weakness may be due to lesions at the level of:

- ♠ **Muscle**

  Weakness of muscles occurs in:

  Facioscapulohumeral dystrophy, dystrophia myotonica

- ♦ **Nerve**

  Nerve lesions occur in:

Motor neurone disease, jugular foremen syndrome

Trapezius

Weakness of the trapezius could be due to:

- ♣ Motor neurone disease, poliomyelitis
- ♥ Jugular foramen syndrome

Ears

Abnormalities may be noted of:

- ♠ Structure
- ♦ Function

Structure

On examination of the structure of the ears one may note:

- ♥ Herpetic vesicles in the Ramsay-Hunt syndrome

Function

Here one would test function of the vestibulocochlear nerve.

Vestibulocochlear Nerve (8ᵗʰ)

One may divide lesions of the vestibulocochlear nerve into:

- ♠ Vestibular lesions
- ♦ Cochlear lesions

Vestibular Lesions

Vestibular lesions present with vertigo, which is described as a sensation of movement (either of the patient or his or her surroundings),

inability to stand, nausea and vomiting, sweating and nystagmus.

The causes of vestibular lesions may be classified as lesions in the:

- ♣ Labyrinth
- ♥ Nerve
- ♠ Central connections

Labyrinth

Lesions of the labyrinth include:

- ♦ Benign paroxysmal vertigo
- ♣ Labyrinthitis
- ♥ Meniere's disease
- ♠ Trauma
- ♦ Otitis media
- ♣ Herpes zoster
- ♥ Drugs: aminoglycosides, quinine, phenytoin,
- ♠ Toxins: alcohol

Nerve Lesions

The 8ᵗʰ nerve may be involved in:

- ♦ Fractures of the skull
- ♣ Vestibular neuronitis
- ♥ Chronic basal meningitis
- ♠ Carcinomatous meningeal infiltration
- ♦ Cerbellopontine angle lesions

Central Lesions

Central lesions that involve the 8ᵗʰ nerve include:

- ♣ Syringobulbia
- ♥ Lateral medullary syndrome
- ♠ Multiple sclerosis
- ♦ Encephalitis
- ♣ Tumours such as glioma

♥ Alcohol

♠ Anticonvulsants

Cochlear Lesions

Cochlear lesions result in abnormalities of hearing.

Deafness

The difference between conductive deafness and perceptive or nerve deafness is made on the basis of the Rinne and Weber test. Normally air conduction is better than bone conduction.

♠ **Rinne Test**

In the Rinne test, a person with normal hearing would hear the sound better when the tuning fork is held in front of the ear rather than when it is held over the mastoid. In conductive deafness the reverse occurs.

♦ **Weber Test**

In the Weber test, conductive deafness would result in the patient hearing the sound better in the affected ear. In nerve deafness the patient would hear the sound better in the normal ear.

Deafness may be due to lesions in the:

♦ **Environment**

Exposure to loud noise

♣ **External Ear**

Impacted wax

♥ **Middle Ear**

Otitis media, damage to the ossicles in Paget's disease of bone, otosclerosis

♠ **Inner Ear**

Meniere's disease

♦ **Nerve**

Compression of the nerve in Paget's disease of bone, acoustic neuroma, basal meningitis, trauma

Drugs: aminoglycosides, aspirin, quinine

♣ **Systemic Factors**

KUS Alport's syndrome

E&M Pendred's syndrome

CVS Long QT syndrome (Jervell-Lange-Nielsen syndrome is an autosomal recessive condition with neural deafness and long QT interval)

LMS osteogenesis imperfecta

Hyperacusis

Hyperacusis refers to abnormally increased hearing. Sounds would be unusually loud and even heard with painful intensity.

♣ Hyperacusis occurs when the stapedius muscle is paralysed in geniculate ganglion lesions

Cortical Deafness

Cortical deafness refers to an inability to recognise spoken language or sounds despite intact hearing. Written text may be understood. Language output is normal. The sites of the lesions are:

♥ Bilateral lesions of the posterosuperior temporal lobe

The causes of cortical deafness are:

♠ Strokes

♦ Prolonged hypotension

♣ Carbon monoxide poisoning

Upper Limbs

The abnormalities that may be detected when the upper limbs are examined in general are those that may be detected:

♦ At rest

♣ Arms raised

At Rest

When looking at the patient's upper limbs as a whole, at rest, one may observe changes in

♥ Structure

♠ Function

Structure

Abnormalities of the structure of the upper limbs are changes in:

♦ Size

♣ Muscle mass

Size

One may observe variations in the size of the upper limbs as a whole.

♦ **Small Limb**. The limb may be small in infantile hemiplegia, childhood poliomyelitis, uncorrected birth trauma

Muscle Mass

When examining muscle mass one may note:

♣ **Atrophy**

Atrophy of muscles may occur in atrophic crural monoplegia, which is rare. The causes are:

Poliomyelitis, motor neurone disease, syringomyelia, brachial plexus lesions

Function of the Upper Limbs at Rest

Functional abnormalities that may be noted with the upper limb at rest are abnormalities of:

♥ Position

♠ Involuntary movements

Position

Abnormalities of the position of the limb at rest would be seen in:

♥ Hemiplegia. Here the limb would be in a state of flexion with flexion at the elbow, the wrist would be flexed and pronated. The fingers would be flexed.

♠ Erb's palsy. This is caused by injury to roots C_5, C_6 and results in weakness of the abductors and lateral rotators of the shoulder and supinators. The arm hangs by the side medially rotated, extended at the elbow and pronated.

Involuntary Movements

Involuntary movements that may be seen with the upper limbs at rest are:

♦ Chorea

♣ Athetosis

♥ Ballism

Arms Raised

When the patient is asked to raise his or her arms one may observe abnormalities of:

- ♠ Power
- ♦ Position
- ♣ Abnormal movements
- ♥ Coordination

Power

An inability to lift the arm or loss of power in the entire upper limb could occur in:

- ♠ Hemiplegia
- ♦ Quadriparesis
- ♣ Monoplegia

Position

Abnormalities of position that may be observed when the patient is asked to raise his or her arms are:

- ♥ Wrist Drop
- ♠ Parietal Drift
- ♦ Pronator Drift

Wrist Drop

Wrist drop is a consequence of radial nerve palsy. Radial nerve palsy may be caused by:

- ♣ Compression (Saturday night palsy, crutch palsy)
- ♥ Trauma due to fracture of the humerus
- ♠ Shoulder dislocation
- ♦ Lead poisoning

Parietal Drift

Parietal drift or an upward drift is caused by:

- ♣ Contralateral parietal lobe lesions

Pronator Drift

Pronator drift (downwards with pronation) occurs in:

- ♥ Upper motor neurone lesions

Involuntary Movements

Involuntary movements that may be observed when the patient is asked to raise his or her arms are:

- ♠ Exaggerated physiological tremor
- ♦ Flapping tremor
- ♣ Chorea
- ♥ Athetosis
- ♠ Ballism

Coordination

The abnormality in coordination that may be noted at this stage of the neurological examination is:

- ♦ **Dysmetria**. In dysmetria when the outstretched arm is tapped, it will dip down and spring back overshooting its original position. This would indicate an ipsilateral cerebellar lesion

Hands

On examination of the hands one may note abnormalities of:

- ♣ Position
- ♥ Muscle mass
- ♠ Involuntary movements
- ♦ Tone
- ♣ Power

Position

Abnormalities that may be observed of the position (shape) of the hands (deformities of the hands) are:

- ♥ Claw hand
- ♠ Ulnar claw hand
- ♦ Simian hand
- ♣ Contractures

Claw Hand

In a claw hand, the fingers are extended at the metacarpophalangeal joints and flexed at the proximal and distal interphalangeal joints. A claw hand may be caused by:

- ♥ Combined median and ulnar nerve lesions
- ♠ T_1 lesions

Ulnar Claw Hand

An ulnar claw hand is a claw hand where only the fourth and fifth fingers are affected. It is caused by lesions of the:

- ♦ Ulnar nerve

Simian Hand

In a Simian hand the hand is ulnar deviated, the index and middle fingers are extended to a greater degree than normal, the thumb lies in the same plane as the other fingers. It is caused by:

- ♣ Complete lesions of the median nerve at the elbow

Contractures

In contractures there is flexion of all the joints, the metacarpophalangeal, the proximal interphalangeal and the distal interphalangeal. Types of contractures that may be observed are:

- ♥ **Dupuytren's Contracture**

  Dupuytren's contracture is caused by fibrosis of the palmar aponeurosis.

- ♠ **Volkmann's Ischaemic Contracture**

  Volkmann's ischaemic contracture refers to contracture of the long flexors of the fingers. Flexion of the fingers becomes greater when the wrist is extended and decreases when the wrist is flexed. Volkmann's ischaemic contracture is caused by ischaemia due to compression by tight plaster casts or it may occur following the formation of haematoma in the forearm muscles.

- ♦ **Stroke**

  In longstanding stroke the patient may develop contractures.

Muscle Mass

Abnormalities that may be detected of the muscle mass of the hand are:

- ♣ Wasting of all the small muscles occurs in T_1 lesions or in combined ulnar and median nerve lesions

- ♥ Wasting of the lateral aspect of the thenar eminence occurs in median nerve lesions

- ♠ Wasting of the hypothenar eminence, the interossei and the medial part of the thenar eminence occurs in ulnar nerve lesions

Involuntary Movements

Involuntary movements that may be observed in the hand are:

- Pill rolling movements in Parkinsonism

Tone

The abnormality of tone that may be observed in the hand is:

Percussion Myotonia

Percussion myotonia refers to slow filling of a depression made in the thenar eminence by percussion. It occurs in:

- Myotonic dystrophy

Power

Abnormalities of power that may occur in the hands are:

- Weakness of all the small muscles of the hand occurs in T_1 lesions or in combined median and ulnar nerve lesions
- Weakness of flexion, abduction and opposition of the thumb occurs in median nerve lesions
- Weakness of the muscles of the hypothenar eminence together with weakness of abduction and adduction of the fingers occurs in ulnar nerve lesions

---

Wrists and Forearms

On examination of the wrists and forearms one may note abnormalities of the following:

- Position
- Muscle mass

- Involuntary movements
- Tone
- Muscle power

Position

- Wrist drop would have been noted already

Muscle Mass

Abnormalities that may be detected of the muscle mass in the forearms are:

- Wasting occurs in peripheral neuropathy
- Wasting of the medial side of the forearm flexor muscle mass occurs in lesions affecting the ulnar nerve at the elbow

Involuntary Movements

Involuntary movements that may occur are:

- Milkmaid's grip. This refers to alternating squeezing and relaxing of the hand when the patient is asked to grip one's fingers. This would be noted in patients with chorea.

Tone

Abnormalities of tone that may be noted are:

- The cogwheel rigidity of Parkinsonism is best noted when performing movements at the wrist joint
- Spasticity occurs in upper motor neurone lesions
- Myotonia may be noted here if one were to shake hands with the

patient. The causes of myotonia are:

Myotonia congenita (this is associated with diffuse muscular hypertrophy)

Dystrophia myotonica

Paramyotonia congenita (refers to episodic myotonia following exposure to cold)

♦ Decreased tone occurs in lower motor neurone lesions

Muscle Power

Abnormalities that may be detected of the power of the muscles involved in movements of the wrists and forearms are:

♣ Weakness of the long flexors and extensors would occur in C_8 lesions

♥ In radial nerve palsy, brachioradialis, supinator and all the forearm extensor muscles would be paralysed. Flexion of the fingers would be normal if the wrist were to be held in a position of dorsiflexion.

♠ In lesions affecting the median nerve in the forearm:

Pronation would be weak. Weakness of the wrist flexors would be evident when tested against resistance. The hand would be ulnar deviated and the tendon of flexor carpi ulnaris would stand out. The index finger cannot be flexed and the middle finger can only be incompletely flexed. The 4th and 5th fingers may be flexed although they are weaker than normal. Flexion at the metacarpophalangeal joints

would be possible in all the fingers through the action of the lumbricals

♦ Lesions affecting the ulnar nerve at the elbow would cause weakness of flexion of the fourth and fifth fingers

Elbows and Upper Arms

When examining the elbows and upper arms one may note abnormalities of:

♣ Position

♥ Tone

♠ Muscle power

♦ Blood pressure

Position

Abnormalities that may be observed of the position of the elbow are:

♣ An increased carrying angle may be the cause of an ulnar nerve lesion

♥ In upper motor neurone lesions the elbow would be flexed

Tone

Abnormalities of tone that may be noted in the upper arm are:

♠ Increased tone of clasp-knife character would be noted in upper motor neurone lesions

♦ Cogwheel rigidity would be noted in Parkinsonism.

Muscle Power

Abnormalities of muscle power that may be detected at the elbow and upper arm are:

♣ Weakness of the triceps and biceps occurs in facioscapulo-humeral dystrophy

♥ Weakness of the triceps with failure to extend the elbow occurs in radial nerve injury caused by lesions in the axilla.

Blood Pressure

The blood pressure may be:

♠ High in cerebrovascular disease

♦ Postural hypotension may occur in autonomic neuropathy

Shoulders

When examining the shoulders one may note changes in:

♥ Structure

♣ Muscle mass

♥ Abnormal movements

♠ Muscle power

Structure

Charcot's joints may occur in:

♦ Syringomyelia

Muscle Mass

Wasting

Wasting may be seen in:

♣ **Muscle Lesions**

Limb girdle muscular dystrophy, facioscapulohumeral muscular dystrophy

♥ **Neuromuscular Junction Lesions**

Eaton-Lambert syndrome

♠ **Lower Motor Neurone Lesions**

Proximal hereditary motor neuronopathy

Abnormal Movements

Abnormal movements that may occur at the shoulder are:

♦ Fasiculation may be seen in proximal hereditary motor neuronopathy

Muscle Power

Weakness

Weakness of the shoulder muscles occurs in:

♣ **Muscle Lesions**

Muscle lesions may be primary myopathies or secondary to systemic causes.

Primary Myopathies

Primary myopathies that present with weakness at the shoulder are:

Limb girdle muscular dystrophy, facioscapulohumeral muscular dystrophy

Systemic Causes

Systemic causes of proximal myopathy have already been discussed in detail

♥ **Neuromuscular Junction Lesions**

Neuromuscular junction lesions that affect the proximal musculature are:

Eaton-Lambert syndrome

♠ **Lower Motor Neurone Lesions**

507

Lower motor neurone lesions that affect the shoulder muscles are:

Proximal hereditary motor neuronopathy

Axillary nerve damage in shoulder injuries causes an almost complete inability to raise the arm at the shoulder.

+ **Upper Motor Neurone Lesions**

Upper motor neurone lesions that affect the shoulder muscles are:

Hemiplegia, quadriplegia

Scapula

On examination of the scapula one may note abnormalities of the following:

♣ Position

♥ Muscle mass

♠ Muscle power

Position

Abnormalities that may be noted in the position of the scapula are:

♣ Elevation

♥ Winging

Elevation

Elevation of the scapula occurs in:

♠ Sprengel deformity. This refers to unilateral or bilateral elevation of the scapula. It is associated with Klippel-Feil syndrome

♦ Facioscapulohumeral muscular dystrophy

Winging

Winging of the scapula may occur in:

♣ Facioscapulohumeral muscular dystrophy

♥ Serratus anterior weakness caused by lesions of the long thoracic nerve, which may be damaged by shoulder injuries, surgery, brachial neuritis.

Muscle Mass

Atrophy

Atrophy of the muscles around the scapula may occur in:

♠ Facioscapulohumeral muscular dystrophy

♦ Limb girdle dystrophy

♣ Neuralgic amyotrophy (brachial neuritis)

Muscle Power

Weakness

Weakness of the scapular muscles occurs in:

♥ Facioscapulohumeral muscular dystrophy

♠ Limb girdle dystrophy

♦ Neuralgic amyotrophy (brachial neuritis)

Reflexes of the Upper Limb

The causes of exaggerated and diminished reflexes have already been dealt with.

♣ **Inverted Supinator Jerk**. This is seen in lesions that occur at spinal segments C_5, C_6. The result is loss of the normal supinator jerk (contraction of the brachioradialis with flexion of the elbow) flexion of the fingers occurs instead. (Lower motor neurone lesion at $C_{5/6}$ upper motor neurone lesion below $C_{5/6}$)

Coordination of Movement in the Upper Limb

Abnormalities of coordination that affect the upper limb could be:

Unilateral

Unilateral abnormalities of coordination are caused by lesions in the:

♥ Ipsilateral cerebellar hemisphere

♠ Connections of the ipsilateral cerebellar hemisphere

Bilateral

Bilateral abnormalities of coordination are caused by:

♦ Bilateral cerebellar lesions

Sensory System

Sensory Loss

The patterns of sensory loss have already been discussed.

A short description of the lesions that affect the hands and nerve lesions of the upper limbs follows.

Hand Lesions

Lesions that may be detected in the hands are the following:

♣ T_1 Lesions

♥ Carpal tunnel syndrome

♠ Ulnar nerve lesions

T_1 Lesions

T_1 lesions cause wasting of the small muscles of the hand; a claw hand would occur if this were advanced. The causes are lesions at the level of:

♦ Anterior horn cell

♣ Root lesions

♥ Brachial plexus lesions

♠ Nerve lesions

Anterior Horn Cells

T_1 lesions that occur at the level of the anterior horn cells are:

♥ Syringomyelia

♠ Motor neurone disease

♦ Distal spinal muscular atrophy

♣ Old polio

♥ Meningovascular syphilis

♠ Cord compression

Root Lesions

Root lesions that occur at the level of T_1 are:

♦ Tumour such as neurofibroma

Remember cervical spondylosis does not cause a claw hand, as it does not affect T_1

Brachial Plexus Lesions

Brachial plexus lesions that affect T_1 may be caused by:

- ♣ Cervical rib
- ♥ Thoracic outlet syndrome. Here the subclavian artery may be compressed and then the radial pulse would be decreased or absent. This may only be apparent when traction is applied to the arm.
- ♠ Pancoast's syndrome
- ♦ Trauma

Nerve Lesions

Nerve lesions that affect T_1 are:

- ♣ Combined ulnar and median nerve lesions

Carpal Tunnel Syndrome

Carpal tunnel syndrome causes wasting of the muscles of the lateral part of the thenar eminence. It results in weakness of flexion, abduction and opposition of the thumb. There would be loss of sensation over the first (lateral) three and a half fingers. Tinel's sign and Phalen's sign may be positive.

The causes of carpal tunnel syndrome are:

- ♥ Idiopathic
- ♠ Excessive use of hands
- ♦ **Systemic Factors**

    Conditions affecting the:

    RAG pregnancy

    E&M myxoedema, acromegaly

    LMS osteoarthrosis, rheumatoid arthritis, gout

    HS amyloidosis

    RS tuberculosis, sarcoidosis

    KUS patients on long-term dialysis

Ulnar Nerve Lesions

Ulnar nerve lesions may occur at the:

- ♣ Wrist
- ♥ Elbow

The features of ulnar nerve lesions are wasting and weakness of the small muscles of the hand except the muscles of the lateral part of the thenar eminence. An ulnar claw may be seen. An ulnar claw hand is hyper-extension of the metacarpopha-langeal joints and flexion of the interphalangeal joints of the fourth and fifth fingers. There is sensory loss over the medial one and a half fingers. The causes of ulnar nerve lesions are:

- ♠ Fracture or dislocation at the elbow
- ♦ Osteoarthrosis at the elbow
- ♣ Occupational trauma
- ♥ Increased carrying angle
- ♠ Wrist or palm injury
- ♦ Mononeuritis multiplex
- ♣ Leprosy

Ulnar Paradox

Lesions of the ulnar nerve at the elbow cause weakness of the ulnar half of flexor digitorum profundus. This weakness of flexion of the 4th and 5th fingers results in straighter fingers. Hence, the paradox is that clawing of the fingers is less marked in high ulnar nerve lesions.

Nerve Lesions of the Upper Limb

Nerve lesions that may occur in the upper limb are those involving the:

♥ Axillary nerve

♠ Radial nerve

♦ Musculocutaneous nerve

♣ Ulnar nerve

♥ Median nerve

Axillary Nerve

The features of axillary nerve lesions are the following:

♠ **Motor Deficit**

Weakness of shoulder abduction

♦ **Sensory Deficit**

Small area of anaesthesia over the lower part of the deltoid

♣ **Causes**

Shoulder dislocation, fracture of the humerus, misplaced injection

Radial Nerve

The radial nerve may be injured at the:

♥ Humerus

♠ Axilla

Humerus

The features of radial nerve lesions at the humerus are the following:

♦ **Motor Deficit**

Wrist drop

♣ **Sensory Deficit**

Small area overlying the first dorsal interosseus

♥ **Causes**

Fracture of the shaft of the humerus, Saturday night palsy

Axilla

The features of radial nerve lesions at the axilla are the following:

♠ **Motor Deficit**

Triceps paralysis as well as wrist drop

♦ **Causes**

Saturday night palsy (pressure on the nerve from sleeping with the arm over a chair when in a state of diminished consciousness), crutch palsy

Musculocutaneous Nerve

The features of lesions of the musculocutaneous nerve are the following:

♣ **Motor Deficit**

Weakness of the biceps, coracobrachialis and brachialis

♥ **Sensory Deficit**

Sensory loss over the lateral aspect of the forearm

♠ **Causes**

Rare alone but may be damaged along with the brachial plexus

Ulnar Nerve

This has been discussed

Median Nerve

The median nerve may be damaged in the:

♦ Carpal Tunnel

♣ Forearm

Carpal Tunnel Syndrome

This has been discussed

Forearm

The features of median nerve damage in the forearm are as follows:

♥ **Motor Deficit**

In addition to carpal tunnel syndrome, wasting of the front of the forearm, paralysis of pronator teres, paralysis of the radial flexors of the wrist, paralysis of the long finger flexors except the ulnar part of the deep flexors.

♠ **Sensory Deficit**

As for carpal tunnel syndrome

♦ **Causes**

Trauma

Remember mononeuritis multiplex may result in any of the above lesions.

Chest

Lesions that may be detected on examination of the chest are as follows:

Chest Wall

Lesions that may occur in the chest wall are:

♣ Gynaecomastia may be seen in dystrophia myotonica

Respiratory System

Lesions that may occur in the respiratory system in relation to neurological disease are the following:

♥ **Ventilatory Insufficiency**

Ventilatory insufficiency may occur in Guillain-Barre syndrome and in myasthenia gravis when a crisis occurs

♠ **Respiratory Infections**

Respiratory infections occur in dystrophia myotonica

♦ **Ondine's Curse**

Ondine's curse refers to failure of the automatic control of respiration by the brainstem. Whilst awake the patient is able to breathe but when the patient falls asleep hypoventilation or even apnoea occur. The cause may be congenital or occur following stroke, multiple sclerosis, tumour compression, surgery, infection.

♣ **Cheyne-Stokes Respiration**

Cheyne-Stokes respiration may indicate:

Bilateral cerebral damage (long cycle)

Damage at the level of the medulla (short cycle)

♥ **Central Pontine Hyperventilation**

Central pontine hyperventilation refers to the rapid, deep breathing seen in pontine lesions. It may be due to episodic switching on and off (abruptly) of the pontine respiratory centre.

♠ **Ataxic Respiration**

Ataxic respiration refers to shallow, irregular respiration. This occurs in damage to the medullary respiratory centre. It is frequently a pre-terminal event.

- ♦ **Carcinoma of the bronchus** may cause:

  Secondary deposits, para-neoplastic effects

- ♣ **Pneumonia** may be associated with:

  Cerebral abscess, meningitis

Cardiovascular System

Lesions that may occur in the cardio-vascular system in relation to neuro-logical disease are the following:

- ♦ Cardiomyopathy and conduction defects occur in dystrophia myotonica

- ♣ Hypertrophic cardiomyopathy occurs in Friedrich's ataxia

- ♥ Valvular lesions, atrial fibrillation, carotid stenosis may be associated with cerebrovascular disease

- ♠ Prosthetic valves may be associated with cerebrovascular disease

- ♦ Right to left shunts may be detected in relation to cerebral abscess

- ♣ Subacute bacterial endocarditis may result in embolic phenomena

- ♥ Dissecting aneurysm of the aorta may involve the spinal arteries and cause spinal cord infarction

Nervous System

Lesions of the nervous system that may be noted in the chest are:

- ♥ Sensory loss occurs in spinal cord lesions

Abdomen

Lesions that may occur in the abdomen in relation to neurological disease are:

- ♠ Weakness of the abdominal muscles occurs in spinal cord lesions

- ♦ Beevor's sign refers to a lesion at T_{10} causing the umbilicus to move upwards when the head is raised.

- ♣ Phrenic nerve palsy causes paradoxical respiration

- ♥ Abdominal reflexes are absent in upper motor neurone lesions

- ♠ Sensory loss occurs in spinal cord lesions

Genitals

Testicular atrophy occurs in:

- ♦ Dystrophia myotonica

Cremasteric Reflex

The cremasteric reflex would be lost in:

- ♣ Spinal cord lesions at the level of L_1, L_2

Lower Limbs

Abnormalities that may be detected on examination of the lower limbs are as follows:

General Examination of the Lower Limbs

On general examination of the lower limbs one may note abnormalities of the following:

- ♥ Size
- ♠ Position
- ♦ Muscle mass
- ♣ Involuntary movements
- ♥ Muscle power

Size

Unequal Size

Inequality in the size of the limbs may be due to:

- ♥ **Lower Motor Neurone Lesions**

  Childhood polio

- ♠ **Upper Motor Neurone Lesions**

  Infantile hemiplegia

Position

When examining the position of the lower limb one may note:

- ♦ A spastic limb would be held in extension with extension of the hips, knees, ankles and toes.

Muscle Mass

Abnormalities that one may note are:

- ♦ Wasting occurs in lower motor neurone lesions
- ♣ A distinctive shape would be observed in hereditary motor sensory neuropathy. Here there is distal wasting with preserved thigh muscles resulting in an inverted champagne glass appearance.
- ♥ Hypertrophy occurs in pseudohypertrophic muscular dystrophy (Duchenne, Becker)

Involuntary Movements

The usual involuntary movements may be observed

Muscle Power

Decreased power in the entire lower limb may be observed in:

- ♦ Crural monoplegia, which is rare
- ♣ Hemiplegia
- ♥ Paraplegia
- ♠ Quadriplegia.

Hips

On examination of the hips one may note abnormalities of the following:

- ♦ Muscle mass
- ♣ Tone
- ♥ Muscle power

Muscle Mass

Wasting

Wasting of the proximal muscles may occur in:

♠ Becker muscular dystrophy, limb girdle dystrophy, proximal hereditary motor neuronopathy

Tone

Abnormalities of muscle tone have been discussed earlier

Muscle Power

Weakness

Reduced power of the muscles of the hip girdle may be noted in:

♣ Becker muscular dystrophy, limb girdle dystrophy, systemic causes of proximal myopathy

♥ Eaton-Lambert syndrome

♠ Diabetic amyotrophy

♦ Proximal hereditary motor neuronopathy

♣ Weakness of adduction and internal rotation of the hip occurs in obturator nerve palsy, which can be caused by pelvic malignancies or by injury during labour.

Thighs

When examining the thighs one may note abnormalities of:

♥ Muscle mass

♠ Muscle power

Muscle Mass

Abnormalities that may occur are:

♥ Wasting occurs in dystrophia myotonica, diabetic amyotrophy

♠ Wasting of the quadriceps occurs in femoral nerve lesions

Muscle Power

Muscle power may be decreased in:

♦ Eaton-Lambert syndrome

♣ Diabetic amyotrophy

♥ Weakness of knee extension occurs in femoral nerve lesions. The femoral nerve may be injured in:

Fractures of the pelvis or femur, dislocation of the hip, surgery on the hip

It may be damaged in psoas abscess, psoas haematomas in haemophiliacs, tumours.

Injuries to the thigh

Knees

Lesions that may occur at the knees are:

Structure

Abnormalities that may be detected are:

♠ Charcot's joints in tabes dorsalis

Function

Tone

Abnormalities of tone have been discussed

Lower Legs

On examination of the lower legs one may note abnormalities of:

♦ Muscle mass

♣ Muscle power

Muscle Mass

Abnormalities that may occur are:

♦ Atrophy of the peronei occurs in hereditary motor sensory neuropathy

♣ Pseudohypertrophy occurs in Becker muscular dystrophy

Muscle Power

Abnormalities of muscle power that may occur are:

♥ Specific decrease in power occurs in hereditary motor sensory neuropathy and in peripheral neuropathy

♠ Sciatic nerve lesions cause weakness of all movement below the knee.

The sciatic nerve may be involved in:

Pelvic tumours, fractures of the pelvis, pressure palsy in intoxicated individuals who fall asleep on a chair with a hard edge.

Ankles

On examination of the ankles one may detect abnormalities of:

Structure

Charcot's joints occur in:

♦ Spina bifida, tabes dorsalis

Function

Tone

Abnormalities of tone have been discussed

Feet

When examining the feet one may note abnormalities of:

♦ Structure

♣ Function

Structure

Abnormalities may be detected of the following:

♥ Shape

♠ Integument

♦ Joints

Shape

Abnormalities that one may note are:

♦ Pes cavus occurs in hereditary motor sensory neuropathy, Friedrich's ataxia, spina bifida

♣ Clawing of the toes occurs in hereditary motor sensory neuropathy

♥ Claw-like deformity of the toes occurs in tibial nerve lesions

Integument

Lesions that could occur are:

♠ Foot ulcers occur in diabetic neuropathy

Joints

Charcot's joints may occur in:

♦ Diabetic neuropathy

Function

Abnormalities that may be detected of the functions of the feet are those affecting:

Muscle Power

Abnormal muscle power may be noted:

- Weakness of plantar flexion and inversion may be due to tibial nerve damage which occurs in penetrating wounds
- ♣ Weakness of plantar flexion occurs in S_1 disc protrusion
- ♥ Weakness of dorsiflexion, eversion and toe extension occurs in common peroneal nerve damage, which may be due to weight loss (loss of the protective fat pad), fractures, plaster cast, leprosy, ganglion, mononeuritis multiplex
- ♠ Weakness of dorsiflexion and eversion occurs in L_5 disc protrusion

Reflexes of the Lower Limb

Abnormalities that may be detected are the following:

- Abnormalities of the tendon reflexes
- ♣ Specific loss of reflexes
- ♥ Up going plantars with absent ankle jerks

Tendon Reflexes

Abnormalities of the tendon reflexes have been discussed earlier.

Specific Loss of Reflexes

Specific loss of reflexes occurs in the following:

- ♥ Knee jerk is absent in femoral nerve lesions
- ♠ Ankle jerk is absent in sciatic nerve lesions

Up Going Plantars with Absent Ankle Jerks

Up going plantars with absent ankle jerks would occur in:

- Subacute combined degeneration of the cord
- ♣ Tabes dorsalis
- ♥ Hereditary cerebellar ataxia (Friedrich's)
- ♠ Motor neurone disease

Coordination

Abnormalities of coordination that affect the lower limb could be:

Unilateral

Unilateral abnormalities of coordination may occur in lesions of the:

- ♥ Ipsilateral cerebellar hemisphere
- ♠ Connections of the ipsilateral cerebellar hemisphere

Bilateral

Bilateral abnormalities of coordination occur in:

- Bilateral cerebellar lesions

Sensation

Sensory lesions have been described earlier. Other lesions that may occur are:

♣ Meralgia paraesthetica causes numbness of the anterolateral aspect of the thigh. It is caused by entrapment of the lateral cutaneous nerve of the thigh.

♥ Common peroneal nerve lesions cause loss of sensation over the lateral aspect of the leg and dorsum of the foot

Nerve Lesions of the Lower Limb

Nerve lesions that may occur in the lower limb are those involving the:

♠ Obturator nerve

♦ Femoral nerve

♣ Lateral cutaneous nerve of thigh

♥ Sciatic nerve

♠ Tibial nerve

♦ Common peroneal nerve

Obturator Nerve

The features of obturator nerve lesions are the following:

♣ **Motor Deficit**

Weakness of adduction and internal rotation of the hip

♥ **Sensory Deficit**

Sensory loss over the medial part of the thigh

♠ **Causes**

Neoplasms of the pelvis, Injuries during parturition

Femoral Nerve

The features of femoral nerve lesions are the following:

♦ **Motor Deficit**

Wasting of the quadriceps, weakness of knee extension.

Proximal lesions may also cause weakness of hip flexion due to paralysis of iliacus

♣ **Reflexes**

Loss of the knee jerk

♥ **Sensory Deficit**

Sensory loss over the front of the thigh and medial aspect of lower leg as far as the medial malleolus

♠ **Causes**

Psoas abscess, psoas haematoma, diabetic amyotrophy, tumours, trauma

Lateral Cutaneous Nerve of Thigh

The features of lesions of the lateral cutaneous nerve of the thigh are the following:

♦ **Sensory Deficit**

Numbness and paraesthesiae over the anterolateral aspect of the thigh (Meralgia Paraesthetica)

♣ **Causes**

It is more common in obese individuals

Sciatic Nerve

The features of sciatic nerve lesions are the following:

♥ **Motor Deficit**

Foot drop, weakness of all muscles below the knee, high lesions also cause weakness of knee flexion

♠ **Reflexes**

Loss of the ankle jerk

♦ **Sensory Deficit**

Sensory loss over the foot except the medial border

♣ **Causes**

Pelvic tumours, fractures of the pelvis and femur, damage in hip replacement operations, pressure palsy.

Tibial Nerve

The features of tibial nerve lesions are the following:

♥ **Motor Deficit**

Weakness of plantar flexion and inversion, weakness of flexion of the toes, claw like deformity of the toes due to paralysis of the interossei

♠ **Sensory Deficit**

Sensation is lost over the sole of the foot

♦ **Causes**

Lesions of the tibial nerve are uncommon

Tarsal tunnel syndrome (compression under the flexor retinaculum) spares the muscles around the ankle

Common Peroneal Nerve

The features of lesions of the common peroneal nerve are the following:

♣ **Motor Deficit**

Foot drop with weakness of dorsiflexion and eversion at the ankle, weakness of toe extension

♥ **Sensory Deficit**

Sensation is impaired over the lateral aspect of the lower leg and the dorsum of the foot

♠ **Causes**

Compression, fractures, ischaemia

Remember mononeuritis multiplex may result in any of the above lesions.

Anal Reflex

The anal reflex would be lost in lesions of the:

♦ Conus medullaris

♣ Cauda equina

Spine

The abnormalities that may be detected on examination of the spine with the patient lying down are the following:

Straight Leg Raising Test

The straight leg raising test would be positive in:

♦ Lesions causing compression of L_4, L_5, S_1

Femoral Stretch

The femoral stretch test would be positive in:

♣ Lesions causing compression of L_1, L_2, L_3

Neck Stiffness

Neck stiffness could indicate:

♥ Meningitis or sub-arachnoid haemorrhage

♠ Tonsillar herniation in posterior fossa tumours

Kernig's Sign

Kernig's sign would indicate:

♦ Meningitis or subarachnoid haemorrhage.

Gait

Abnormalities of gait may be due to:

♦ Sensory lesions

♣ Motor lesions

♥ Cerebellar lesions

♠ Basal ganglia lesions

♦ Frontal lobe lesions

Remember that abnormalities of gait may also be due to abnormalities of the locomotor system.

Sensory Lesions

Proprioceptive loss results in the loss of the ability to appreciate the position of the limbs and thus impairment of gait occurs.

Motor Lesions

Motor lesions that cause abnormal gait are lesions of muscle, neuro-muscular junction lesions, lower motor neurone or upper motor neurone lesions.

Cerebellar Lesions

Cerebellar lesions cause gait abnor-malities as a result of impairment of coordination and balance.

Basal Ganglia Lesions

Basal ganglia lesions cause rigidity and paucity of movement and thus hinder normal gait.

Frontal Lobe Lesions

Frontal lobe lesions interfere with performance of complex tasks

Assessment of Gait

When assessing gait one may note abnormalities of the following:

♣ Posture

♥ Character

♠ Quantity

♦ Rhythm

♣ Associated features

♥ Modifying factors

Posture

When assessing posture one may note abnormalities of the:

♣ Spine

♥ Arms

♠ Lower limbs

Spine

The spine would be stooped in:

♦ Parkinsonism

♣ Proprioceptive loss

Arms

The arms would be:

♥ Held wide apart for balance in cerebellar lesions and in proprio-ceptive loss

♠ Flexed in hemiplegia

Lower Limbs

Abnormal positions that one may detect in the lower limbs would be:

♦ Broad base in: cerebellar lesions, proprioceptive loss, gait apraxia

♣ In hemiplegia the lower limb would be held in extension.

Character of Gait

Note any deviation from the normal character of movement.

Normal Gait

When analysing gait it would be best to begin with a phase of the gait cycle and analyse the phases of the cycle to the beginning of the next cycle. Begin with heel strike.

The heel of the foot strikes the floor and this is followed by the foot being placed in contact with the floor from heel to toe. The foot is externally rotated and pronated during this phase. Next, the heel begins to rise and the forefoot then pushes the foot off the floor. This is followed by a swing phase where the foot swings forward to the next heel strike. The foot is dorsiflexed during this phase to allow it to clear the ground. The contralateral foot is out of phase with these movements. Heel strike with one foot coincides with forefoot push in the other; foot contact in one corresponds to the swing phase in the other.

The knee goes through two flexion and extension phases during a cycle. The knee is extended during initial heel strike and then becomes partially flexed before extending again. As forefoot push begins the knee flexes once more and flexion becomes maximal during the swing phase.

The hip flexes and extends once per cycle.

The trunk twists about a vertical axis with the shoulder girdle rotating in the opposite direction to the pelvis. Pelvic swing is more marked in females than in males. Shoulder movement is more marked in males.

Arm swing is out of phase with the legs. When the right leg swings forward the left arm does so and vice versa.

Types of Abnormal Gait (Abnormal Character)

The types of abnormal gait (abnormal character) that may be encountered are the following:

♥ Parkinsonian

♠ *Marche a petits pas*

♦ High steppage

♣ Scissor

♥ Ataxic

♠ Stamping

♦ Spastic

♣ Hemiplegic

♥ Waddling

♠ Gait apraxia

♦ Painful

Parkinsonian

In Parkinsonism the patient is bent forwards and walks with short, shuffling steps. There is no arm swing.

Marche a petits pas

In *marche a petits pas* the patient walks with short steps but the stance is upright and there is marked arm swing. The steps are rapid and tapping. It occurs in diffuse cerebrovascular disease.

High Steppage

High steppage gait occurs due to foot drop where dorsiflexion of the foot cannot occur. The knee is flexed and raised to allow the foot to clear the ground. It occurs in $L_{4, 5}$ root lesions, common peroneal lesions, peripheral neuropathy. Occasionally it may be due to lesions in the motor cortex.

Scissor Gait

In a scissor gait, the legs cross each other as they move forwards. The toes are pointed inwards. It is seen in paraparesis due to cerebral palsy, multiple sclerosis, cord compression.

Ataxic Gait

In an ataxic gait the patient walks as if they are drunk, veering to the side of the lesion if the lesion is unilateral. Ataxia occurs in cerebellar lesions such as phenytoin toxicity, alcohol toxicity, multiple sclerosis, cerebrovascular disease, tumour.

Stamping Gait

In a stamping gait the patient stamps the feet on the ground. It is seen in sensory loss in peripheral neuropathy, subacute combined degeneration of the cord, tabes dorsalis.

Spastic Gait

In bilateral upper motor neurone lesions, both legs are spastic and cannot be lifted off the ground. The patient walks with stiff lower limbs. Hardly any flexion occurs at the knees.

Hemiplegic Gait

In hemiplegia, there is unilateral spasticity with flexor hypertonia in the upper limbs and extensor hypertonia in the lower limbs. The arm is held in flexion and the lower limb is extended, with extension at the knee and ankle. The patient has to tilt the body to the opposite side and move the lower limb in a semicircle in order to propel it forward. It is seen in stroke.

Waddling Gait

In a waddling gait there is marked rotation of the pelvis and shoulders whilst walking. It is seen in proximal myopathy, bilateral congenital dislocation of the hips.

Gait Apraxia

In gait apraxia, the gait is abnormal as if the patient has forgotten how to walk. It occurs in frontal lobe lesions such as normal pressure hydrocephalus, cerebrovascular disease.

Painful Gait

A painful (antalgic) gait occurs in arthritis, trauma. The painful limb buckles each time it bears weight so that the impact is cushioned. The good limb hurries through to minimise the duration that the painful limb has to bear weight.

Further Analysis of Character of Gait

If there is difficulty in analysing the character of gait, it may be useful to break down the analysis to specific areas. The areas are:

- ♣ Foot
- ♥ Knee
- ♠ Hips
- ♦ Shoulders and Arms

Foot

The abnormalities that may be noted in the foot are:

- ♣ **Broad base**: cerebellar lesions, sensory neuropathy
- ♥ **Shuffle**: Parkinsonism
- ♠ **Foot drop**: high steppage gait
- ♦ **Stamping**: sensory neuropathy
- ♣ **Pointing inwards**: scissor gait, spastic gait, hemiplegia
- ♥ **Extended**: spastic, hemiplegic

Knee

The abnormalities that may be noted are:

- ♠ **High knee lift**: high steppage
- ♦ **Lack of flexion**: spasticity

Hips

The abnormalities that may be noted are:

- ♣ **Marked swing** in waddling gait
- ♥ **Circumduction** in hemiplegia

Shoulders and Arms

The abnormalities that may be noted are:

- ♠ **Lack of arm swing** in Parkinsonism

Quantity

One may note abnormalities in the length of the stride the patient takes.

- ♦ **Small Steps**. The patient would take small steps in Parkinsonism, gait apraxia and in *marche a petits pas*

Rhythm

Variations in the rhythm of gait are:

- ♣ Hesitant in Parkinsonism
- ♥ Drunken in cerebellar lesions

Associated Features

Abnormal associated features that may be observed when analysing gait are:

- ♠ Loss of arm swing, tremor in Parkinsonism
- ♦ Increased arm swing in *marche a petits pas*

Modifying Factors

Gait may be modified by asking the patient to perform:

Heel Toe (Tandem) Walking

Tandem walking would be abnormal in:

- ♣ Midline cerebellar (vermis) lesions

Romberg's Sign

Romberg's sign would be positive in loss of proprioception in:

- ♥ Sensory neuropathy
- ♠ Posterior column lesions

Standing from a Seated or Squatting Position

Standing from a seated or squatting position would be abnormal and the patient would find it difficult in:

♦ Proximal myopathy

Gower's Sign

Gower's sign refers to the patient using his or her upper limbs to climb up his or her lower limbs to rise from the floor. It occurs in any disorder in which the muscles of the pelvic girdle are weak.

Back

On examination of the back one may note changes in the:

Integument

Abnormalities that may be noted are the following:

♣ A tuft of hair in the lumbosacral region could signify spina bifida

♥ A shagreen patch is a flesh-coloured plaque over the lower back. It occurs in tuberose sclerosis

Spine

The abnormalities that may be noted when the spine is examined with the patient standing are the following:

♠ **Kyphoscoliosis**

Kyphoscoliosis is seen in Friedrich's ataxia, muscular dystrophies, syringomyelia, von

Recklinghausen's disease, hereditary motor sensory neuropathy

Lumbar disc disease causes scoliosis with the convexity to the side of the lesion. It is usually maximal at the affected level.

♦ **Lordosis**

Excessive lordosis may occur in muscular dystrophies, congenital hip disease.

♣ **Rigid Spine**

The spine may be rigid due to paravertebral muscle spasm in lumbar spine or disc disease.

♥ **Tender Spine**

A tender spine would occur in bony tumours or infections of the spine

Autonomic Dysfunction

Lesions of the autonomic nervous system have been discussed earlier.

Chapter 17

The Locomotor System

In the locomotor system one will study conditions that affect the bones, joints, tendons, and muscles. In addition clinical features of the causes and effects of conditions that affect the locomotor system but are reflected in other systems will also be studied.

History Taking

One should ask about:

♥ Pain

♠ Swelling

♦ Deformity

♣ Stiffness

♥ Movement

A review of systems should then be performed.

Physical Examination

Physical examination of the locomotor system involves examination of the bones, the joints, the tendons and the muscles. A description of the method of examination of the bones, the joints and the tendons will follow. Examination of the muscles should be performed in the manner described in the chapter on the central nervous system.

A systematic method of examination of the locomotor system follows this initial general description of examination of the bones, the joints, the tendons and the muscles.

Bones

Examine the following aspects of structure of the bones:

♠ Dimensions

♦ Cover

♣ Contents

♥ Connections

Dimensions

One should note the following:

♠ Position

♦ Size

♣ Shape

Position

Note the position of the bone. A bone may not be in its normal position if it has been fractured and displaced or if there has been dislocation or subluxation of a joint. Dislocation refers to total loss of contact between articular surfaces and subluxation to partial loss of contact between articular surfaces.

Size

Note the following aspects:

♥ Length

♠ Width

Length

Note the length of the bone. Compare this with the other side.

Width

Note the width of the bone. Compare this with the other side.

Shape

Note the shape. If deformity of bone is observed, note whether it is a localised deformity or whether there are generalised deformities of bone.

Cover

Examine the state of the overlying integument.

Contents

Examine the contents of the bone. Palpate the bone and note any tenderness or warmth. Crepitus may be inadvertently felt during examination of a fractured bone.

Connections

Examine the connections of the bone. They are the:

♦ Joint above

♣ Joint below

Note any abnormality of the joint above and the joint below.

Joints

Examination of the joints may be divided into:

♠ Examination of structure of the joint

♦ Examination of function of the joint

Structure of the Joint

Examine the following aspects:

♣ Dimensions

♥ Cover

♠ Contents

Dimensions

Note the following:

♦ Position

♣ Size

♥ Shape

Position

Make a note of the position of the joint at rest. If a joint is inflamed the limb would assume a position that would maximise the joint space.

Size and Shape

Next, assess the size and shape of the joint.

Cover

Assess the state of the integument overlying the joint.

Contents

Note the following aspects:

♠ Warmth

♦ Tenderness

♣ Consistency

Place a hand over the joint. Note the temperature; this is best felt with the back of one's hand. Compare the temperature over the joint with the surrounding skin and with the opposite joint. Note whether there is any tenderness. If the joint is swollen, determine the consistency of the swelling. The swelling may be due to fluid, synovial thickening or bone overgrowth.

Fluid is fluctuant and moves within the joint

Synovial thickening feels soft and spongy

Bone feels hard and does not move

Function of the Joint

Examine function of the joint by noting the following:

- ♥ Position
- ♠ Range of movement
- ♦ Character of movement
- ♣ Associated features
- ♥ Modifying factors
- ♠ Rate
- ♦ Rhythm

Position

Note the position of the joint at rest.

Range of Movement (Quantity)

Next, quantify the range of movement of the joint. Assess this by asking the patient to perform movements of the joint actively and then proceed to put the joint through its full range of movements. That is, test active and passive movements of the joint. Look for the ability to perform the normal range of movement and observe if there are any abnormal movements. This is done by making a rough assessment visually. A goniometer may be used for more accurate assessment.

Character

If a change occurs in the range of movement of a joint, characterise this change. The changes that may occur are the following:

- ♣ The presence of a detached fragment within the joint causes restriction of movement when the direction of movement is towards the detached fragment.

- ♥ If the synovium, cartilage or bone is involved, movement is restricted in all directions.

- ♠ If the capsule or a ligament is damaged movement towards the affected structure relieves any pain whilst movement away from the damaged structure aggravates the pain. Any abnormal movement that occurs would be away from the damaged area.

Associated Features

When assessing joint movement, make a note of any associated features such as pain or crepitus.

Modifying Factors

When testing active movements, note any manoeuvres the patient may employ to facilitate movement of the joint.

Rate

The rate of movement would be slow if there is pathology affecting the joint.

Rhythm

The normal smooth rhythm of movement would be lost if there is any form of pathology affecting the joint.

Tendons

Examine the tendons by noting the following:

◆ Dimensions

♣ Cover

♥ Contents

♠ Connections

Dimensions

Note the following:

◆ Position

♣ Size

♥ Shape

Position

Make a note of the position of the tendon.

Size and Shape

Examine the size and shape of the tendon. Pay particular attention to any localised deformity.

Cover

Carefully note the following:

♠ Integument

◆ Effusion

♣ Crepitus

Examine the skin overlying the tendon. Palpate the tendon and note any effusions in relation to the tendon sheath. Feel for tendon sheath crepitus, which is a grating or creaking sensation that occurs on movement of the tendon.

Contents

Note the following:

♥ Warmth

♠ Tenderness

◆ Consistency

Palpate the tendon and note any warmth or tenderness. Feel the consistency of the tendon.

Connections

Note whether the connections or attachments of the tendon are intact.

Muscles

Examination of the muscles should be performed using the method described in the chapter on the central nervous system.

Examination of the Locomotor System

When examining a patient with a condition related to the locomotor system, one should commence as usual with a general examination and then proceed to perform regional examination.

General Examination

The most important observation is the posture of the patient. A quick assessment should be made at this point. A more formal assessment will be made when examining the spine. Next, assess the state of growth and development and the metabolic state of the patient. Note any marked changes in the integument. Note the body temperature. (Posture, Height and Proportions, Weight and Shape, Integument, Body Temperature)

Regional Examination

Examination is best begun with the patient seated on the edge of the examination couch or bed.

Head

Make a note of the mental state. Assess the dimensions of the head and movement of the head. Then examine the nose, the eyes, the face (scalp, forehead, malar region, chin).

Examine the structure of the jaw. Next, examine the tempero-mandibular joint. Place one's fingers over the tempero-mandibular joint, ask the patient to open the mouth and assess the range of movement on opening the mouth. Enquire about pain and palpate for clicks on opening the mouth.

Complete examination of the mouth (lips, teeth, gums, buccal mucosa, tongue, palate, fauces, salivary glands). Then examine the ears.

Upper Limbs

Now examine the upper limbs. Begin with a general examination of the upper limbs. Observe the position of the limbs at rest and look for any

obvious change in size and shape. Note any change in the integument.

Hands

One should examine:

- ♣ Structure
- ♥ Function

Structure

Begin with the dorsal aspect. Note the overall dimensions. Pay particular attention to the overall shape of the hands. Look at the nails and skin. Assess the size and shape of the thumb and each of the fingers. Following this, carefully inspect the bones, joints and tendons of the thumb, the second, third, fourth and fifth fingers and then the bones joints and tendons of the dorsum of the hands and wrists. Evaluate the muscle mass.

Ask the patient to turn the hands over and repeat the process, that is, inspect the palmar aspect. Inspect the skin and then the bones, joints, tendons and muscles of the palmar aspect of the hand. Next, palpate the fingers, the palms and dorsum of the hands and the wrists and note any warmth, tenderness or swelling of the bones and joints. Palpate the tendons and note any warmth, tenderness, swelling or thickening. Note any tendon sheath crepitus. To do this, place the palmar aspects of one's fingers against the palm of the patient's hand whilst gently flexing and extending the metacarpopha-langeal joints. Inflamed tendons may be felt creaking in their sheaths and nodules may be palpated. Some clinicians prefer to elicit tendon sheath crepitus later when performing passive movements of the metacarpophalangeal joints.

Feel the hands and ascertain the state of the peripheral circulation and palpate the radial pulse.

Function

After examining the structure of the hands, proceed to evaluate function of the locomotor system of the hands. This will entail examining:

♦ Movements of the hands and wrists (active and passive)

♣ Overall function of the hand

Movements of the Hand and Wrist

The movements that are tested are movements at the:

♥ Interphalangeal joints

♠ Metacarpophalangeal joints

♦ Movement of the hand as a whole

♣ Movements at the wrist joint

Assessment

One should assess:

♥ Active movements

♠ Function of the hands

♦ Passive movements

Active Movements

Test active movements. Begin by asking the patient to pretend to play a piano. Then ask the patient to touch each finger in turn with the thumb of the same hand. Ask the patient to make a fist. Ask the patient to place the hands in the prayer position (Do not say, "Pray for me," as this might prompt the reply, "Too late for that!") Next, ask the patient to place the hands in the reversed prayer position with the backs of the hands touching each other. (Pray in Australia! This is very amusing unless one happens to be from Australia or worse in a professional examination the examiner is an Australian.)

Aide Memoire

Active movements of the hands may be remembered as:

Play, Pinch, Punch, Pray

Function of the Hands

Test the following:

♣ Hand grip

♥ Pincer grip (between the thumb and the index finger)

♠ Simple functions

Hand Grip

Ask the patient to grip one's fingers as tight as they can. Remember to place one's fingers as close to the wrist as possible as this will prevent the patient using too much force. It is preferable to place one's fingers in the depression between the thenar and hypothenar eminences.

Pincer Grip

Ask the patient to place the tips of the thumb and index finger together and attempt to separate them.

Simple Functions

Assess simple functions. Ask the patient to pick up an object, do up a button, pretend to comb his or her hair and observe any limitation of activity. Remember this assesses function of several joints.

Passive Movements

Perform passive movements at the wrist, the metacarpophalangeal and the interphalangeal joints. Note the range of movement and observe if there are any abnormal movements.

If one wishes one may examine passive movements when examining structure of the hand. However, examining active movements first will enable one to determine the degree of limitation of movement and enable one to note whether movements are painful.

To complete examination of the hands perform neurological examination of the hands if required.

Forearms

Next, examine the structure of the forearm. Then test function. Test pronation and supination movements.

Elbows

Ask the patient to extend the elbow and examine the flexor aspect. Note the position at rest. Feel for tenderness over the epicondyles. Ask the patient to flex the elbow, pay particular attention to the integument over the extensor aspect of the elbow, note the range of movement. Next, examine the upper arms and shoulders.

Shoulders

Examine the following:

♦ Structure

♣ Movements at the shoulder

♥ Scapula

♠ Glenohumeral movement

Structure

Pay attention to the size and shape of the shoulder. Note any abnormality of the structure of the glenohumeral, the acromioclavicular and the sternoclavicular joints. Palpate for tenderness over the sternoclavicular joints, the acromioclavicular joints, the subacromial bursa, the supraspinatus tendon and the biceps tendon.

Movements at the Shoulder

The movements at the shoulder are a combination of scapulothoracic, glenohumeral, acromioclavicular and sternoclavicular movements.

Note the position of the shoulder at rest.

Now ask the patient to clasp the hands at the back of the head. Next, ask the patient to clasp the hands behind his or her back and brace the shoulders back. Note any restriction of movement.

Alternatively one may ask the patient to touch (scratch) the back of his or her head with the fingers and then touch (scratch) his or her back.

Move behind the patient to examine the scapula and assess glenohumeral movement of the shoulder.

Scapula

Examine the dimensions of the scapula. Assess the muscle mass and palpate for tenderness.

Glenohumeral Movement

Hold the scapula to fix it and prevent scapulothoracic movement and thus allow examination of glenohumeral movement. To fix the patient's right scapula one should use one's left hand and to fix the patient's left scapula one should use one's right hand. Hold the patient's forearm with one's other hand, flex the elbow and use the forearm as a pointer. Examine movements at the gleno-humeral joint. Examine flexion, extension, abduction, adduction, internal and external rotation.

As one is now behind the patient, it would be best to take this opportunity to examine the neck from behind.

Neck

Examine:

♦ Structure

♣ Function (Movements of the neck)

Structure

Inspect the neck and palpate. Feel for spasm of the sternocleidomastoid muscle and the paracervical muscles. Feel for tenderness over the occiput, the spinous processes of the vertebrae and the facet joints. Palpate for enlarged lymph nodes if required.

Front of Neck

Move to the front of the patient. Examine the neck in the usual fashion (dimensions, integument, thyroid, sternocleidomastoid, jugular venous pressure, carotids, trachea, lymph nodes). Note the dimensions in particular.

Movements of the Neck

Examine the range of movement of the neck. The movements are flexion, extension, rotation to the right and then to the left and finally lateral flexion in both directions.

Ask the patient to bend his or her head forward and touch the chest with the chin. Then ask the patient to look up as far as possible. Ask the patient to turn the chin to the right and then to the left. Then ask the patient to move his or her left ear towards the left shoulder and then move his or her right ear towards the right shoulder. Apply pressure to the top of the head whilst the patient performs lateral flexion as this may expose features of nerve root compression.

In practice, if required, one should perform neurological examination of the upper limbs.

Chest

In practice one should examine the chest in the usual fashion. That is, one should examine the chest wall and the contents of the chest; the heart and the lungs. Remember that pathological processes that involve the costovertebral joints may restrict chest expansion. One may measure chest expansion at the lowest part of the fourth intercostal space first in maximum exhalation and then in maximum inspiration. A difference of approximately five centimetres should be expected.

Back

In practice one should examine the back of the patient at this point. The usual method as described in the earlier chapters should be followed.

Abdomen

In practice one should examine the patient's abdomen at this point. Ask the patient to assume the supine position and then proceed to examine the abdomen in the usual fashion.

When examining the abdominal wall one should, in particular, note the distance between the lower ribs and the iliac crest.

Lower Limbs

It would be best to initially examine the structure of the lower limbs and then examine function as a series of movements that will examine the function of all the joints. This is more convenient for the patient.

Structure

Examine the structure of the lower limb in general and then examine the regions.

General examination of the Lower Limbs

Make a note of:

- ♣ Position
- ♥ Length
- ♠ Integument
- ♦ Muscle wasting

Note the dimensions. Pay particular attention to the position of the lower limbs at rest. Measure the apparent length and true length of the lower limbs. The apparent length is the distance between the umbilicus and the medial malleolus. The true length is the distance between the anterior superior iliac spine and the medial malleolus. Before measuring true length both limbs should be placed in comparable positions. For example if one limb is fixed in adduction then the other limb too should be positioned in adduction before measurements are made. A decrease in apparent length occurs due to tilting of the pelvis. The true length would be decreased in disease of the hip joint. Note the state of the integument. Note any wasting of the muscles.

Hips

Note the position of the hips at rest. Next, determine the position of the greater trochanters. To do this place one's thumbs on the anterior superior iliac spines. Feel the greater trochanters with one's fingers. If one is higher than the other, that is the abnormal side. Palpate inferior to the mid-point of the inguinal ligament to feel for tenderness over the joint

Thighs

Note the dimensions. Quadriceps wasting is an early sign of disease.

Knees

Examine the structure of the knees in detail. Make a note of the position of the knees at rest. Note any swelling, change in shape or redness. Palpate gently and note any warmth or tenderness. Determine the consistency of any swelling that may be present.

Fluid in the Knee

The tests that may be used to detect fluid in the knee are:

♣ Patellar tap

♥ Cross-fluctuation

♠ Bulge test

Patellar Tap

If the knee is swollen perform patellar tap to see if this is due to fluid in the knee joint.

Place one's left palm over the suprapatellar bursa and compress any fluid within it so that it enters the knee joint. With the thumb, index and middle fingers of one's right hand dip the patella. If fluid is present within the joint, this fluid will be displaced and the patella will be felt to tap the underlying bone.

Cross-fluctuation

Another approach to detect the presence of fluid in the knee joint is to test for cross-fluctuation. Compress the suprapatellar bursa with one's left hand. Place the thumb and index fingers of one's right hand on either side of the knee joint near the inferior margin of the patella. Alternately compress and release the left hand and the thumb and fingers of the right hand to elicit cross-fluctuation.

Bulge Test

For small effusions one may perform the bulge test. Empty the medial parapatellar fossa by exerting pressure with the flat of the examining hand. Alternatively, one may use a firm wiping movement of the hand. Now compress the suprapatellar bursa by exerting pressure with the palm of one's left hand. If there were fluid in the knee, the medial parapatellar fossa would be seen to bulge out. Alternatively one may compress the lateral parapatellar fossa to demonstrate filling of the medial parapatellar fossa.

One may palpate the popliteal fossa at this stage or leave examination of this till later.

Lower Legs

Examine the structure of the lower legs in detail.

Ankles and Feet

Note the dimensions. Look in particular at the shape of the feet. Examine the dorsum of the feet. Look at the nails and skin. Assess the size and shape of the big toe and each of the toes. Examine the bones, joints, and tendons of the big toe and each of the toes in turn and then examine the bones, joints, tendons of the foot and the ankle joint. Assess the muscle mass. Palpate for tenderness over the joints and tendons especially the Achilles tendons. Examine the plantar aspect similarly starting with the skin and then the bones, joints, tendons and muscles. Palpate for tenderness over the plantar fascia. Feel the skin and assess the state of the peripheral circulation and palpate the dorsalis pedis and posterior tibial pulses.

Examination of Function of the Lower Limbs

After completing general and regional examination of the lower limbs, one should proceed to examine function of the lower limbs.

Movements of the Lower Limbs

The joints that are tested are the following:

♥ Sacroiliac Joints

Springing is employed to test for inflammation. Movement is not tested at the sacroiliac joint.

♠ Hips

Movements at the hip joint are tested first with the knee in flexion and then with the knee in extension.

Extension of the Hip

This is not a true extension of the hip joint as extension of the hip joint is prevented by the strong anterior capsule. The movement of extension is produced by rotation of the pelvis and extension of the spine.

♦ Knees

Movements at the knee joints are all in one plane. A small degree of extension may be noted in some. Compare the degree of extension with the other side.

♣ Ankles and Feet

Ankle and foot movements are movements at the ankle joint, the subtalar joint, the midtarsal joint, the tarsometatarsal joints and the interphalangeal joints.

Method of Examination of Function of the Joints of the Lower Limbs

One should begin proximally. Start with the sacro-iliac joints. After examining the sacroiliac joints, examine function of the right lower limb. Complete examination of function of the right lower limb and then proceed to examine function of the left lower limb.

Sacroiliac Joints

Place both hands over the patient's iliac crests with one's thumbs overlying the anterior superior iliac spines. Perform compression and distraction and look for evidence of pain.

Right Lower Limb

Next, examine the right lower limb. Examine the following aspects:

♥ Position

♠ Movements

535

Position

With the lower limb at rest note the position of the:

♦ Right lower limb in general

♣ Hip

♥ Knee

♠ Ankle and foot

Movements

As it is not possible to examine movements at individual joints without moving the other joints it is best to group examination of the joints of the lower limb. Thus one will examine:

♦ Hip and Knee

♣ Ankle and Foot

Hip and Knee Movements

One should examine the following:

♥ Flexion of the hip and knee

♠ Thomas' test

♦ Hip movements with the knee in flexion

♣ Knee movements

♥ Hip movements with the knee in extension

Flexion of Hip and Knee

With one's left palm over the patient's right patella and one's right hand holding the patient's leg just above the ankle, ask the patient to flex the knee and hip as much as he or she can. Note the range of movement and feel for crepitus.

Thomas' Test

Place one's left hand underneath the patient's spine. Press on the patient's right knee with one's right hand, flex the hip and knee as much as possible and obliterate the lumbar lordosis. Observe if there is any flexion of the contralateral hip. If the contralateral limb rises off the couch or bed, it indicates a fixed flexion deformity of the contralateral hip.

Hip Movements with the Knee in Flexion

Place one's left hand on the patient's right knee and with one's right hand supporting the patient's lower leg just above the ankle, flex the patient's knee and perform movements of the hip with the knee in flexion; that is internal and external rotation, abduction and adduction. In the normal limb one should be able to flex, abduct and externally rotate the hip so that the foot (of the limb being examined) may be placed on the contralateral knee and the knee (of the limb being examined) comes to lie on or near the couch. (FABER flexion, abduction, external rotation)

Knee

Next, place the patient's foot on the bed with the knee still flexed. Sit on the bed or couch with one's buttocks by the patient's foot so that it prevents the foot from moving. Grasp the patient's tibia with both hands with one's thumbs anteriorly. Gently test for forward and backward motion. If movement is detected this would indicate that the cruciate ligaments are damaged.

Now ask the patient to straighten the knee. Note the degree of extension. With one's left hand by the side of the knee and one's right hand just above the ankle test for medial and lateral laxity of the knee.

Hip Movements with the Knee in Extension

Next, test movements of the hip with the knee in extension. When testing abduction and adduction, use one's right hand to move the limb. Hold the limb with the right hand just above the ankle. Place the thumb of one's left hand on the contralateral anterior superior iliac spine so that movement of the pelvis would be detected at the end of the range of movement of the hip. When testing external and internal rotation use the position of the patella or foot to monitor movement. Test abduction, adduction, internal rotation, external rotation.

Ankle and Foot

Now test movements at the ankle joint, the foot and the toes. First ask the patient to perform the movements actively and then perform passive movements. One should test movements at the ankle joint, the subtalar joint, the midtarsal joint, the tarsometatarsal joints and the interphalangeal joints. These movements are discussed below.

If one finds it difficult to raise the patient's foot off the bed for examination, then one may place the patient's foot over the contralateral leg with the knee flexed and the hip abducted and externally rotated, in a position similar to that adopted when testing the ankle jerk.

Movements at the Ankle and Foot

The movements that are tested are as follows:

- ♣ Ankle movement
- ♥ Subtalar movement
- ♠ Midtarsal movement
- ♦ Tarsometatarsal and interphalangeal movement

Ankle Movement

Grasp the patient's midfoot with one hand and the lower leg with the other hand, test dorsiflexion and plantar flexion. These are movements at the ankle joint.

Subtalar Joint

Grasp the patient's heel with one hand and the tibia with the other, move the heel inwards and outwards. (Medially and laterally)

Midtarsal Movement

Grasp the patient's heel with one hand and the forefoot with the other. Move the forefoot inwards and outwards. (Medially and laterally)

Tarsometatarsal and Interphalangeal Movement

Examine movements of the toes. The toe movements are flexion and extension.

This concludes examination of the right lower limb with the patient in the supine position.

Left Lower Limb

Now go to the other side of the examination couch or bed and repeat the procedure for the left lower limb. The technique will have

537

to be the converse of that used for the right lower limb. In places where one used one's right hand one should use the left and vice versa.

In practice, if required, neurological examination of the lower limbs may be performed at this point.

Spine

Examination of the spine may be carried out with the patient in the:

♣ Supine position

♥ Prone position

♠ Standing

Supine Position

The test that is carried out with the patient in the supine position is the straight leg raising test.

Straight Leg Raising Test

To begin with ask the patient to raise the right lower limb off the bed or couch with the knee extended. Ask the patient to raise the lower limb off the bed as far as possible. Once the maximum has been reached grasp the patent's heel with one's right hand and placing the left hand over the knee to maintain the position of the limb, raise the lower limb as far as possible. This is the straight leg raising test. If the patient has a positive response noted by pain radiating down the back of the lower limb, lower the limb slightly and dorsiflex the ankle. The pain should be reproduced. Note the angle at which pain was initially induced.

Repeat the test on the other side.

Prone Position

Ask the patient to turn over and lie prone and examine each limb in turn. Take the opportunity to palpate the popliteal fossa and examine for a Baker's cyst.

Spine in the Prone Position

The main aspect of examination of the spine that is performed with the patient in the prone position is the femoral stretch. However, one should bear in mind that very rarely power of the muscles of the spine may be tested.

Muscle Power

The power of the erector spinae muscles is rarely tested. If required test this by asking the patient to lift his or her head off the examination couch or bed and observe contraction of the erector spinae. One may also ask the patient to lift his or her lower limbs off the examination couch or bed and observe contraction of the erector spinae.

Femoral Stretch

Perform the femoral stretch test. With the patient lying in the prone position one should flex the patient's knee (extending the hip joint will increase tension on the femoral nerve roots). A positive sign is pain radiating down the front of the thigh.

This concludes examination with the patient lying down.

Patient Standing

Now ask the patient to stand and examine the spine, and assess gait. If required one should perform the Trendelenburg test and assess the patient's ability to stand from a seated or squatting position.

Spine

When examining the spine with the patient standing, one should assess the following:

- ♦ Structure
- ♣ Function

Structure

One should examine:

- ♥ Dimensions
- ♠ Contents

Dimensions

Look at the spine and note the shape of the spine. Define any deformity.

Contents

Gently palpate the spine and note any localised tenderness.

Function

One should examine:

- ♦ Position
- ♣ Movements

Position

Observe the posture of the patient. Ask the patient to stand against a wall. The patient's heels, buttocks and occiput should touch the wall.

To objectively assess this measure the wall to tragus distance.

Movements of the Spine

Assess movements of the spine. One should assess:

- ♥ Flexion
- ♠ Extension
- ♦ Lateral Flexion
- ♣ Rotation

Flexion (Schober Test)

Draw a line across the dimples overlying the sacroiliac joints. Measure 10 cms from this point and draw another line parallel to the first. Ask the patient to bend and attempt to touch his or her toes. Measure the distance between the two lines that have been drawn and note any increase in this distance. The normal should be an increase to over 15 cms.

Extension, Lateral Flexion, Rotation

Now ask the patient to lean back and assess extension of the spine. Ask the patient to bend sideway and assess lateral flexion. Stand behind the patient and hold the patient's hips with one's index fingers on the patient's anterior superior iliac spines. Now ask the patient to turn his or her head and shoulders to the right and then to the left and assess the degree of rotation achieved. One's hands on the patient's hips detect and prevent any rotation of the pelvis.

Gait

Ask the patient to walk and assess gait. The method described in the chapter on the nervous system should be used.

Trendelenburg Test

Perform the Trendelenburg test.

Observe the patient from behind. Ask the patient to raise one foot off the ground and stand on one leg. In health the hip with the leg raised should tilt upwards. If there is disease in the weight-bearing hip, the contralateral hip dips downwards.

Standing from the Seated or Squatting Position

Observe the patient standing up from the seated position. Asking the patient to squat and stand up is a better test but it is not always practical.

Lesions of the Locomotor System

One should consider lesions that affect:

- ♥ Bones
- ♠ Joints
- ♦ Tendons
- ♣ Bursae
- ♥ Muscles

Bones

When considering disorders of bone, think of those that affect:

- ♠ Bone cells
- ♦ Connective tissue of bones
- ♣ Periosteum
- ♥ All elements of bone
- ♠ Disorders secondary to systemic disease

Disorders of Cells

Abnormalities that occur in relation to bone cells are:

- ♠ Primary neoplasms
- ♦ Secondary neoplasms
- ♣ Dysplasia

Primary Neoplasms

Primary neoplasms of bone may be:

- ♥ Osteoma
- ♠ Osteoblastoma
- ♦ Osteosarcoma
- ♣ Chondroma
- ♥ Chondroblastoma
- ♠ Chondrosarcoma
- ♦ Osteoclastoma
- ♣ Giant Cell Tumour
- ♥ Ewing's sarcoma

Secondary Neoplasms

Secondary neoplasms could be those arising from the:

- ♠ **RS** bronchus
- ♦ **RAG** breast, prostate
- ♣ **E&M** thyroid

♥ **KUS** kidney

♣ **HS** multiple myeloma

Dysplasia

Dysplasia of bone could be:

♣ Inherited Skeletal Dysplasia

♥ Paget's disease of bone

Inherited Skeletal Dysplasia

Inherited skeletal dysplasia may affect:

♥ Cartilage

♠ Bone

♦ Osteoclasts

♣ Fibrous tissue

Dysplasia of Cartilage

The types of dysplasia that affect cartilage are:

♥ Achondroplasia

♠ Spondyloepiphyseal dysplasia

♦ Multiple hereditary exostoses

Dysplasia of Bone

Dysplasia of bone gives rise to a rare group of disorders, the sclerosing bone dysplasias, which result in multiple deformities of bone.

Osteoclasts

Disorders of osteoclasts result in an inability to reabsorb bone. This results in osteopetrosis or marble bone disease. The types are:

♣ Severe osteopetrosis

♥ Mild osteopetrosis

♠ Carbonic anhydrase II deficiency

Fibrous Dysplasia

Fibrous dysplasia refers to conditions in which areas of immature fibrous tissue are found in the skeleton. The types are:

♦ Monostotic Fibrous Dysplasia

♣ Polyostotic Fibrous Dysplasia

Disorders of Connective Tissue of Bone

The connective tissue of bone may be affected by:

♠ Osteomalacia and rickets

♦ Osteoporosis

♣ Osteogenesis imperfecta

♥ Hypophosphatasia (alkaline phosphatase deficiency resulting in defective mineralisation of bone)

Periosteum

The periosteum may be affected by:

♠ Osteomyelitis, which may be caused by pyogenic bacteria, tuberculosis

♦ Hypertrophic pulmonary osteoarthropathy

All Elements of Bone

All elements of bone may be affected by:

♣ Avascular necrosis

♥ Fracture

Avascular Necrosis of Bone

Avascular necrosis of bone may be secondary to:

Definite:

♥ **LMS** fracture of the femoral neck, hip dislocation

♠ **HS** sickle cell disease

♦ **RS** decompression sickness

♣ **E&M** Gaucher's disease

♥ **Physical agents** radiotherapy

♠ **Drugs** corticosteroids, heparin

Possible:

♦ **LMS** systemic lupus erythematosus, gout

♣ **IS** psoriasis

♥ **HS** polycythaemia rubra vera

♠ **E&M** Cushing's syndrome, diabetes mellitus

♦ **GIT** pancreatitis, pancreatic cancer, fatty liver

♣ **KUS** renal transplant

♥ **CVS** atherosclerosis

♠ **Drugs** cytotoxic chemotherapy

♦ **Toxins** alcohol abuse

Fracture

Fractures of bones may be:

♣ Traumatic

♥ Pathological

Pathological Fractures

Pathological fractures may be caused by:

♠ Neoplasms (primary or secondary)

♦ Inflammation (osteomyelitis)

♣ Metabolic conditions (osteomalacia, osteoporosis)

♥ Dysplasia (Paget's disease of bone)

Systemic Disorders

Systemic disorders result in pathological processes in bones by causing:

♠ Osteoporosis

♦ Osteomalacia

♣ Avascular necrosis

♥ Hypertrophic pulmonary osteoarthropathy

Osteoporosis

Osteoporosis is characterised by a reduction in bone mass and disruption of the architecture of bone. Risk factors for osteoporosis are:

♠ **Internal Factors**

Increasing age, female gender, Caucasian or Asian race, family history of osteoporosis

♦ **External Factors**

Dietary factors such as a low calcium intake

♣ **Systemic Factors**

Conditions affecting the:

RAG secondary amenorrhoea, primary hypogonadism, premature menopause

E&M acromegaly, hyperthyroidism, hyperparathyroidism, Cushing's syndrome, diabetes mellitus

KUS chronic renal failure

> **LMS** rheumatoid arthritis, prolonged immobilisation
>
> **GIT** nutritional failure, inflammatory bowel disease
>
> **Drugs** steroid therapy
>
> **Toxins** cigarettes, alcohol
>
> **Surgery** organ transplantation

Growing Bones

Disorders of growing bones result in:

- ♦ Short stature
- ♣ Tall stature
- ♥ Sclerosing bone dysplasia

Short Stature

Short stature may be due to:

- ♠ Primary disorders of bone
- ♦ Secondary to systemic disease

Primary Disorders of Bone

Primary disorders of bone would result in either:

- ♣ Disproportionate short stature
- ♥ Proportionate short stature

Disproportionate Short Stature

Disproportionate short stature would manifest either as:

- ♠ Short limbs
- ♦ Short trunk

Short Limbs

Short limbs are caused by:

- ♣ Achondroplasia

- ♥ Achondroplasia like dwarfs (a variety of rare syndromes exist)
- ♠ Hypophosphatasia
- ♦ Osteogenesis imperfecta

Short Trunk

Short trunk is caused by:

- ♠ Spondyloepiphyseal dysplasia

Proportionate Short Stature

Proportionate short stature occurs in:

- ♦ Rickets
- ♣ Hypophosphataemic rickets
- ♥ Mucopolysaccharidoses

Systemic Disorders

Systemic disorders that result in short stature are:

- ♠ Nutritional failure
- ♦ Chronic childhood disease affecting any system
- ♣ Precocious puberty

Tall Stature

Tall stature may be:

- ♥ Tall stature with normal proportions
- ♠ Tall stature with eunuchoid proportions

Tall Stature with Normal Proportions

Tall stature with normal proportions may be due to:

- ♦ Normal variation
- ♣ Gigantism

Tall Stature with Eunuchoid Proportions

Tall stature with eunuchoid proportions may be due to:

- ♥ Primary disease of connective tissue
- ♠ Hypogonadism

Primary Diseases of Connective Tissue

Primary diseases of connective tissue that result in tall stature with eunuchoid proportions are:

- ♦ Marfan's syndrome
- ♣ Homocystinuria

Sclerosing Bone Dysplasia

Sclerosing bone dysplasia gives rise to multiple deformities of bone. Several rare syndromes have been described.

Joints

Conditions that occur in the joints may be disorders affecting:

- ♥ Internal Factors
- ♠ Synovium
- ♦ Capsule
- ♣ Articular Cartilage
- ♥ Systemic Factors

Internal Factors

Internal factors usually result in inflammation of the joints. They are:

- ♠ Infections
- ♦ Crystals

- ♣ Loose Bodies

Infections

Infections that result in inflammation of the joints are:

- ♥ Septic arthritis (the causes are: *Staphylococcus aureus, Streptococcus pneumoniae, Haemophilus influenzae,* less commonly gram-negative bacilli such as *Escherichia coli.* Many other organisms have been reported.)
- ♠ Tuberculous arthritis
- ♦ Meningococcal arthritis
- ♣ Gonococcal arthritis
- ♥ Salmonella
- ♠ Lyme disease
- ♦ Infective endocarditis
- ♣ Viral infections
- ♥ Fungal infections

Crystals

Crystals that cause inflammation of the joints are:

- ♠ Uric acid crystals
- ♦ Pyrophosphate crystals

Loose Bodies

Loose bodies refer to fibrous, bony, cartilaginous or osteocartilaginous fragments within a synovial joint. The causes of loose bodies are:

- ♣ Osteochondritis dissecans
- ♥ Synovial chondromatosis
- ♠ Osteophytes
- ♦ Fractured articular surfaces
- ♣ Damaged menisci

Synovium

The synovium may be affected by:

♥ Arthritis

Rheumatoid arthritis, systemic lupus erythematosus, juvenile chronic arthritis (juvenile idiopathic arthritis /Still's disease), rheumatic fever

♠ Osteochondromatosis

♦ Pigmented villonodular synovitis

Capsule

The capsule may be affected by:

♣ Trauma

♥ Periarthritis

♠ Calcific periarthritis

♦ Hypermobility syndrome. This may be primary or associated with Ehlers-Danlos syndrome, Marfan's syndrome

Articular Cartilage

The articular cartilage may be affected by:

♣ Osteoarthritis

♥ Wilson's disease

♠ Haemochromatosis

♦ Relapsing polychondritis

♣ Osteochondritis dissecans

Systemic Factors

Systemic factors that result in disorders of the joints are conditions affecting the:

♥ **GIT** enteropathic synovitis, autoimmune hepatitis, primary biliary cirrhosis, haemochro-matosis, Whipple's disease, pancreatitis

♠ **HS** leukaemia (gout), haemophilia (haemarthroses), sickle cell disease, arthritis in acute leukaemia, amyloidosis

♦ **IS** psoriasis, erythema nodosum

♣ **CNS** Charcot's joints (in syringomyelia the shoulder is involved, in tabes dorsalis the knees and ankles, in diabetes mellitus the foot)

♥ **E&M** acromegaly, hypothy-roidism, combined hyperlipi-daemia, familial hypercholesterolaemia, diabetes mellitus in childhood causes joint contractures

♠ **KUS** azotaemic arthropathy

Tendons

Conditions that affect the tendons are:

♦ Enthesopathy

♣ Tenosynovitis

Enthesopathy

Enthesopathy refers to a pathological process affecting the specialised area at the junction of tendons or ligaments and bone. It is usually due to:

♥ Repetitive strain injury

♠ It may be a feature of spondy-loarthropathy

Tenosynovitis

Tenosynovitis refers to inflammation of the tendon sheaths. It may be due to:

545

- Friction syndromes
- Inflammatory disease such as rheumatoid arthritis

Bursae

Bursitis refers to inflammation of bursae. Bursitis may be due to:

- Trauma
- Repetitive strain
- Gout
- Arthritis
- Infection

Muscle

Disorders of the muscles have been discussed in the chapter on the nervous system.

Presentation of Arthropathy

Arthropathy may present as:

- Monoarthropathy
- Polyarthropathy
- Spondyloarthropathy

Monoarthropathy

Monoarthropathy may affect:

- Large joints
- Small joints

Large Joint Monoarthropathy

Monoarthropathy of a large joint may be due to:

- Pseudogout
- Osteoarthritis

- Haemarthroses
- Septic arthritis

Small Joint Monoarthropathy

Monoarthropathy of a small joint is usually due to:

- Gout
- Septic arthritis (rare)

Polyarthropathy

Polyarthropathy may predominantly affect:

- Large joints
- Small joints

Large Joint Polyarthropathy

Polyarthropathy predominantly affecting large joints may be due to:

- Rheumatic fever
- Osteoarthrosis
- Septic arthritis (rare)

Small Joint Polyarthropathy

Polyarthropathy predominantly affecting small joints may be due to:

- Rheumatoid arthritis
- Psoriatic arthropathy
- Other connective tissue disorders
- Gout
- Osteoarthrosis

Spondyloarthropathy

Spondyloarthropathy refers to a group of inflammatory diseases that predominantly affect the axial skeleton, peripheral joints and entheses.

Spondyloarthropathy may be due to:

- ♠ Ankylosing spondylitis
- ♥ Reactive arthritis
- ♠ Psoriasis
- ♦ Enteropathic arthritis (in inflammatory bowel disease)

Reiter's syndrome refers to a triad of arthritis, conjunctivitis and urethritis/cervicitis

Findings on History

The findings that may be obtained on taking a history are as follows:

Bone Pain

Bone pain may be due to conditions affecting the:

♣ Bone Marrow

Leukaemia, myeloma, secondary deposits

♥ Bone

Bone tissue may be affected by the following pathological processes:

Metabolic :osteomalacia, osteoporosis

Tumours: primary or secondary tumours

Dysplasia: Paget's disease of bone

Inflammation: osteomyelitis

Ischaemia :avascular necrosis

Stiffness

Variations in the timing of stiffness would help to differentiate the type of arthropathy.

- ♠ If stiffness is increased in the morning it usually indicates rheumatoid arthritis
- ♦ If stiffness increases as the day goes on it is more likely to be osteoarthritis

Findings on Examination

The abnormalities that may be detected on physical examination are as follows:

General Examination

The abnormalities that may be detected on general examination of the patient are those in relation to the following:

- ♥ Dimensions
- ♠ Integument
- ♦ Body temperature

Dimensions

The abnormalities that may be detected would be in relation to:

- ♣ Posture
- ♥ Height
- ♠ Size and shape of bones
- ♦ Weight

Posture

The posture of the patient would give clues to the underlying disorder.

- ♣ A stooped posture would be a feature of ankylosing spondylitis
- ♥ Kyphosis would be a feature of severe osteoporosis

Height

Variations in height that may be of significance are the following:

- ♠ Tall stature
- ♦ Short stature
- ♣ Loss of height

Tall Stature

Tall stature could be either:

- ♠ Tall stature with normal proportions
- ♦ Tall stature with eunuchoid proportions

The conditions in which the above occur have been discussed earlier.

Short Stature

Short stature could be either:

- ♣ Short stature with normal proportions
- ♥ Short stature with abnormal proportions

These conditions have been discussed earlier.

Loss of Height

Loss of height may occur due to destruction of bone in:

- ♠ Paget's disease of bone
- ♦ Osteoporosis
- ♣ Hyperparathyroidism

When loss of height occurs, arm span would be greater than height.

Abnormal Size and Shape of Bones

Abnormal size and shape of bones may be due to:

- ♥ Congenital Disorders
- ♠ Acquired Disorders

Congenital Disorders

Congenital disorders that cause abnormal size and shape of bones are:

- ♦ Engelman-Camurati syndrome (a type of sclerosing bone dysplasia)
- ♣ Other rare inherited bone dysplasias

Acquired Disorders

Acquired disorders that result in abnormal size and shape of bones are:

- ♥ Paget's disease of bone

Weight

Body weight may be:

- ♠ **Increased** :osteoarthrosis
- ♦ **Decreased**: cachexia due to long standing inflammatory disease

Integument

When assessing the integument one may note changes in:

- ♣ Colour
- ♥ Surface
- ♠ Consistency
- ♦ Circulation

Colour

Changes in the colour of the skin that are of significance are:

- ♣ Pigmentation of the skin would be a feature of haemochromatosis, Whipple's disease

Surface

Abnormalities that may be noted on the surface of the skin are:

♥ Skin rashes

Skin rashes may be due to:

Psoriasis, secondary syphilis, brucella, Lyme disease, septicaemia

Drug induced: gold, penicillamine

♠ An evanescent, pink, maculopapular rash occurs in juvenile chronic arthritis

♦ Erythema marginatum occurs in rheumatic fever

♣ Erythema nodosum occurs in polyarteritis nodosa, rheumatoid arthritis, rheumatic fever, sarcoidosis

♥ Vasculitis

Palpable purpura due to vasculitis may be caused by:

Rheumatoid arthritis, systemic lupus erythematosus, Henoch-Schonlein purpura, Churg-Strauss syndrome, Wegener's granulomatosis, polyarteritis nodosa

Drugs such as penicillin, sulphonamides

♠ Purpura could be due to treatment with gold, penicillamine

♦ Ecchymoses may be due to steroids

Consistency

When examining the consistency of the skin one may note:

♥ Loose skin. This occurs in pseudoxanthoma elasticum, Ehlers-Danlos syndrome

Circulation

When assessing the blood vessels of the skin, lesions that may be observed are:

♠ Livedo reticularis. This occurs in polyarteritis nodosa, systemic lupus erythematosus

Body Temperature

Fever may be a feature of:

♥ Still's disease

♠ Septic arthritis

Regional Examination

The abnormalities that may be detected on regional examination are as follows:

Head

On examination of the head one may detect abnormalities in relation to:

♠ Size

♦ Shape

♣ Movement

Size

Changes in the size of the head that may be observed are:

♥ An increase in size and change in shape of the skull would be observed in Paget's disease of bone.

♠ Moon face could be iatrogenic following steroid treatment

Shape

Variations in the shape of the head that would be significant are:

♦ Frontal bossing would be a feature of Paget's disease of bone

Movement

Abnormalities of movement of the head that may be observed are:

♣ In ankylosing spondylitis when the patient is asked to turn his or her head to look to a side, he or she has to move the body as a whole.

Nose

On examination of the nose one may note:

♥ Saddle nose in relapsing polychondritis

♠ Rash in systemic lupus erythematosus

Eyes

On examination of the eyes one may detect abnormalities of the following:

Orbits

Abnormalities may be noted of:

♦ Site

♣ Shape

Site

The site of the orbits in relation to one another may alter in certain states.

♦ Widely spaced orbits may occur due to enlargement of the sphenoid bone. This is known as hypertelorism and may occur in osteogenesis imperfecta.

Shape

Variations in the shape of the orbits that are of significance are the following:

♣ Prominent supraorbital ridges may occur in acromegaly.

♥ Localised changes in shape may occur due to underlying lesions such as granulomata or histiocytosis

♠ Replacement of bone by fibrous vascular tissue occurs in polyostotic fibrous dysplasia or Albright's syndrome.

Eyelids

Abnormalities that may occur in the eyelids are:

♦ Heliotrope rash occurs in dermatomyositis

♣ A rash may occur in systemic lupus erythematosus

Conjunctiva

Lesions that may be noted in the conjunctiva are:

♠ Conjunctivitis is a feature of inflammatory arthropathies

♦ Episcleritis is an intense hyperaemia of the superficial vessels it causes minor discomfort, no pain. It occurs in rheumatoid arthritis

♣ Keratoconjunctivitis sicca is a condition in which the eyes are dry due to destruction of lacrimal tissue. It occurs in Sjogren's syndrome.

The test used to confirm this is Schirmer's test where a filter paper is hooked over the lower eyelid. In normal lacrimation, 15 mm should be wet in 5 minutes. In keratoconjunctivitis sicca less then 5 mm would be wet.

Sjogren's Syndrome

Sjogren's syndrome is a syndrome caused by destruction of exocrine glandular tissue as a result of inflammation. It may be:

♥ **Primary Sjogren's syndrome**

Where the condition exists on its own

♠ **Secondary   Sjogren's syndrome**

Where it is associated with other diseases such as rheumatoid arthritis, systemic lupus erythematosus, scleroderma, polymyositis, primary biliary cirrhosis. A similar condition may be associated with HIV, hepatitis C and HTLV 1 infection.

Sclera

Abnormalities that may be detected are:

♠ Blue sclerae are seen in Marfan's syndrome,   Ehlers-Danlos syndrome, osteogenesis imperfecta

♦ Scleritis. This is a painful condition that results in a deep, purple hue of the sclera due to dilatation of the deep scleral vessels. It occurs in rheumatoid arthritis

♣ Scleromalacia perforans. This refers to thinning of the sclera with resultant perforation. It may occur in rheumatoid arthritis

♥ Pigmentation of the sclera may be seen in ochronosis (alkaptonuria)

Anterior Chamber

When examining the anterior chamber one may note:

♠ Hypopyon, pus in the anterior chamber, may complicate anterior uveitis

♦ Synechiae occur as a sequel to episodes of anterior uveitis. Synechiae are adhesions between the iris and the lens (posterior synechiae) or between the iris and the cornea (anterior synechiae)

Iris

Lesions that may occur in the iris are:

♣ Anterior uveitis may occur in Reiter's syndrome, ankylosing spondylitis, rheumatoid arthritis, Behcet's disease

♥ Tremor of the iris may be seen due to lens dislocation in Marfan's   syndrome, homocystinuria

Lens

On examination of the lens one may note:

♠ Cataract. This may occur following treatment with steroids, chloroquine

♦ Dislocation of the lens may occur in:

Marfan's syndrome (upward dislocation)

Homocystinuria (downward dislocation)

Fundus

Lesions that may be observed in the fundus are the following:

♣ Optic atrophy may occur in Paget's disease of bone

♥ Papilloedema may occur in systemic lupus erythematosus

♠ Chloroquine may cause a retinopathy, which is dose dependent. It results in a bull's eye appearance and is associated with a permanent reduction in central vision.

♦ Angioid streaks are seen in Paget's disease of bone, pseudoxanthoma elasticum

♣ Fundal haemorrhages occur in systemic lupus erythematosus

♥ Cytoid bodies are white exudates that occur in systemic lupus erythematosus

♠ Retinal detachment may occur in Marfan's syndrome

3rd, 4th and 6th Nerves

Pupils

Abnormalities that may be noted are:

♦ The pupils may be irregular due to previous episodes of uveitis.

Face

On examination of the face one may detect abnormalities in relation to the following:

Scalp

Features of note would be:

♣ Alopecia would be a feature of systemic lupus erythematosus.

♥ Psoriatic plaques may be seen in the scalp

♠ Rheumatic nodules occur at the back of head. They are a feature of rheumatic fever

Malar Region

In the malar region one may note abnormalities of the:

♦ Surface

♣ Circulation

Surface

One may note:

♦ Butterfly rash in systemic lupus erythematosus

♣ Heliotrope rash in dermato-myositis

Circulation

Lesions that may occur in relation to the blood vessels in the malar region are:

♥ Telangiectasiae occur in scleroderma

Mouth

The abnormalities that may be detected are those in relation to the following:

Jaw

Involvement of the temperomandibular joint occurs in:

♠ Temperomandibular arthrosis. This causes pain, clicking or limitation of movement. It is more common in young women.

♦ Rheumatoid arthritis

♣ Osteoarthrosis

Lips

Abnormalities that may be noted in the lips are:

♥ Microstomia occurs in scleroderma

♠ Perioral skin puckering or pseudorhagades occurs in scleroderma

♦ Ulceration of the lips may occur in Behcet's disease, inflammatory bowel disease

Buccal Mucosa

The buccal mucosa would be:

♣ Dry in Sjogren's syndrome

Palate

The palate would be:

♥ High arched in Marfan's syndrome

Salivary Glands

Abnormalities that may be noted are:

♥ Parotid enlargement may occur in Sjogren's syndrome

Speech

Abnormalities of speech that may be significant are:

♠ A hoarse voice may occur in rheumatoid arthritis (due to cricoarytenoid joint involvement)

Ears

On examination of the ears one may detect abnormalities of the following:

♦ Structure

♣ Function

Structure

Abnormalities that may be noted are the following:

♦ Tophi may be seen in gout

♣ Psoriatic plaques may be seen behind the ears

♥ Relapsing polychondritis causes redness, swelling and pain. Later it results in a floppy ear. It is associated with synovitis mainly of the large joints.

Hearing

Decreased hearing may occur in:

- ♠ Paget's disease of bone
- ♦ Osteogenesis imperfecta

In Paget's disease of bone, deafness may be due to auditory nerve compression in the internal auditory canal due to overgrowth of bone resulting in nerve deafness or changes in the ossicles could cause a conduction defect.

Hands

On examination of the hands one may note abnormalities of the following:

Size

The size of the hands may be:

- ♣ **Increased**: acromegaly
- ♥ **Apparent Decrease**: scleroderma

Shape

The overall shape of the hands may differ from normal. The change may be:

- ♠ Squaring in osteoarthrosis
- ♦ Narrow in scleroderma

Nails

Lesions that may be observed in the nails are the following:

- ♣ Pitting of the nails is seen in psoriatic arthropathy
- ♥ Clubbing occurs in inflammatory bowel disease, Whipple's disease, hypertrophic pulmonary osteoarthropathy

- ♠ Nail fold infarcts occur in rheumatoid arthritis, dermatomyositis
- ♦ Dilated nail fold vessels are seen in dermatomyositis. In this condition, the cuticles may be ragged.
- ♣ Nail fold capillary dilatation occurs in systemic sclerosis

Skin

On examination of the skin over the hands one may note abnormalities of the following:

- ♥ Surface
- ♣ Consistency
- ♦ Circulation

Surface

Lesions that may occur on the surface of the skin over the hands are the following:

- ♥ Red plaques with silvery scales occur in psoriasis
- ♣ Tophi occur in gout
- ♦ Calcinosis occurs in scleroderma
- ♣ Gottron's papules, which are violaceous papules with a flat top, may be found over the interphalangeal joints in dermatomyositis.

Consistency

Variations in the consistency of the skin of the hands are:

- ♥ Diabetic stiff hands (cheiroarthropathy). In this condition tight, waxy skin mainly affecting the dorsum of the fingers would be noted. It is associated with joint stiffness that affects extensor movements.

♠ In the early stages of systemic sclerosis the skin may be oedematous and puffy. This stage may be accompanied by stiff, painful joints and tendon sheath crepitus may be felt.

♦ In the later stages of systemic sclerosis the skin over the fingers becomes shiny, smooth, tight and bound to the underlying structures.

Circulation

Circulatory changes that may occur in the skin of the palms of the hands are:

♣ Palmar erythema may be seen in rheumatoid arthritis

Locomotor System

When examining the locomotor system of the hands one may note abnormalities of the following:

Thumb

Abnormalities that may be noted are:

♥ Z deformity (fixed flexion and subluxation of the metacarpophalangeal joint with hyperextension of the interphalangeal joint) occurs in rheumatoid arthritis

♠ Squaring of the carpus may be seen as a result of subluxation at the carpometacarpal joint. This occurs in osteoarthrosis

Fingers (Overall)

One may note that the fingers are abnormal in shape. The abnormalities could be:

♦ Swan neck deformity. This refers to hyperextension at the proximal interphalangeal joint with flexion at the metacarpophalangeal and distal interphalangeal joint. It occurs in rheumatoid arthritis.

♣ Spindle shaped fingers are caused by swelling of the proximal interphalangeal joints in rheumatoid arthritis

♥ Sausage shaped fingers, where uniform swelling of the whole digit occurs, would be seen in dactylitis which may occur in Reiter's syndrome, psoriatic arthropathy, sarcoidosis, tuberculosis

♠ Mallet finger refers to a flexion deformity of the terminal interphalangeal joint caused by rupture of the extensor tendon

♦ Boutonnière deformity refers to a flexion deformity of the proximal interphalangeal joint with extension at the metacarpophalangeal and terminal interphalangeal joints. It is caused by rupture of the insertion of the extensor tendon to the middle phalanx.

♣ Trigger finger refers to the inability to extend the fingers following flexion. It is caused by a nodule in the flexor tendon. The examiner may extend the finger passively and a characteristic give is felt as the nodule enters the tendon sheath

555

♥ Telescoping of the fingers is seen in the destructive, mutilating arthropathy that can occur in psoriasis

♠ Tapering of the fingers is seen in scleroderma.

Metacarpophalangeal Joints

At the metacarpophalangeal joints one may note:

♦ Ulnar deviation which is a feature of rheumatoid arthritis

Proximal Interphalangeal Joints

At the proximal interphalangeal joints one may note:

♣ The proximal interphalangeal joints are commonly affected in rheumatoid arthritis

♥ Bouchard's nodes are bony nodules at the proximal interphalangeal joints

Distal Interphalangeal Joints

The distal interphalangeal joints are usually affected in:

♠ Osteoarthrosis

♦ Psoriatic arthropathy

♣ Gout

Heberden's nodes are bony nodules at the distal interphalangeal joints

Activity of Disease

Features that would indicate active disease are:

♥ Swelling, warmth and tenderness would indicate active disease

♠ Soft tissue swelling would indicate synovitis

♦ Redness or erythema usually indicates crystal arthropathy or infection.

Hypermobile Joints

Hypermobile joints occur in:

♣ Ehlers-Danlos syndrome

♥ Marfan's syndrome

♠ Benign joint hypermobility syndrome

Tendons of the Fingers

Lesions of the tendons would result in:

♣ Trigger finger

♥ Boutonnière deformity

♠ Mallet finger

♦ Tendon sheath crepitus occurs in the early stages of systemic sclerosis and in rheumatoid arthritis

Aponeurosis

Lesions of the aponeurosis may cause:

♣ Dupuytren's contracture

Wrists

Lesions that may be noted at the wrists are:

♥ The wrist is involved in rheumatoid arthritis and in osteoarthrosis

♠ De Quervain's tenosynovitis refers to tenosynovitis of the extensor tendon of the thumb

Other Lesions that may present as Arthropathy of the Hands

Other lesions that may present as arthropathy of the hands are the following:

♦ Pancreatic arthropathy. Pancreatic disease may be associated with a synchronous arthritis and panniculitis or it may predate clinical evidence of pancreatic disease.

♣ Azotaemic arthropathy occurs after several years of dialysis. It affects the interphalangeal joints in particular and causes synovitis.

♥ Diabetic cheiroarthropathy complicates childhood diabetes mellitus

Muscles

On examination of the muscles one may notice muscle wasting.

Muscle Wasting

Muscle wasting would be a feature of:

♣ Rheumatoid arthritis

Circulation

Conditions that may affect the peripheral circulation of the hands are:

♥ Reflex Sympathetic Dystrophy Syndrome (RSDS)/Complex Regional Pain Syndrome Type I (Sudek's atrophy)

♣ Raynaud's Phenomenon

♦ Erythromelalgia

Reflex Sympathetic Dystrophy Syndrome (RSDS)/Complex Regional Pain Syndrome Type I (Sudek's atrophy)

This may present as:

♣ An acute phase with burning pain, tenderness, hyperaesthesia, allodynia (usually non-painful stimuli cause pain), oedema, Raynaud's phenomenon, vasodilatation, altered sweating

♥ Dystrophic stage with skin atrophy

♠ Atrophic stage with cutaneous atrophy and development of contractures

The causes are:

♦ Trauma

♣ Central nervous system lesions such as strokes

♥ Idiopathic

Complex Regional Pain Syndrome Type II (Causalgia)

Complex regional pain syndrome type II refers to a burning pain that may occur following nerve section or amputation.

Raynaud's Phenomenon

In Raynaud's phenomenon, the phases are; initially the fingers go cold and white and then become blue due to stasis and finally red due to hyperaemia.

The causes of Raynaud's phenomenon are conditions affecting the:

♠ **LMS** systemic sclerosis, systemic lupus erythematosus, dermatomyositis, rheumatoid arthritis, mixed connective tissue disease

Thoracic outlet syndrome

- **HS** cold agglutinins, cryoglobulins
- **CVS** atherosclerosis
- **Drugs** beta blockers, ergot alkaloids

Erythromelalgia

Erythromelalgia refers to a painful, inflammatory, vasodilatation of the extremities. It may be:

- Idiopathic

Or due to:

- Thrombocythaemia
- Drug induced: calcium channel antagonists

Radial Pulse

On examination of the radial pulse one may note:

- The radial pulse would be diminished or absent in the thoracic outlet syndrome
- A bounding pulse may occur in Paget's disease of bone

Elbow

Lesions that may occur at the elbow are the following:

- Plaques occur in psoriasis
- Nodules occur in rheumatoid arthritis. They are firm nodules that are frequently attached to the perosteum. They reflect high levels of disease activity and severity.

- Olecranon bursitis results in pain and swelling over the olecranon bursa. It may occur in rheumatoid arthritis, ankylosing spondylitis, gout, repetitive injury
- Lateral epicondylitis causes pain and tenderness over the lateral epicondyle. This is increased by extension of the wrist against resistance. The cause is overuse.
- Medial epicondylitis causes pain and tenderness over the medial epicondyle. This is increased by flexion of the wrist against resistance. It is caused by overuse.
- Hypermobile joints occur in Ehlers-Danlos syndrome
- Charcot's joints may occur in syringomyelia

Upper Arms

Abnormalities that may be detected in the upper arms would be in relation to:

Blood Pressure

One may note:

- The blood pressure may differ on the two sides in the thoracic outlet syndrome

Shoulder

Lesions that may occur at the shoulder are the following:

- Adhesive capsulitis causes restriction of movement and pain in the shoulder. It results in pain and limitation of movement in all directions (active and passive movements). It is associated with diabetes mellitus, myocardial infarction, thyroid disease and pulmonary disease.

♣ Rotator cuff tendinitis causes pain, which is maximum in the deltoid region. It results in a painful arc of abduction from 60-120 degrees. Passive movements are full. The pain is increased by movement against resistance. It is associated with repetitive movement, diabetes mellitus

♥ Calcific tendinitis causes acute pain at the tip of the shoulder and results in limitation of both active and passive movement.

♠ Bicipital tendinitis causes pain in the anterior aspect of the shoulder.

♦ Rotator cuff rupture causes pain in the deltoid area and results in an inability to abduct the shoulder if the rupture is complete.

♣ Stiffness and pain in the shoulders occurs in polymyalgia rheumatica

♥ Charcot's joints may occur in syringomyelia

♠ Weakness of the muscles of the shoulder girdle occurs in polymyositis

Neck

In the neck one may note abnormalities of the following:

♦ Skin

♣ Joints

♥ Arteries

♠ Lymph nodes

Skin

Abnormalities that one may detect in the skin over the neck are:

♦ Tight skin occurs in systemic sclerosis

♣ Loose skin occurs in Pseudoxanthoma elasticum

Joints

Lesions of significance that occur in the neck are:

♥ Cervical spine disease in rheumatoid arthritis affects the upper cervical spine

Arteries

Abnormalities that may be detected are:

♠ A bruit may occur over the subclavian artery in the thoracic outlet syndrome

Lymph Nodes

When examining the lymph nodes one may detect:

♦ Generalised lymphadenopathy. This occurs in juvenile chronic arthritis

Chest Wall

One may observe:

♣ Rickety rosary (swelling of the costochondral junctions), Harrison's sulcus (a linear depression of the lower ribs, just above the costal margins) are seen as sequelae of childhood rickets

Respiratory System

Lesions of relevance to the locomotor system that may be detected are:

♥ Decreased chest expansion occurs in ankylosing spondylitis

♠ Pulmonary fibrosis occurs in rheumatoid arthritis, systemic lupus erythematosus, sarcoidosis

♦ Pulmonary hypertension occurs in systemic sclerosis

♣ Ankylosing spondylitis causes apical fibrosis

♥ Pleural effusion occurs in rheumatoid arthritis, systemic lupus erythematosus

♠ Pleurisy occurs in juvenile chronic arthritis

Cardiovascular System

Lesions of relevance that may be detected are:

♦ Carey Coombs murmur may be heard in acute rheumatic fever

♣ Aortic incompetence occurs in ankylosing spondylitis, tertiary syphilis

♥ Libmann-Sachs endocarditis occurs in systemic lupus erythematosus

♠ Cardiac failure may occur in Paget's disease of bone

♦ Myocarditis may occur in rheumatoid disease

♣ Atrioventricular block may occur in ankylosing spondylitis

♥ Systemic sclerosis may cause pulmonary hypertension, congestive cardiac failure, cardiac arrhythmias, pericardial effusion

♠ Pericarditis occurs in rheumatoid disease, juvenile chronic arthritis

Marfan's syndrome is associated with spontaneous pneumothorax, bullae, apical fibrosis, aspergilloma, bronchiectasis, mitral valve prolapse, coarctation of the aorta

Abdominal Wall

On examination of the abdominal wall one may observe:

♦ Decreased distance between the lower costal cartilages and the iliac crest in osteoporosis

♣ Prominent Abdomen

Loss of chest expansion in ankylosing spondylitis causes predominantly abdominal breathing and this results in a protuberant abdomen.

Abdominal protuberance is also a feature of osteoporosis

♥ Transverse furrow. In severe osteoporosis, a transverse furrow may be seen across the abdomen

♠ Psoriatic plaques may be seen in the umbilicus

Contents of the Abdomen

In relation to the contents of the abdomen, abnormalities that may be detected are the following:

Liver

Lesions that may occur in the liver are:

- ◆ Hepatosplenomegaly may occur in amyloidosis, autoimmune hepatitis, juvenile chronic arthritis
- ♣ Myeloproliferative disorders may cause gout

Spleen

Lesions that may occur in the spleen are:

- ♥ The spleen would be enlarged in Felty's syndrome.

Kidneys

Lesions that may be detected in the kidneys are:

- ♠ The kidneys may be enlarged due to amyloidosis

Hernial Orifices

On examination of the hernial orifices one may detect the following:

- ◆ Inguinal and femoral hernias are common in Marfan's syndrome

Genitals

Lesions that may occur in the genitals are:

- ♣ Ulceration may be seen in Behcet's syndrome
- ♥ Circinate balanitis occurs in Reiter's syndrome
- ♠ Urethral discharge may occur in Reiter's syndrome, gonorrhoea

General Examination of the Lower Limbs

On general examination of the lower limbs one may note abnormalities of:

Position

Variations in the position of the lower limbs that would be of note are:

- ◆ External rotation and shortening of the lower limb occurs in disease of the hip
- ♣ Apparent shortening of the lower limb occurs in pelvic tilting secondary to spinal disease
- ♥ Flexion deformity would occur in disease of the knee

Sacroiliac Joints

The sacroiliac joints are affected in:

- ♠ Reiter's syndrome
- ◆ Ankylosing spondylitis
- ♣ Reactive arthropathy
- ♥ Psoriasis

Hips

The hips may be affected in:

- ♠ Osteoarthrosis. Osteoarthrosis of the hip causes pain in the groin, the front of the thigh and in the knee. Later stiffness may occur. Early findings on examination are limitation of internal and external rotation. Later all movements are impaired but a good range of flexion is often preserved.

561

- Avascular necrosis. Avascular necrosis of the hip presents with severe hip pain. The underlying causes have been documented earlier

♣ Weakness of the muscles of the pelvic girdle occurs in polymyositis

♥ Pain and stiffness occurs in polymyalgia rheumatica

Knees

Lesions that affect the knees are the following:

♠ **Swollen knee**

A swollen knee may be due to:

- Fluid
- Synovial thickening
- Bone overgrowth

Fluid the causes of accumulation of fluid in the knee are: trauma, haemorrhage (which may be due to an underlying coagulopathy), inflammation (which may be caused by infection, crystal arthropathy, loose bodies, immune mediated)

Synovial thickening occurs in arthritis such as rheumatoid arthritis

Bone overgrowth occurs in osteoarthrosis, Paget's disease of bone

♦ **Genu valgum and genu varum**

Genu Valgum or knock-knee refers to angulation of the knee medially with the tibia being abducted in relation to the femur.

Genu Varum or bow-legs refers to bowing of the knee and leg outwards. There is medial angulation of the tibia

The causes are:

Malunion of fractures, osteoarthrosis (varus usually), rheumatoid arthritis (valgus usually), Paget's disease of bone, rickets

However, in most instances there is no underlying cause

♣ Pre-patellar bursitis may occur due to repetitive trauma (housemaid's knee, clergymen's knee)

♥ Baker's cyst is a cyst in the popliteal fossa. This is caused by the flow of fluid from an effusion in the knee into the gastrocnemius-semimembranous bursa. It results in pain and stiffness and a swelling at the posterior aspect of the knee. It is associated with inflammatory arthritis.

♠ Charcot's joints may occur in tabes dorsalis. Charcot's joints are neuropathic joints, which are caused by loss of the protective sensations. They are not usually painful and present with swelling and instability. The findings are a deformed, swollen joint with abnormal, painless, movement with loud crepitus and associated neurological features.

♦ Enteropathic arthritis may affect the knee

♣ Hyperextensible joints occur in Ehlers-Danlos syndrome, Marfan's syndrome. Genu recurvatum may occur.

Lower Leg

Lesions that may occur are:

♥ Erythema nodosum may occur in rheumatoid arthritis

♣ Pyoderma gangrenosum may occur in rheumatoid arthritis

♦ Vasculitis results in palpable purpura. It occurs in connective tissue disease

♣ Sabre tibia

Sabre tibia may be:

True sabre tibia A true sabre tibia occurs due to softening of the bone in Paget's disease, rickets

Apparent sabre tibia An apparent sabre tibia is caused by periostitis, which occurs in syphilis, yaws

♥ Ruptured Baker's cyst (popliteal cyst) may give the appearance of a deep vein thrombosis. The presence of a crescent shaped bruise below the medial malleolus is an useful clue to popliteal cyst rupture or calf haematoma.

Ankles

Lesions that may be detected at the ankle are the following:

♥ Ankle oedema may occur in the nephrotic syndrome, which may be due to:

Amyloidosis in long standing rheumatoid arthritis, ankylosing spondylitis

Drugs such as gold and penicillamine

♠ Valgus deformity refers to outward tilting of the heel due to subtalar joint damage. This may occur in rheumatoid arthritis

♦ Charcot's joints may occur in spina bifida, tabes dorsalis

♣ Achilles tendinitis occurs in Reiter's syndrome

Feet

Lesions that may occur in the feet are the following:

♥ Pes cavus refers to an increase in the concavity of the longitudinal arch of the foot. It is caused by neurological disorders and there would be associated clawing of the toes.

♠ Pes planus refers to a decrease in the longitudinal arch of the foot so that on standing the medial border of the foot is close to or touches the ground. It is usually congenital but may be associated with muscular weakness. It also occurs in Ehlers-Danlos syndrome, Marfan's syndrome.

♦ The arches of the foot may be flattened in rheumatoid arthritis.

♣ Keratoderma blenorrhagica causes reddish-brown macules, which may progress to pustules and then to crusted lesions. It occurs in Reiter's syndrome.

♥ Chronic tophaceous gout causes asymmetrical swelling and deformity of the small joints. Tophi formation occurs in the periarticular tissues.

♠ Plantar fasciitis occurs in Reiter's syndrome

563

- Charcot's joints may occur in diabetes mellitus

Toes

Lesions that may occur in the toes are the following:

- The first metatarsophalangeal joint is commonly affected in gout. This causes pain, swelling and redness.
- Hallux valgus refers to lateral deviation of the great toe. It is usually caused by incorrect footwear but it may also occur in rheumatoid arthritis, osteoarthrosis
- Hallux rigidus causes pain at the base of the great toe whilst walking. The metatarsophalangeal joint is thickened due to osteophyte formation and flexion and extension are restricted. It is caused by osteoarthrosis.
- Pain and swelling of the metatarsophalangeal joints are early manifestations of rheumatoid arthritis.
- Subluxation of the metatarsophalangeal joints is common in rheumatoid arthritis
- Hammer toe refers to a fixed flexion deformity of an interphalangeal joint. It may occur in rheumatoid arthritis.
- Claw toes refer to fixed flexion deformities of the interphalangeal joints. They occur in rheumatoid arthritis.

Nervous System

Lesions of the nervous system that are of relevance to joint disease are the following:

- Peripheral neuropathy may occur in rheumatoid arthritis
- Mononeuritis multiplex causing foot drop may occur in rheumatoid arthritis
- Cauda equina syndrome may occur in advanced ankylosing spondylitis

Spine

On examination of the spine one may note abnormalities of:

- Structure
- Function

Structure

Abnormalities that may be observed are:

- Kyphosis may be due to ankylosing spondylitis, osteoporosis
- Spondyloarthropathy may occur in inflammatory bowel disease
- Kyphoscoliosis occurs in Ehlers-Danlos syndrome, Marfan's syndrome
- An angular kyphosis (gibbus) occurs in tuberculosis of the spine
- A localised scoliosis would be seen in intervertebral disc lesions

Function

Abnormalities may be detected in relation to:

- ♠ Position
- ♦ Movements

Position

Wall to occiput (wall to tragus) distance would be:

- ♠ Increased in ankylosing spondylitis

Movements of the Spine

When examining spinal movements one may detect:

- ♦ Restriction of spinal movements. This occurs in spondyloarthropathy

Ankylosing Spondylitis

The clinical features of ankylosing spondylitis may be remembered as a number of A's. They are:

- ♣ **LMS**

  Aching and **A**rcing of the spine

  Attachments **A**ffected: attachments of tendons and ligaments to bone (entheses)

- ♥ **CVS**

  Aortitis

  Aortic Regurgitation

  Atrioventricular Block

- ♠ **RS**

  Apical fibrosis

  Apical cavitation (superinfection with **A**spergillus)

- ♦ **KUS**

  Amyloidosis

- ♣ **CNS**

  Anterior uveitis

  Anaesthesia (cauda equina syndrome)

- ♥ **GIT**

  Abdominal protuberance

Gait

Lesions would be as described in the chapter on the nervous system.

Trendelenburg Test

The Trendelenburg test would be positive in:

- ♣ Osteoarthrosis of the hip

Standing from a Seated or Squatting Position

Standing from a seated or squatting position would be difficult for patients who have:

- ♠ Proximal myopathy. In relation to the locomotor system one should consider polymyositis, dermatomyositis, drug induced proximal myopathy (steroids, chloroquine)

Chapter 18

Communication and Ethics

Basis of Assessment

Before considering the specific features of the communication and ethics station, it would be wise to pause and consider how a candidate is assessed by the examiners. This would apply to any type of professional examination.

When examining a patient, one would examine structure and function of the human body as a whole and structure and function of the various organs and organ systems that make up the human body and thereby one would detect clues that lead to a diagnosis.

When evaluating a candidate, the examiners undertake a similar process. Although it would be politically incorrect to say so, it is highly likely that aspects of structure are taken into consideration. Function or performance is definitely being evaluated.

In addition, one must remember that in day-to-day practice one is being constantly assessed by patients, their relations and friends, one's colleagues and other staff. The basis of their assessment is the same as that of a set of examiners at a formal professional examination. Hence, studying the following aspects of professional enhancement and applying them in day-to-day practice is not only a good way of preparing for examinations, it is an essential part of being a competent physician.

Structure

External appearance is important. Remember that a book is initially judged by its cover. It is the attraction of the cover that makes a reader, buyer or thief pick up a book and without doing so they will not glance through it and make the decision to borrow, buy or steal it. In marketing, a great deal of time and effort is spent on designing packaging as advertising and sales executives are well aware of the effects that external appearances have on the sales of a product. In nature, millions of years of evolution have produced striking external appearances in both plants and animals as this is of the utmost importance for their survival. In the field of medicine, clinicians devote years of training to develop the ability to judge the state of health or identify disease in an individual by the presence or absence of external physical signs that denote underlying pathology. Thus, one would be unwise to dismiss external appearance as unimportant. It is very likely that the appearance of the candidate would make the examiners in a professional examination form an initial opinion that would most likely influence their ultimate judgement. The same would apply in day-to-day practice with regard to the initial opinion formed of the physician by patients, their relations and friends, colleagues and other staff.

Most aspects of structure or external appearance cannot be changed but, there are certain aspects that are amenable to change and attention should be paid to these. They are:

- ♥ Clothing and Grooming
- ♠ Physical Fitness

Clothing and Grooming

In a professional examination, a smart, dark suit should be worn whatever the sex of the candidate. In some centres ladies may wear sari or other dress in keeping with their traditions. Shoes should be well polished; jewellery and make-up should be kept to the minimum. Male candidates would be advised to dispense with the latter two items. Hair should be well groomed.

For day-to-day practice one should follow a similar dress code. It would be best to dress smart and simple.

Physical Fitness

In addition to a healthy body allowing one to present oneself in a favourable light, one should remember that a healthy body is an essential pre-requisite for a healthy mind. This is important in preparation for professional examinations and clinical practice and for enhanced performance in professional examinations and clinical practice.

Function

Examiners wish to assess how well a candidate functions as a clinician. Their method of assessment of function is the same as that employed in assessment of function of an organ or organ system. This should not be surprising as every human being, even a candidate at examinations, is a collection of organs and organ systems!

Examination of Function

The method of examination of function follows the usual form, which is examination of:

- ♦ Position
- ♣ Character
- ♥ Quantity
- ♠ Transmission (Associated Features)
- ♦ Modifying Factors
- ♣ Rate
- ♥ Rhythm

Position

This is important. An air of confidence, but not overconfidence, should be projected. When standing, one should do so in an erect, yet relaxed, posture. Drooping shoulders and bent head will definitely give a negative impression. Look people straight in the eye. Avoidance of eye contact is an easy way to convey an incorrect impression to the examiners.

When seated, do so with one's feet placed firmly on the ground, maintain the spine in an erect position, the shoulders should be relaxed but should not droop. Maintain eye contact with the person with whom one communicates.

It would be best not to fold one's arms across one's chest when speaking to either the subject or the examiners.

Character (Quality)

The character (quality) of knowledge possessed by the candidate will be assessed although this is difficult. The examiners will attempt to evaluate whether the candidate is regurgitating knowledge that has been hastily swallowed or whether it is knowledge that has been carefully chewed over, ingested, digested and absorbed and has become an integral part of the individual. In other words, the examiners will try and ascertain whether the candidate's knowledge of clinical features is based on an understanding of pathogenesis and pathophysiology and whether he or she understands the rationale behind the relevant investigations and treatment. Hence, it is important to demonstrate that one's knowledge has been acquired on this basis. Being methodical is the best way to do this.

Similarly, when demonstrating skills, it is important to show that one's skills have been developed and mastered by years of dedicated practice rather than hastily learned a few weeks prior to the examination.

Quantity

The quantity of knowledge possessed by the candidate is fairly easy to judge and this is probably the easiest part of examining.

Transmission (Associated Features)

Transmission refers to non-verbal communication. This is an important means of communication but should be used judiciously. Some actions may unwittingly convey a bad impression and should be avoided These include scratching one's head or other parts of one's anatomy, looking up at the ceiling for divine inspiration, irritating use of gestures with one's hands such as those used by politicians.

Modifying Factors

Always be prepared to modify your answers according to the response of the examiners. However, one should be careful and avoid changing answers that one is confident are right. Some examiners may attempt to modify the candidate's performance by aggressive behaviour or on the other hand a condescending attitude. This type of challenge should be welcomed by the candidate who has worked hard as it will show off one's ability to work in stressful situations.

Rate

The rate of presentation of knowledge and demonstration of skill is important. This should be moderate. Neither too slow, which will give the impression of incompetence, nor too fast which will convey the impression of carelessness. This applies to both speech and actions.

Rhythm

Maintain a rhythm in both speech and actions. Hesitation and being disjointed does not convey the impression of ability and professionalism.

Communication

The art of effective communication should not be restricted to professional examinations. It is part-and-parcel of daily life and should be developed on a continuing basis. Two aspects of communication that should be developed are:

♥ Subject matter (Content)

♠ Technique

Subject Matter (Content)

The biggest problem faced by the candidate at the communication station, is not the ability to communicate. It is unlikely that one would have progressed to this stage of a career in medicine if one were unable to communicate. The problem is where one is faced with a situation in which one does not know what to communicate. Knowledge of subject matter is essential. Without this one would be completely lost. Imagine that one were to be asked to explain the intricacies of Buddhist metaphysics or the Abidhamma. It is unlikely that many would succeed.

Hence, the most important preparation for the communication station is to develop a large knowledge base.

Technique

Next, one should analyse the technique of communication more closely. The function of speech may be divided into three phases. The first phase is where one listens and analyses what is said. The second is a planning phase where one plans an appropriate response. The third is a delivery phase where the response is delivered. Thus, one derives the following aspects of communication:

♦ Listen

♣ Plan

♥ Convey (Delivery)

Listening

The ability to listen is very important. This is an active process. One must not allow one's mind to wander but instead one should constantly maintain an awareness of what the patient or subject is saying. This is difficult, as one's mind will wander especially in stressful situations. However, developing the skill of active listening is very important and should be practiced diligently. Remember that appropriate verbal and non-verbal prompting is very important as it shows the patient or subject that one is maintaining interest and encourages him or her to talk. However, remember that one should carefully direct the interview and not allow the patient or subject to ramble on unchecked.

Details to be Obtained

The details that one should obtain whilst listening are those details that one would obtain whilst taking a history without the details pertaining to the diagnosis, as these details would be already known in the communication and ethics station. Thus, they would be the patient or subject's:

- ♠ **Beliefs**
- ♦ **Expectations**
- ♣ **Anxieties (Concerns)**

  Regarding:

  Causes

  Effects

  Survival

However, if one feels that aspects of the history need clarifying then one may do so.

Planning

Planning is one of the vital components in achieving success in this situation. One should prepare a strategy for this beforehand. Apart from history taking there are other aspects of communication skill that are required in practice and that may be tested in a professional examination. They are; discussing and communicating strategy for investigation, discussing and communicating strategy for management of disease, explaining to patients and their carers the various aspects of diagnosis, investigation, management and prognosis. Ethics is an integral part of all these aspects. Hence, in planning one should consider:

- ♥ Planning Investigation
- ♠ Planning Management
- ♦ Planning Explanation

- ♣ Ethics

Planning Investigation

The scenarios that one may face in a professional examination are the same as those that one is faced with every day when dealing with patients. How does one investigate a patient in a particular clinical situation? With experience and development of clinical sense, one almost automatically thinks of the appropriate investigation to document the initial clinical diagnosis. But, when learning, and at times when difficulty arises, it is good to have a system that one may refer to. The simplest system would be to have a list of investigations and refer to the list for selection of the relevant tests. Very much like a menu in a restaurant. This may appear too simplistic but it is reliable. However, it would be more desirable to have a formal plan.

Formal Plan for Investigation

When formulating a plan for investigation of a patient one should define:

- ♥ Objectives
- ♠ Methods
- ♦ Risks and Benefits
- ♣ Cost

Objectives

The objectives of investigation are to confirm and document the four components of diagnosis; Anatomical Diagnosis, Pathological Diagnosis, Physiological Diagnosis, Aetiological Diagnosis.

Methods

The methods are probably the easiest aspect of planning investigation. Have a list of investigations and pick the relevant investigations from this list.

Risks and Benefits

Some investigations carry a risk whilst others may be unpleasant. One should take these aspects into account and decide on the balance of risk to benefit for each individual.

Cost

Cost should be taken into account. The reality of life is that someone must pay for all the investigations that are carried out on a patient whatever the type of service provided.

Available Investigations (Methods)

The investigations that are usually used are the following:

- ♥ Analysis of Body Fluids
- ♠ Imaging
- ♦ Nuclear Medicine
- ♣ Electrophysiology
- ♥ Physiological Assessment
- ♠ Endoscopy
- ♦ Surgery
- ♣ Tissue Diagnosis

Body Fluids

The most commonly used investigations are the analysis of body fluids. The body fluids that are analysed are blood, urine, faeces, saliva, cerebrospinal fluid, pleural fluid, ascitic fluid, joint aspirate and semen.

The methods of analysis may be conveniently divided into:

- ♥ Physical methods
- ♠ Chemical methods
- ♦ Biological methods

Physical Methods

The physical methods usually begin with a measurement of quantity. This would include volume of fluid and the pressure, which the fluid is under. Visualisation both with the naked eye and the use of magnification is performed. Analysis of characteristics such as viscosity too may be performed.

Chemical Methods

The chemical methods used analyse the presence of and quantify the amount of simple ions and more complex molecules. Samples used may be random or timed.

Biological Methods

These methods involve the analysis of cellular components of the fluids, assessment of components derived from the immune system such as antibodies and microbiological assessment. Microbiological assessment would involve bacteriology, virology, mycology and parasitology.

Analysis of Body Fluids

In practice, analysis of body fluids would be carried out by different departments and recall would be easier if one were to think of analysis of body fluids in terms of:

♣ Haematology

♥ Biochemistry

♠ Microbiology

♦ Immunology

♣ Cytology

♥ Genetics

Imaging

The next commonly used modality is imaging. Various modes of imaging are available. The commonest used are the different types of:

♣ Radiology

♥ Ultrasonography

Radiology

The types of radiological investigations used are the following:

♠ Plain X-ray

♦ Contrast studies

♣ Computerised tomography

♥ Magnetic resonance imaging (included here for ease of classification)

Ultrasound

Ultrasound includes:

♠ Standard regional ultrasound scanning

♦ Echocardiography

♣ Doppler

Nuclear Medicine

Another type of investigation is the use of radioactive isotopes to study structural and functional changes in organs or organ systems.

Electrophysiology

This is commonly used. Electrocardiography is the most common type of electrophysiological study used. Dynamic testing with exercise should be included. Electroencephalography and electromyography should also be borne in mind.

Physiological Assessment

This method is also commonly used. Examples are the use of Oesophageal Function Tests or Intestinal Motility Testing. Pulmonary Function Tests and Urinary Flow Studies should also be considered.

Endoscopy

Visualisation of internal structures with the use of endoscopes should be included although strictly speaking this should be considered as a more advanced method of examination rather than an investigation.

Surgery

The use of surgery in diagnosis must not be forgotten. Diagnostic laparoscopy or laparotomy, thoracoscopy, mediastinoscopy and invasive biopsy are important modalities of investigation.

Tissue Diagnosis

The use of histopathology in the investigation of a patient is quite often the most important determinant of treatment especially in the case of malignant disease.

Aide Memoire

The acronym **FINE PEST** *may be used as an aide memoire.* **F**luids, **I**maging, **N**uclear medicine,

Electrophysiology, **P**hysiological tests, **E**ndoscopy, **S**urgery, **T**issue diagnosis.

Management

By this stage of one's career it would have become obvious that very few illnesses can be cured. Cure is limited to a few diseases caused by infections or some cancers that may be eradicated completely from the body. All the rest of human illness is controlled. One should have realised by now that it is the individual patient that is managed, not the illness. Hence, a management plan must be tailored to suit the individual's needs. Blind adherence to a protocol or guideline is not in the best interests of the patient.

Planning Management

It would be wise to consider the principles underlying management of patients. A rational approach to this would greatly simplify one's strategy. This will help in professional examinations as well as in practice. After analysing the principles underlying management one may formulate a management plan.

Principles of Management

The first principle in managing patients is to arrive at a diagnosis. This diagnosis should be as complete as possible. That is one should define the four components of diagnosis:

- ♥ Anatomical Diagnosis
- ♠ Pathological Diagnosis
- ♦ Physiological Diagnosis
- ♣ Aetiological Diagnosis

On the basis of this it is easy to see how one would devise a management plan for an individual patient.

Aetiological Diagnosis

If the aetiology is known then one would plan to deal with this and thus hope to **Cure** the illness. A classic example would be the treatment of the aetiological agent, the malaria parasite, thus achieving a cure for malaria. The same would apply to most infectious diseases although at the present moment this cannot be said for some infections notably viral infections such as HIV.

Pathological Diagnosis

If the aetiology is unknown but the pathology is defined then one would plan to **Control** the disease process. Examples of this are the chronic inflammatory diseases of unknown origin such as inflammatory bowel disease and inflammatory arthropathy of unknown aetiology such as rheumatoid disease. Here one would hope to use agents to achieve and then maintain remission.

Physiological Diagnosis

If a physiological abnormality were to be defined this would enable one to plan **Support** for that particular dysfunction. Good examples are respiratory or nutritional support for respiratory or nutritional failure.

Anatomical Diagnosis

If a deficit or deformity in anatomy were to be defined then one may use **Surgery** in an attempt to repair or reconstruct this. Repair of an atrial septal defect or a ventricular septal defect would be examples of this approach.

Some may argue that this approach is too simplistic but if one were to analyse it carefully one would realise that it is quite rational and robust.

A good example to illustrate this would be the change that has occurred in the management of peptic ulcer. When only the pathology and physiological dysfunctions were defined, numerous approaches to management were used incorporating various types of surgical techniques. When one of the main aetiological agents, *Helicobacter pylori*, was identified, the entire approach changed and these surgical techniques have become obsolete.

To conclude one would advise using a Rational Approach to Medicine (RAM) rather than slavish adherence to protocols and guidelines.

Do not follow like a sheep, be a RAM instead!

Management Plan

The components of a management plan may be defined as:

- ♥ Objectives of Management
- ♠ Methods of Management
- ♦ Risks and Benefits
- ♣ Cost

Objectives of Management

The objectives of management are:

- ♥ Cure
- ♠ Control
- ♦ Symptom Relief
- ♣ Support
- ♥ Prevention

These objectives are quite easy to understand.

Cure

If possible one should attempt to cure the patient; that is eradicate the illness and thus cure the patient.

Control

If a cure is not possible than one should control the disease process.

Symptom Relief

Symptomatic relief should be provided whilst cure or control is being achieved or if cure or control is not possible.

Support

Support may be classified as:

- ♠ System Support
- ♦ Discharge Support

System Support

During the period of the patient's illness one should provide support to the various organs and organ systems by either treating or preventing failure of these organs or organ systems and thus one would support the patient in toto.

The organ systems that should be supported include Respiratory, Nutritional, Renal, Cardiac, Mobility (LMS), and Skin Care (IS). Psychological support is an important area that should not be neglected.

Discharge Support

Discharge support would concentrate on:

- ♣ Housing
- ♥ Support by Ancillary Workers

Housing

The patient's own home would be the preferred option and if this is not possible one should consider the options available in the society in which one practices. This would include protected environments such as long-stay hospital facilities, nursing homes and supervised housing. Palliative care institutions may be required in terminally ill patients.

Support by Ancillary Workers

This is an important aspect of discharge planning. The ancillary workers who should be involved include nursing staff, home help or servants depending on the society in which one practices and the provider of supplies and meals. Other staff who would be involved are physiotherapists, occupational therapists and social workers.

Prevention of Illness

Prevention of illness includes the patient, his or her family and society in general.

Prevention may be:

- ♠ Prevention of disease
- ♦ Prevention of recurrence of disease
- ♣ Prevention of complications of disease

Methods of Management

There are a variety of methods by which one would be able to achieve the above objectives of management. When considering these methods one should take into account the risks and benefits of each method and be prepared to discuss them. The methods are:

- ♠ Drugs
- ♦ Surgery
- ♣ Radiation therapy
- ♥ Biological agents
- ♠ Lifestyle Adjustments
- ♦ Staff
- ♣ Equipment
- ♥ Accommodation (Residence)

Drugs

Drugs refer to the pharmaceutical agents available.

Surgery

Surgery refers to the surgical techniques available.

Radiation Therapy

Radiation therapy refers to the use of therapeutic radiation such as radiotherapy, use of ultraviolet light, photodynamic therapy.

Biological Agents

This refers to the use of agents such as blood and blood products, antibodies, probiotics, stem cells

Lifestyle Adjustments

The main lifestyle adjustments are in relation to:

- ♥ Diet

- ♠ Exercise
- ◆ Abuse (substances such as alcohol, cigarettes, drugs)

Staff

In the provision of these methods of management one should remember the role of ancillary staff such as nursing staff, physiotherapists, occupational therapists, dieticians, pharmacists.

Equipment

When managing patients, specialised equipment may be required in certain situations. Examples are ventilators, dialysis machines, syringe pumps.

Accommodation (Residence)

Specialised types of accommodation may be required for patients under certain circumstances. As examples one may think of intensive care beds, high-dependency units, acute medical beds and long-stay beds.

This would also apply to discharge planning.

Aide Memoire

As an aide memoire to the objectives of management one may use the formula $C_2 S_2 P$. This stands for **C**ure, **C**ontrol, **S**ymptom relief, **S**upport, **P**revention.

As an aide memoire to the methods of management one may use the mnemonic **Poison, Cut, Burn, Biological Agents and LASER**.
Here poison refers to drugs, cut to surgery, burn to radiation therapy. Biological agents have been described. **LASER** stands for **L**ifestyle **A**djustments, **S**taff, **E**quipment (referring to specialised equipment)

and **R**esidence (referring to accommodation of the patient). As these are similar to the agents used in warfare, one may describe this as aggressive management!

Objectives	Methods
Cure	Poison
Control	Cut
Symptom Relief	Burn
Support (System Support and Discharge Support)	Biological Agents
Prevention	Lifestyle Adjustments
	Staff
	Equipment
	Residence (Accommodation)

Risks and Benefits

When each method of management is considered the risks and benefits that may accrue to each individual patient should be assessed.

Costs

The costs of each method of management must be taken into account if a management plan is to be sustainable.

Explanation

In practice and in professional examinations one may be called upon to explain a wide variety of topics in varied situations.

The common topics one may be called upon to deal with are an explanation of:

- ♣ Diagnosis
- ♥ Prognosis
- ♠ Bad news
- ♦ Investigations
- ♣ Management
- ♥ Lifestyle adjustments
- ♠ Consent

Planning Explanation

This is not a daunting task but it should be approached methodically. In planning explanation one should plan to address the beliefs, expectations, and anxieties (concerns regarding causes, effects and survival) of the patient or subject with whom one is dealing. The simplest way of doing this is to tell them what one's own beliefs and expectations are regarding the topic being discussed and what one's own thoughts are regarding the causes, effects and chances of survival. This would apply to any of the topics listed above.

Hence in providing an explanation one should address:

- ♦ Beliefs
- ♣ Expectations
- ♥ Causes
- ♠ Effects
- ♦ Survival

Beliefs

One should explain to the subject, in appropriate language, what one's beliefs (knowledge and views) are regarding the topic of discussion.

Expectations

One should explain to the subject in appropriate language what one's expectations are regarding the topic of discussion.

Causes

One should explain to the subject what one's thoughts are regarding the cause of the illness that is being discussed. If it is investigation or treatment that is being discussed, explain the reasons why the investigation or treatment is deemed necessary.

Effects

One should explain what one's thoughts are regarding the effects of the topic under discussion, be it illness, investigation, therapy, lifestyle adjustment. This may need to include, where appropriate, effects on relatives, colleagues or society.

Survival

One should explain to the subject what one's thoughts are regarding survival in relation to the topic of discussion.

Ethics

Ethics is a difficult area. Although in reality there are definite rights and wrongs many do not accept reality and wish to debate these issues as if they can change reality through debate. Hence, in these situations ethics depend on many factors including one's ethnic and cultural background, religion, philosophy and experiences in life. Remember that this makes it equally difficult for the examiners to assess as political correctness also comes into play.

Three principles must be maintained. They are:

- ♣ Duty
- ♥ Respect
- ♠ Law

Duty

One is bound by one's duty to the patient. Duties are manifold but in short one should do what is in the best interests of the patient and avoid harm.

Respect

Respect the individual as one would like to be respected.

Law

Remember laws vary in different countries. One should be aware of the laws of the country in which one is practising or being examined in. Stick to the law where applicable. If not use common sense.

> Accept reality,
>
> Reject rhetoric

Issues in Ethics

Four issues should be considered in particular. They are issues of:

- ♦ Confidentiality
- ♣ Competence
- ♥ Consent
- ♠ Controversy

Confidentiality

Any information that the patient divulges to the physician should be kept in confidence. One is duty bound to do so. Exceptions to this occur. One may divulge this information to colleagues for the purpose of managing the patient but this remains in the course of one's duty to the patient. The other instance where one may divulge information about the patient is where one's duty to society outweighs one's duty to the patient. This is in relation to:

♦ **Infectious Disease**

If the patient suffers from severe communicable disease

♣ **Work**

Where the patient's line of work may cause danger to society

♥ **Driving**

Where the patient may cause danger to society by driving a motor vehicle.

♠ **National Security**

Where national security is threatened usually by terrorism.

♦ **Court Order**

When one is required to do so by a court order. This is however outside one's control.

Competence

Competence refers to the ability of the patient to understand the nature of his or her illness and make a rational decision regarding this.

Consent

The mentally competent patient may give consent to, or refuse, investigation or treatment. It is the duty of the doctor to abide by the patient's decision. The decision may be made at the time or it may have been made earlier in the form of an advance directive. An advance directive may be a contentious issue in certain countries where the law regarding it is not clear and if circumstances have changed since the directive was made.

In most countries relations or friends may not give or withhold consent regarding a patient's management. Hence, in mentally incompetent patients the doctor should act in the best interests of the patient.

In instances where controversy arises in a patient unable to give consent one may make an application for the patient to be made a ward of court and then a judge would deal with the matter.

In psychiatric patients the relevant mental health act of the country in which one is practising may be evoked.

Following death, the next of kin have legal possession of the body. Hence, their consent is required for post-mortem examination or organ donation.

Controversy

Two issues are of particular relevance here. Both relate to patients who are mentally incompetent to make decisions for themselves. They are:

♣ Feeding or nutritional support

♥ Life Support

These are particularly difficult issues. One should always bear in mind that duty is paramount. All actions should be taken with the patient's best interests in mind.

The following aphorism has been used by many to guide their decisions, "One's duty is to prolong life, not postpone death." However, it is not one's duty to assess the quality of life of another being. This would allow abuse of power. One's duty as a physician is to decide on the benefits of treatment. Hence, assess whether the intervention would be of benefit to the patient.

Convey (Delivery)

The third aspect of the technique of communication is to convey one's plans (delivery). In practice the effectiveness of delivery would determine compliance on the part of the patient. In professional examinations this is the aspect of communication that can be assessed by the examiners.

Delivery of the plan to the patient or subject involves:

♠ Verbal communication

♦ Non-verbal communication

Verbal Communication

Where verbal communication is concerned, the language used should be appropriate to the intellectual level of the patient or subject. Erudite language should be avoided in most instances, however one should avoid using language that is too simple as this would come across as being patronising.

Non-Verbal Communication

Non-verbal communication would include the use of appropriate gestures and facial expressions and the use of diagrams or available literature.

Method of Conveying (Delivery)

One should avoid a monologue and interact with the patient or subject. Look for signs of misunderstanding on the part of the patient or subject and enquire whether he or she understands. Do not do this too often, as it would appear patronising. Allow the patient or subject to interrupt but if this becomes too frequent, one should tactfully ask him or her to allow one to finish.

Remember that people do what they perceive is in their best interests. Hence, at all times try and show how the suggestions will benefit them. In addition, do try and show that the patient has been involved in the decision making process.

Procedure for Facing the Communication and Ethics Station

To face the communications and ethics station one should go through the following steps:

♣ Plan

♥ Introduce/Identify

♠ Listen

♦ Modify

♣ Convey (Deliver)

Plan

Read the scenario carefully. The scenario may be to communicate a plan for investigation, which may even be the performance of a post mortem examination, or discuss a plan of management or explain a topic. Use the methods outlined earlier to formulate a plan, write down this interim plan and use it for reference.

Introduce/Identify

On entering the station the steps one should follow are:

♦ Introduce oneself to the patient or subject.

♣ Clarify the identity of the patient or subject

♥ If the subject is not the patient, clarify the relationship of the subject to the patient.

♠ If the subject is not the patient clarify that consent has been obtained to discuss the patient's condition with the subject.

Listen

♣ Listen to what the patient or the subject has to say.

♥ Maintain a state of awareness and do not let one's mind wander whilst the person speaks.

Objectives Of Listening

In this situation, the objectives of listening are to ascertain the person's:

♠ **Beliefs**

Beliefs may be divided into:

Knowledge of the Subject

Define what they already know

Views on the Subject

Define their views (opinions) on the subject

◆ **Expectations**

Define their expectations

♣ **Anxieties (Concerns)**

Define their concerns regarding:

Causes

Effects

Survival

Modify

Reassess the plan and modify it on the basis of any new information that has been obtained.

Convey (Deliver)

One should then communicate the plan bearing in mind that one is being assessed and the basis on which one's performance is being assessed. Remember, the process should be interactive and not a monologue.

Finally:

Look before you leap,

You will not fall in too deep,

Analysis before action,

Will bring success and satisfaction.

Appendix

Summary of History Taking and Physical Examination

As an aide memoire for candidates taking professional examinations, a summary of history taking and physical examination techniques follows:

History Taking

Identification

Introduce oneself, identify patient

Analysis of Symptoms

- ♠ **Position**: Site and Radiation
- ♦ **Character**: Nature
- ♣ **Quantity**: Severity
- ♥ **Transmission**: Associated features
- ♠ **Modifying Factors**: Precipitating, Aggravating and Relieving Factors
- ♦ **Rate**: Onset, Duration, Cessation
- ♣ **Rhythm**: Periodicity

Analysis of Systems

Endocrine and Metabolism

- ♦ Height
- ♣ Size of Extremities
- ♥ Weight
- ♠ Body Temperature
- ♦ Sweating
- ♣ Energy

Integumental System

- ♥ Rash
- ♠ Sweating
- ♦ Dry Skin
- ♣ Pigmentation
- ♥ Itching
- ♠ Hair
- ♦ Nails

Cardiovascular System

- ♥ Chest pain
- ♠ Palpitations

♦ Dyspnoea (with effort or at rest and associated orthopnoea or paroxysmal nocturnal dyspnoea)

♣ Swelling (of the ankles, the abdomen and the genitalia)

♥ Claudication

♠ Cold extremities

♦ Cyanosis

♣ Fatigue

♥ Syncope

Respiratory System

Upper Respiratory Tract

♥ Sneezing

♠ Blocked nose

♦ Nasal discharge

♣ Postnasal drip

♥ Epistaxis

♠ Facial pain

♦ Hoarseness

♣ Aphonia

Lower Respiratory Tract

♥ Dyspnoea

♠ Wheeze

♦ Cough

♣ Sputum

♥ Haemoptysis

♠ Chest pain

Gastrointestinal System

Digestive Tract

♥ Appetite

♠ Mastication

♦ Pain or soreness of the mouth

♣ Swallowing:

Enquire about difficulty in swallowing or pain.

♥ Heartburn

♠ Reflux

♦ Belching

♣ Abdominal Pain

♥ Early Satiety

♠ Bloating or Distension

♦ Swelling

♣ Bowel Movements:

Number of motions

Consistency

Blood

Mucous

♥ Evacuation of Faeces:

Enquire about rectal sensation, continence and adequacy of evacuation (complete or incomplete evacuation). Ask about ease of commencement of evacuation or the need to strain.

♠ Prolapse of rectum

♦ Perianal Problems:

Discharge, pain, lump

Hepato-Biliary System

♣ Pain

♥ Jaundice

♠ Itch

♦ Discoloration of Urine

♣ Colour of Stool

♥ Lack of Energy

♠ Swelling (of the abdomen and limbs)

Kidneys and Urinary System

- ♦ Micturition:

  Frequency

  Quantity

  Quality

- ♣ Act of Micturition:

  Sensation of fullness of the bladder

  Initiation of micturition

  Straining

  Force of the urinary stream

  Interruption to the passage of urine

  Terminal dribble

  Sensation of incomplete emptying of the bladder

  Burning sensation on passage of urine

- ♥ Swelling of the Body

- ♠ Abdominal Pain

Reproductive and Genital System

Male

- ♥ Erectile function
- ♠ Ejaculation
- ♦ Pain in the genitalia
- ♣ Swelling of the genitalia
- ♥ Rash
- ♠ Ulceration
- ♦ Discharge

Female

- ♣ Menstrual periods:

  Frequency

  Number of days the period lasts

  Quantity of menstrual flow

  Pain during menstruation

- ♥ Vaginal discharge
- ♠ Pain
- ♦ Irritation
- ♣ Rash
- ♥ Ulceration
- ♠ Dyspaerunia (pain or discomfort during sexual intercourse)

Obstetric History

- ♦ Number of pregnancies
- ♣ Number of deliveries
- ♥ Types of delivery
- ♠ Complications of pregnancy, labour and puerperium

Sexual History (Males and Females)

- ♦ Partners
- ♣ Contraception

Haematological System

- ♥ Breathlessness
- ♠ Lack of energy
- ♦ Recurrent infections
- ♣ Bleeding tendency
- ♥ Swelling of the lymph nodes
- ♠ Swelling of the abdomen
- ♦ Bone pain

Central Nervous System

Cortex

- ♥ Dominant side (whether the patient is right or left handed)
- ♠ Fits
- ♦ Loss of consciousness
- ♣ Mood
- ♥ Sleep

Cranium

- ♠ Headaches

Cranial Nerves

Nose

- ♥ Changes in the sense of smell

Eyes

- ♠ Visual disturbances

Face

- ♦ Weakness
- ♣ Sensory disturbance

Mouth

- ♥ Speech
- ♠ Swallowing
- ♦ Taste

Ears

- ♣ Vertigo
- ♥ Hearing

Cord and Connections

- ♠ Abnormal movements
- ♦ Weakness
- ♣ Incoordination
- ♥ Sensory disturbance

- ♠ Gait
- ♦ Bowel function
- ♣ Bladder function

Canal (spine)

- ♥ Backache

Locomotor System

- ♥ Pain
- ♠ Swelling
- ♦ Deformity
- ♣ Stiffness
- ♥ Movement

Elicit Details

- ♥ Past Illnesses
- ♠ Drug History
- ♦ Drug Intolerance
- ♣ Allergies
- ♥ Personal History:

  Diet

  Exercise

  Alcohol Intake

  Smoking
- ♠ Family History
- ♦ Social History:

  Family

  Work

  Housing

  Activities of Daily Living (Washing, Dressing, Eating, Going to the Toilet, Shopping, Preparation of Food)

  Support (Patients may receive support from family, friends, neighbours, Religious

Organisations, Non-Governmental Organisations, Social Services)

Leisure Activities

Sexual History (where appropriate). This may be included here or in the review of the reproductive and genital system

♣ Beliefs:

Thoughts (Views)

Knowledge

♥ Expectations

♠ Anxieties (Concerns):

Causes

Effects

Survival

Template

In the PACES examination, it would be wise to write down a template (using the above) on a sheet of paper in the intermission between stations and use this to jot down notes whilst taking the history.

Endocrine and Metabolism

General Examination

♥ Position

♠ Height and Proportions

♦ Weight and Shape

♣ Integument

♥ Body Temperature

Head

♠ Mental state

♦ Dimensions

♣ Nose

♥ Eyes

♠ Face (scalp, forehead, eyebrows, malar region, chin) Chvostek's sign if required

♦ Mouth (jaw, lips, teeth, gums, buccal mucosa, tongue, palate, fauces, salivary glands)

♣ Ears

Hands

♥ Dimensions

Dorsum of the hands

IS

♠ Nails and skin

LMS

♦ Bones, joints, tendons and muscles

Palms

IS

♣ Skin

LMS

♥ Bones, joints, tendons and muscles

CVS

♠ Peripheral circulation

♦ Radial pulse

CNS

♣ Tremor

♥ Flapping tremor

Forearms, Upper Arms, Shoulders and Axillae

♠ Quick examination, detailed examination only if indicated.

Neck

♦ Dimensions

♣ Integument

♥ Thyroid gland

♠ Sternocleidomastoid muscles

♦ Jugular venous pressure

♣ Carotids

♥ Trachea

♠ Lymph nodes

(Quick look, detailed examination only if required)

Thyroid Gland

From Front

♦ Inspect the neck

♣ Look for enlargement of the gland

♥ Ask the patient to swallow and see whether the gland moves upwards. A glass of water should be provided for this purpose.

From Behind

♠ Perform palpation, stand behind the patient who should be seated comfortably in an upright chair

♦ Note the dimensions, the cover (surface), the contents and the connections

♣ Ask the patient to swallow, define the lower margins of the gland

♥ Palpate the carotids and the cervical lymph nodes

Front of the Patient

♠ Palpate the trachea

♦ Auscultate for bruits over each lobe and listen for stridor.

♣ Look for Pemberton's sign

Chest

♥ Examine the chest wall and the contents of the chest, heart and lungs. Only if indicated

Abdomen

♠ Ask the patient to lie supine and examine the abdomen. Only if indicated

Lower Limbs

♦ General

♣ Hips

♥ Thighs

♠ Knees

♦ Lower legs

♣ Feet

Only if indicated

Integumental System

Skin and Mucosa

Inspect

♥ Size (contraction of the skin or conversely the skin being redundant)

♠ Shape (reflection of the state of the underlying tissue together with either contraction or redundancy of the skin)

♦ Colour of the skin

♣ Sweat

♥ Sebum

♠ Blood vessels

Palpate

♦ Surface (rash, sweat, sebum)

♣ Consistency

♥ Temperature

♠ Tenderness

♦ Skin elasticity

♣ Mobility of the skin over underlying structures

♥ Capillary refill

Skin Rashes

♣ Type

♥ Arrangement

♠ Distribution

Hair

Inspection

- ◆ Site
- ♣ Quantity of hair
- ♥ Pattern of distribution
- ♠ Shape
- ◆ Colour of the hair
- ♣ Surface (sheen, foreign bodies)

Palpation

- ♥ Easy pluckability
- ♠ Brittle hair

Nails

Inspection

- ◆ Site
- ♣ Size
- ♥ Shape
- ♠ Margins.
- ◆ Colour
- ♣ Surface
- ♥ Attachment
- ♠ Blood vessels

Palpate

- ◆ Early clubbing
- ♣ Tender areas
- ♥ Capillary pulsations in aortic regurgitation
- ♠ Capillary refill time in vascular insufficiency

Cardiovascular System

General Examination

- ♥ Position
- ♠ Height and Proportions
- ◆ Weight and Shape
- ♣ Integument
- ♥ Body Temperature

Head

- ♠ Mental state
- ◆ Dimensions, integument, movement
- ♣ Nose
- ♥ Eyes
- ♠ Face (scalp, forehead, eyebrows, malar region, chin)
- ◆ Mouth (jaw, lips, teeth, gums, buccal mucosa, tongue, palate, fauces, salivary glands)
- ♣ Ears

Hands

- ♥ Dimensions

Dorsum of hands

IS

- ♠ Nails and skin

LMS

♦ Bones, joints, tendons and muscles

Palms

IS

♣ Skin

LMS

♥ Bones, joints, tendons and muscles

CVS

♠ Peripheral circulation

♦ Radial pulse:

Condition of the vessel wall

Transmission (left radial, femoral)

Rate

Rhythm

Volume

Character

CNS

♣ Tremor

♥ Flapping tremor

Forearms and Upper Arms

Quickly inspect the forearms and upper arms

Brachial Artery

♠ Inspection

♦ Palpation (character of the pulse, brachio-radial delay)

♣ Auscultation (mention measurement of blood pressure)

Neck

♦ Dimensions

♣ Integument

♥ Thyroid gland

♠ Sternocleidomastoid muscles

♦ Jugular venous pressure:

Height

Character

Transmission

Modifying Factors

♣ Carotids:

Inspection

Palpation

Auscultation (usually left to be performed in conjunction with auscultation of the heart)

♥ Trachea

Chest

Examine the chest wall and heart

Chest Wall

♠ Deformity (chest wall in general and the praecordium in particular)

♦ Integument:

Scars

Gynaecomastia

Pacemaker

♣ Respiratory distress

Heart

Examine the heart

Semi-Recumbent Position

Inspection

- ♥ Position of the apex beat
- ♠ Pulsations over the praecordium and elsewhere in the chest

Palpation

- ♥ Apex beat:

  Position

  Rate and Rhythm (not an important point at which rate and rhythm are analysed)

  Quantity

  Character

  Transmission

  Modifying factors
- ♠ Left parasternal heave
- ♦ Pulsations over the praecordium or elsewhere in the chest
- ♣ Palpable heart sounds
- ♥ Thrills

Percussion

- ♠ When indicated percuss the left and right cardiac border.

Cardiac Auscultation

- ♥ Count the rate of the heart sounds
- ♠ Note the rhythm of the heart sounds
- ♦ Listen to the first heart sound. Define whether it is normal in intensity, loud or soft. Ascertain whether the intensity of the sound varies between beats. Define its character. Define whether it is single or split and if split whether the split varies with respiration.

- ♣ Repeat for the second heart sound.
- ♥ Listen in early diastole for an opening snap, opening click or tumour plop
- ♠ Listen in mid diastole for the presence of a third heart sound or pericardial knock.
- ♦ Listen in late diastole for the presence of a fourth heart sound.
- ♣ Listen in early systole for an opening or ejection click.
- ♥ Listen in mid systole for the presence of a mid-systolic click
- ♠ Listen in systole for any murmurs. If a murmur is heard define it.
- ♦ Listen in diastole for any murmurs. If a murmur is heard define it.
- ♣ Listen for any extra-cardiac sounds.

Left Lateral Position

Repeat palpation, auscultation

Patient seated up and leaning forward

Repeat palpation and auscultation (breath held in expiration)

_____

Back

- ♥ Spine
- ♠ Scapula

- Sacral oedema
- Lung bases
- Murmurs

Ask to examine the abdomen and lower limbs. Usually not required.

Respiratory System

General Examination

- Position
- Height and Proportions
- Weight and Shape
- Integument
- Body Temperature

Head

- Mental state
- Dimensions
- Integument
- Nose
- Eyes
- Face (scalp, forehead, eyebrows, malar region, chin)
- Mouth (jaw, lips, teeth, gums, buccal mucosa, tongue, palate, fauces, salivary glands)
- Ears

Hands

- Dimensions

Dorsum of the hands

IS

- Nails and skin

LMS

- ◆ Bones, joints, tendons and muscles

Palms

IS

- ♣ Skin

LMS

- ♥ Bones, joints, tendons and muscles

CVS

- ♠ Peripheral circulation
- ◆ Radial pulse

CNS

- ♣ Tremor
- ♥ Flapping tremor

Neck

- ◆ Dimensions
- ♣ Integument
- ♥ Thyroid gland
- ♠ Sternocleidomastoid muscles
- ◆ Jugular venous pressure
- ♣ Carotids (not usually required)
- ♥ Trachea:

  Position

  Length

  Movement

  Stridor

- ♠ Lymph nodes (say that they will be examined when the patient sits up to examine the back)

Chest

Chest Wall

Inspection

- ◆ Size
- ♣ Shape
- ♥ Skin
- ♠ Breasts
- ◆ Blood vessels
- ♣ Movements

Palpation

- ♥ Consistency
- ♠ Circulation (direction of blood flow)

Lungs

Move to the foot end of the bed

Respiration

- ♥ Position
- ♠ Rhythm
- ◆ Volume
- ♣ Character
- ♥ Transmission

Move back to the side of the patient

- ♠ Rate

Palpation

- ♥ Position of the Apex Beat
- ♠ Respiratory Movements
- ◆ Tactile Vocal Fremitus

Percussion

- ♣ Direct percussion over the clavicles

♥ Proceed downwards and outwards:

Upper zones

Mid zones

Lower zones

♠ Cardiac dullness

♦ Liver dullness

Auscultation

Listen over the chest and analyse:

Breath Sounds

♥ Position

♠ Character

♦ Quantity

♣ Transmission:

Vocal resonance

Aegophony

Whispering pectoriloquy

Added Sounds

♠ Crepitations (crackles)

♦ Rhonchi (wheeze)

♣ Squawks

♥ Stridor

♠ Pleural rubs

Back

♥ Neck:

Lymph nodes

♠ Spine

♦ Scapula

♣ Posterior aspect of Chest Wall

♥ Posterior aspect of Lungs

Abdomen

General Examination

♥ Position

♠ Height and Proportions

♦ Weight and Shape

♣ Integument

♥ Body Temperature

Head

♠ Mental state

♦ Dimensions

♣ Nose

♥ Eyes

♠ Face (scalp, forehead, eyebrows, malar region, chin)

♦ Mouth (jaw, lips, teeth, gums, buccal mucosa, tongue, palate, fauces, salivary glands)

♣ Ears

Hands

♥ Dimensions

Dorsum of the hands

IS

♠ Nails and skin

LMS

♦ Bones, joints, tendons and muscles

Palms

IS

♣ Skin

LMS

♥ Bones, joints, tendons and muscles

CVS

♠ Peripheral circulation

♦ Radial pulse

CNS

♣ Tremor

♥ Flapping tremor

Neck

♠ Dimensions

♦ Integument

♣ Look for elevation of the jugular venous pressure

♥ Mention to the examiners that one would perform a thorough examination of the lymph nodes when the patient is asked to sit up to examine the back of the patient.

Chest

♦ Dimensions

♣ Integument

♥ Gynaecomastia

Abdomen

♠ Position the patient

♦ Expose the abdomen correctly

♣ Ask the patient to keep the mouth partially open and breathe gently

♥ The patient's arms should rest by his or her side.

♠ One should be satisfied that the patient is comfortable prior to commencing examination

♦ An enquiry should be made whether the patient has any pain and note the location of the pain.

Abdominal Wall

♣ Size

♥ Shape

♠ Integument (scars, stoma)

♦ Umbilicus

♣ Distended veins (ascertain the direction of blood flow in these vessels)

♥ Look for herniae (ideally, herniae are examined with the patient standing)

♠ Respiratory movements

♦ Peristaltic movement

♣ Visible pulsation

Contents of the Abdomen

Examine the contents of the abdomen:

Initial palpation

S shape

♥ Left hypochondrium

♠ Epigastrium

♦ Right hypochondrium

♣ Right lumbar region

♥ Central abdomen (umbilical region)

♠ Left lumbar region

♦ Left iliac fossa

♣ Hypogastric region (suprapubic)

♥ Right iliac fossa

Followed by

♥ Liver

♠ Spleen

♦ Kidneys

♣ Epigastrium for any masses

♥ Aorta and para-aortic nodes

♠ Left iliac fossa

♦ Suprapubic region for enlargement of the bladder and for masses arising from the pelvis

♣ Right iliac fossa

Percussion

♥ Define any lump that has been detected

♠ Percuss the liver

♦ Percuss the spleen

♣ Percuss the centre of the abdomen

♥ Percuss the flanks

♠ Percuss the suprapubic region

♦ Demonstrate shifting dullness if flank dullness is detected

♣ Demonstrate fluid thrill if possible

Auscultation

♥ Succussion Splash

♠ Bowel Sounds

♦ Bruits

♣ Venous hum

Mention that one would wish to examine the neck and back, the inguinal region, the genitals and perform a rectal examination

Central Nervous System

Dress

♥ Assess the way the patient is dressed

General Examination

♥ Position

♠ Height and Proportions

♦ Weight and Shape

♣ Integument

♥ Body Temperature

Examination of the Cerebral Hemispheres

♦ Level of Consciousness

♣ Speech:

Phonation, Comprehension, Articulation, Repetition, Identification, Expression

♥ Frontal Lobe:

Orientation, Attention or concentration, Thoughts

♠ Temporal Lobe:

Memory, Mood

♦ Dominant Parietal Lobe:

Calculation, Writing, Identification or recognition

♣ Non-Dominant Parietal Lobe:

Visual and Sensory Inattention, Spatial Neglect, Dressing Apraxia, Constructional Apraxia

♥ Occipital Lobe:

Visual agnosia

♠ Mental Score

Cranium

♦ Note any structural abnormalities of the head

Cranial Nerves

Olfactory Nerve

♣ Ask about the sense of smell

Eyes

Examine structure and function

Structure

♥ Note any structural abnormality

Optic Nerve

♠ Visual acuity

♦ Visual fields

♣ Sensory inattention

♥ Visual agnosia (if required)

♠ Fundus

Third, Fourth and Sixth Nerves (Occulomotor, Trochlear, Abducent)

♦ Position (eyelids, eyeballs)

♣ Eye movements:

Range of movement

Nystagmus

Pupillary constriction during convergence

♥ Pupils:

Assess any structural abnormalities of the iris and note the colour

Size

Shape

Pupillary Light Reflexes

Swinging Light Test

Accommodation Reflex

Ciliospinal Reflex

Face

♣ Note any abnormality of structure of the scalp, the forehead, the eyelids, the malar region, the chin

Seventh Nerve

♠ Position

♦ Size

♣ Power:

Raise the eyebrows and wrinkle the forehead

Shut the eyes tightly

Puff the cheeks out

Say "eee"

♥ Reflexes:

Corneal reflex

Glabella tap

♠ Buccofacial Apraxia

♦ Taste Sensation

Jaws

♣ Structure of the jaws

Motor Component of the Trigeminal Nerve (Muscles of Mastication)

♦ Size

♣ Power:

Clench teeth

Open mouth against resistance

♥ Reflexes:

Jaw jerk

Sensory Component of the Trigeminal Nerve

♣ Only if required

Corneal reflex

♥ Test the corneal reflex if required

Mouth

♠ Examine the structure of the mouth

Cranial Nerves Nine, Ten and Twelve (Glossopharyngeal, Vagus and Hypoglossal)

Soft Palate

♦ Position

♣ Movement

♥ Reflexes:

The gag reflex is not tested in professional examinations

Tongue

♦ Size

♣ Involuntary movements (as it sits on the floor of the mouth)

♥ Tone (as it sits on the floor of the mouth)

♠ Power (protrude tongue, move it from side to side)

Taste sensation

♦ Not usually tested in professional examinations

Neck and Shoulders

♣ Look for any abnormality of structure of the neck and shoulders.

Eleventh Cranial Nerve (Accessory)

♥ Position (of the neck)

♠ Size

♦ Power:

Turn the chin to one side and then to the other against resistance

Shrug the shoulders against resistance

Ears

♣ Examine the structure of the ears.

Eighth Cranial Nerve (Vestibulocochlear)

Cochlear Component (Hearing)

♥ Test hearing:

Whispered voice

Rubbing fingers

♠ **Weber's test**

♦ **Rinne's test**

Examination of Upper Limbs

Examine structure and function of the upper limbs

Examination of Structure

♥ Size

♠ Shape

♦ Integument

♣ Muscle mass

Motor Function

♠ Position

♦ Involuntary Movements

♣ Tone

♥ Power

♠ Reflexes

♦ Coordination

Summary of Examination of Muscle Power in the Upper Limbs

♥ **Raise Arms**

Palms downwards

Palms upwards

Close eyes

Tap palms

♠ **Thumbs**

Abduction (T_1)

Opposition (T_1)

♦ **Fingers**

Abduction (T_1)

Adduction (T_1)

Flexion (C_8)

Extension (C_7)

♣ **Wrist**

Flexion (C_6)

Extension (C_7)

♥ **Elbow**

Flexion (C_6)

Extension (C_7)

♠ **Shoulder**

Abduction (C_5)

Adduction (C_6)

♦ **Scapula**

Serratus anterior

Supraspinatus

Infraspinatus

Reflexes

♠ Tendon reflexes (biceps, triceps, supinator)

♦ Hoffman reflex

♣ Grasp reflex

Reinforce if no reflex can be elicited

Coordination

♥ Finger nose test

♠ Dysdiadochokinesis

♦ Dysmetria

Sensory System of the Upper Limbs

♦ Touch

♣ Light touch

♥ Pain

♠ Temperature

♦ Vibration sense

♣ Proprioception

Tinel's sign and Phalen's sign if required

Higher Sensory Function

♥ Stereognosis

♠ Agraphaesthesia

♦ Two Point Discrimination

♣ Sensory Inattention

Chest, abdomen and inguinal region are not usually examined in professional examinations

Lower Limbs

Structure

♥ Size

♠ Shape

♦ Integument

♣ Muscle mass

Motor Function

♥ Position

♠ Involuntary Movements

♦ Tone

♣ Power

♥ Reflexes

♠ Coordination

Summary of Examination of Muscle Power in the Lower Limbs

♦ **Hips**

Flexion ($L_{1,2}$)

Extension (L_5)

Abduction (L_4)

Adduction (L_3)

♣ **Knees**

Flexion (L_5)

Extension (L_3)

♥ **Ankles**

Dorsiflexion (L$_4$)

Plantarflexion (S$_2$)

♠ **Big Toes**

Extension (L$_5$)

Flexion (S$_1$)

Reflexes

♦ Tendon reflexes:

Knee Jerk

Ankle Jerk

♣ Plantar Response

Reinforcement

♥ If no reflex is elicited

Clonus

♠ If exaggerated reflexes are observed, look for clonus

Coordination

♦ Test coordination using the heel-shin test

Sensation

♦ Touch

♣ Light touch

♥ Pain

♠ Temperature

♦ Vibration sense

♣ Proprioception

Higher Sensory Function

♥ Stereognosis

♠ Agraphaesthesia

♦ Two Point Discrimination

♣ Sensory Inattention

Spine

♥ Truncal ataxia

Gait

♠ Gait

♦ Heel toe (tandem) walking

Romberg's Sign

♠ Look for Romberg's sign

Standing from a Seated or Squatting Position

♥ Observe the patient standing from a seated or squatting position

Apraxia

♠ Dressing Apraxia

♦ Reading

♣ Writing

♥ Constructional Apraxia

Locomotor System

General Examination

- ♥ Position
- ♠ Height and Proportions
- ♦ Weight and Shape
- ♣ Integument
- ♥ Body Temperature

Head

- ♠ Mental state
- ♦ Dimensions, movement
- ♣ Nose
- ♥ Eyes
- ♠ Face (scalp, forehead, malar region, chin)
- ♦ Examine the structure of the jaw
- ♣ Examine the tempero-mandibular joint
- ♥ Mouth (lips, teeth, gums, buccal mucosa, tongue, palate, fauces, salivary glands)
- ♠ Ears

Hands

Structure

Dorsum

- ♦ Dimensions. Pay particular attention to the overall shape of the hands

- ♣ Nails and skin
- ♥ Overall size and shape

    Bones, joints and tendons

    Thumb

    Second, third, fourth and fifth fingers

    Hands and wrists

- ♠ Muscle mass

Palms

- ♦ Repeat the process for the palmar aspect
- ♣ Palpate the fingers, the hands and the wrists and note any warmth, tenderness or swelling
- ♥ Palate the tendons and note any warmth, tenderness or swelling
- ♠ Note any tendon sheath crepitus (may be done whilst assessing passive movements)
- ♦ Peripheral circulation
- ♣ Radial pulse

Movements of the Hand and Wrist

- ♥ Pretend to play a piano
- ♠ Touch each finger in turn with the thumb of the same hand
- ♦ Make a fist
- ♣ Prayer position
- ♥ Reversed prayer position

Function of the Hands

- ♣ Hand grip
- ♥ Pincer grip (between the thumb and the index finger)
- ♠ Simple functions (pick up object, do up buttons, comb hair)

603

Passive Movements

◆ Perform passive movements:

    Range of movement

    Abnormal movements

If one wishes, one may perform examination of passive movements when one examines structure of the hand.

Forearm

♣ Structure of the forearm

♥ Pronation and supination movements

Elbow

Ask the patient to extend the elbow and examine the flexor aspect:

♠ Position at rest

◆ Tenderness over the epicondyles

Ask the patient to flex the elbow and examine:

♣ Integument over the extensor aspect of the elbow

♥ Range of movement

Shoulder

Examine structure and function of the shoulder

Structure

♠ Shape

◆ Abnormalities of structure:

    Glenohumeral joints

    Acromioclavicular joints

    Sternoclavicular joints

♣ Tenderness:

    Sternoclavicular joints

    Acromioclavicular joints

    Subacromial bursa

    Supraspinatus tendon

    Biceps tendon

Movements of the Shoulder

♥ Position of the shoulder at rest

♠ Clasp the hands at the back of the head

◆ Clasp the hands behind his or her back and brace the shoulders back

Alternatively

♣ Touch the back of the head

♥ Scratch the back

Scapula

♣ Dimensions

♥ Muscle mass

♠ Tenderness

Glenohumeral Movement

◆ Fix scapula

♣ Flexion

♥ Extension

♠ Abduction

◆ Adduction

♣ Internal rotation

♥ External rotation

Neck

Examine structure and function of the neck

Structure

- ♠ Spasm of the sternocleidomastoid muscle and the paracervical muscles
- ♦ Tenderness over the occiput, the spinous processes of the vertebrae and the facet joints
- ♣ Palpate lymph nodes if required

Front of Neck

Examination of structure in full is not required in professional examinations. Note any abnormality of the dimensions and integument.

Movements of the Neck

- ♦ Flexion
- ♣ Extension
- ♥ Rotation to the right and then to the left
- ♠ Lateral flexion in both directions

Examination of the chest and abdomen is not usually required in professional examinations

---

Lower Limbs

Structure

General

- ♣ Position
- ♥ Length (measure true and apparent length if required)
- ♠ Muscle wasting
- ♦ Integument

Hips

- ♣ Position of the greater trochanters

♥ Tenderness over the joint

Thighs

- ♠ Dimensions

Knees

- ♠ Position
- ♦ Swelling
- ♣ Redness
- ♥ Warmth
- ♠ Tenderness

Fluid in the Knee

- ♦ Patellar tap
- ♣ Cross-fluctuation
- ♥ Bulge test

Lower Leg

- ♠ Structure

Ankle and Foot

- ♦ Dimensions

Dorsum of the foot

IS

- ♣ Nails and skin

LMS

- ♥ Overall size and shape
  Bones, joints, and tendons
    Big toe
    Each of the toes in turn
    Foot
    Ankle joint
- ♠ Muscle mass
- ♦ Tenderness over the joints and the tendons

Plantar Aspect

IS

♣ Skin

LMS

♥ Bones, joints, tendons

♠ Muscles

♦ Tenderness over the plantar fascia

CVS

♣ Peripheral circulation

♥ Dorsalis pedis and posterior tibial pulses

Examination of Function of the Lower Limbs

Examine function of the lower limbs as a sequence of movements.

Sacroiliac Joints

♠ Compression

♦ Distraction

Right Lower Limb

Examine the right lower limb then move to the other side of the bed or couch and examine the left lower limb.

Position

♦ Right lower limb in general

♣ Hip

♥ Knee

♠ Ankle and foot

Movements

Examine movements of the joints

Hip and Knee Movements

♥ Flexion of the hip and knee

♠ Thomas' test

♦ Hip movements with the knee in flexion (internal and external rotation, abduction and adduction)

♣ Knee movements (forward and backward motion, degree of extension, medial and lateral laxity)

♥ Hip movements with the knee in extension (abduction, adduction, internal rotation, external rotation)

Movements of the Ankle and Foot

♣ Ankle movement

♥ Subtalar movement

♠ Midtarsal movement

♦ Tarsometatarsal and interphalangeal movement

Left Lower limb

Repeat the examination on the left side. Use the converse of the method used on the right side.

Spine

Examine the spine with the patient supine, prone and then standing

Supine Position

♣ Straight leg raising test

Spine in the Prone Position

♥ Femoral stretch

♠ Rarely power of the erector spinae muscles

Patient Standing

Ask the patient to stand and examine structure and function

Structure

Examine structure

Dimensions

♦ Shape

Contents

♣ Tenderness

Function

Examine function

Position

♥ Stand against a wall (heels, buttocks and occiput should touch the wall)

Movements of the Spine

♠ Flexion (Schober test)

♦ Extension

♣ Lateral Flexion

♥ Rotation

Gait

♠ Assess gait

Trendelenburg Test

♦ Perform the Trendelenburg test.

Standing from a Seated or Squatting Position

♣ Observe the patient standing from a seated or squatting position

Communication and Ethics

Procedure for Facing the Communication and Ethics Station

♣ Plan

♥ Introduce/Identify

♠ Listen

♦ Modify

♣ Convey (Deliver)

Plan

♥ Read the scenario carefully

♠ Formulate a plan

♦ Write down this interim plan and use it for reference

Introduce/Identify

On entering the station the steps one should follow are:

♠ Introduce oneself to the patient or subject.

♦ Clarify the identity of the patient or subject

♣ If the subject is not the patient, clarify the relationship of the subject to the patient.

♥ If the subject is not the patient clarify that consent has been obtained to discuss the patient's condition with the subject.

Listen

♠ Listen to what the patient or the subject has to say.

♦ Maintain a state of awareness and do not let one's mind wander whilst the person speaks.

Objectives of Listening

In this situation, the objectives of listening are to ascertain the person's:

♣ Beliefs:

Knowledge of the Subject

Views (thoughts) on the Subject

♥ Expectations

♦ Anxieties (Concerns):

Causes

Effects

Survival

Modify

♦ Reassess the plan

♣ Modify it on the basis of any new information that is obtained

Convey (Deliver)

♥ Communicate the plan

♠ Bear in mind that one is being assessed

♦ Basis on which one's performance is being assessed

♣ Communication process should be interactive

♥ Not a monologue

Plans

Plan for Investigation

♥ Objectives

♠ Methods

- ◆ Risks and Benefits
- ♣ Cost

Methods

- ♥ Analysis of Body Fluids
- ♠ Imaging
- ◆ Nuclear Medicine
- ♣ Electrophysiology
- ♥ Physiological Assessment
- ♠ Endoscopy
- ◆ Surgery
- ♣ Tissue Diagnosis

Plan for Management

Objectives

- ♥ Cure
- ♠ Control
- ◆ Symptom Relief
- ♣ Support (Systems support and discharge support)
- ♥ Prevention

Methods

- ♥ Poison
- ♠ Cut
- ◆ Burn
- ♣ Biological agents
- ♥ LASER

Risks/Benefits

Cost

Planning Explanation

Address:

- ◆ Beliefs
- ♣ Expectations
- ♥ Causes
- ♠ Effects
- ◆ Survival

Template

In the PACES examination, it would be wise to write down a template (using the above), on a sheet of paper, in the intermission between stations and use this to jot down notes whilst one discusses the problem with the patient or subject.

Index

Printed in the United Kingdom
by Lightning Source UK Ltd.
117812UK00001B/7-12